Tiny You

Tiny You

A WESTERN HISTORY
OF THE ANTI-ABORTION MOVEMENT

Jennifer L. Holland

UNIVERSITY OF CALIFORNIA PRESS

University of California Press
Oakland, California

© 2020 by Jennifer L. Holland

Chapter 5 was published in a slightly altered version as "'Survivors of the Abortion Holocaust': Children and Young Adults in the Anti-Abortion Movement," *Feminist Studies* 46, no. 1 (2020).

Library of Congress Cataloging-in-Publication Data

Names: Holland, Jennifer L., 1981– author.
Title: Tiny you : a western history of the anti-abortion movement |
    Jennifer L. Holland.
Description: Oakland, California : University of California Press, [2020] |
    Includes bibliographical references and index.
Identifiers: LCCN 2019049758 (print) | LCCN 2019049759 (ebook) |
    ISBN 9780520295865 (cloth) | ISBN 9780520295872 (paperback) |
    ISBN 9780520968479 (ebook)
Subjects: LCSH: Pro-life movement—West (U.S.)—Case studies. |
    Pro-life movement—West (U.S.)—History—20th century.
Classification: LCC HQ767.5.U5 H65 2020 (print) | LCC HQ767.5.U5 (ebook) |
    DDC 362.1988/80978—dc23
LC record available at https://lccn.loc.gov/2019049758
LC ebook record available at https://lccn.loc.gov/2019049759

Manufactured in the United States of America

28 27 26 25 24 23 22 21 20
10 9 8 7 6 5 4 3 2 1

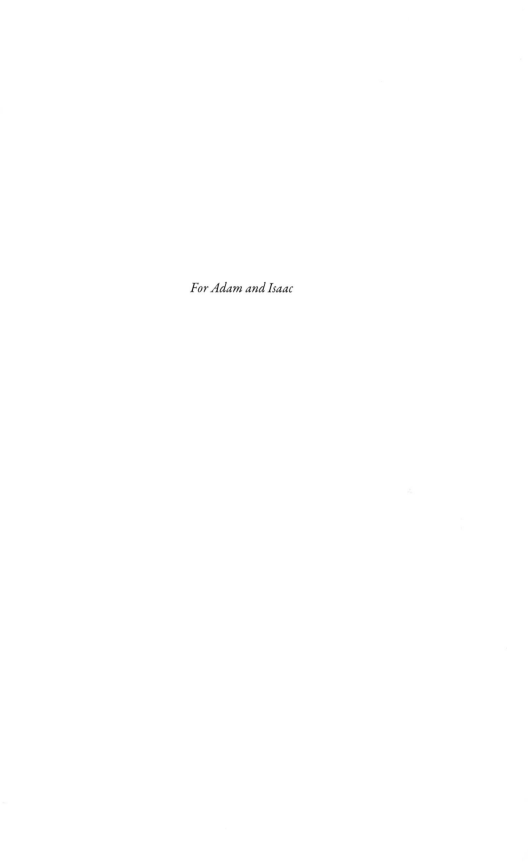

For Adam and Isaac

CONTENTS

ILLUSTRATIONS

ACKNOWLEDGMENTS

I have accumulated over ten years' worth of debts while writing this book. I cannot repay those debts but I must acknowledge at least some of the incredible people who made this book possible. This book would not have been written or finished without the financial support of a variety of institutions. The University of Wisconsin History Department, the Charles Redd Center for Western Studies, the Arthur and Elizabeth Schlesinger Library on the History of Women in America at Radcliffe, the Center for Research on Gender and Women at the University of Wisconsin, the American Association of University Women (AAUW), and Office of Vice Presidential Research at the University of Oklahoma have all contributed to this project.

This book depended on the labor and insights of archivists and librarians across the country. I want to thank the staff of the Center for Southwest Research at the University of New Mexico, University of New Mexico School of Law Library, the Denver Public Library, Arizona State University's archives, the State of Arizona Research Library, the J. Willard Marriott Library at the University of Utah, the John Hay Library at Brown University, the L. Tom Perry Special Collections at Brigham Young University, the New Mexico State Records Center, Merill-Cazier Library Special Collections and Archives at Utah State University, New Mexico State University Special Collections and Archives, the Schlesinger Library, and the Wisconsin Historical Society. I am also grateful to Laurie Scrivener for all her help.

I finished this book while at the University of Oklahoma (OU). My colleagues and students helped me reach the finish line. In the last few years, nothing propelled me more than their confidence in me and this book. Committee G offered me tireless support, while the counsel of Miriam Gross, Judith Lewis Phillips, and Elyssa Faison shaped the text in important ways. Katy Schumaker and Ronnie Grinberg were great friends and a great writing group, offering suggestions on large parts of this manuscript. In the History Research Workshop, OU graduate students and colleagues gave generous comments on a particularly difficult chapter. Rachel Shelden, Andy Shelden, Marc Levine, Rhona Siedelman, Tina Warinner, Anne Gibson, Jess Pearson, Elyse Singer, Anne Hyde, Kathy Brosnan, David Wrobel, Jamie Hart, and Warren Metcalf have all sustained me in their own ways. Andy Shelden edited much of this book when it (and I) needed it most. Thanks as well to Toryn Sperry for her research assistance and Chelsea Burroughs for her work on the index.

Niels Hooper at the University of California Press has nurtured this project over the last couple of years. I am honored to have him as my editor. Thanks also to Robin Manley at the Press. Rickie Solinger and two anonymous reviewers provided careful and thorough comments on different versions of this manuscript. Karissa Haugeberg was my reader superhero. All their expert comments have improved this book immeasurably.

This book began in Logan, Utah in conversations about gender and history with Mike Lansing. He has stuck with me—and this project—since then. He is a gifted mentor and a model of how to be in this profession. This book came into being in Madison, Wisconsin, among an amazing cohort of advisors, mentors, and colleagues. Haley Pollack and Ari Eisenberg made much of this book better with their comments and possible through their friendship. I do not know how I would have gotten through graduate school without them. Libby Tronnes, Crystal Moten, Megan Raby, Doug Kiel, Meridith Beck Sayre, Andrew Case, and Charles Hughes were the best dissertation writing group a person could ask for. A wider UW community carried me forward through graduate school. A special thanks to Simon Balto, Meggan Billotte, Scott Burkhardt, Trudy Fredericks, Mark Goldberg, Brenna Greer, Marian Halls, Michel Hogue, Jennifer Hull, the late Doria Johnson, Faron Levesque, Jessie Manfrin, Jillian Jacklin, Stacey Smith, Tyina Steptoe, Maia Surdam, Naomi Williams, Keith Woodhouse, and Tom Yoshikami, in addition to those named above. In Ann Arbor, Logan, Madison, Buffalo, and beyond, a host of other mentors gave me their time and intellectual energy: the late Jeanne Boydston, Cindy Cheng, Philip Deloria, Finn Enke, Nan Enstad, the late Camille Guérin-Gonzales, David Herzberg, Judy Houck, Will Jones, David Rich Lewis, Maria Montoya, Jennifer Ratner-Rosenhagen, Jennifer Ritterhouse, and Ona Siporin. I am especially grateful to Michelle Nickerson, who offered essential support at critical moments. Susan Cahn saved the day more than once, while being a truly wonderful friend. Thank you.

This book would not have the merits it does without the guidance of Susan Lee Johnson. She took a chance on me and gently schooled me in the histories of place and race, straightforward prose, and professionalism. Generous with her time and emotional support, Susan always made me a priority, not just my work. Her intellectual rigor, political commitments, attention to detail, and overall good-heartedness have made my work infinitely better and me a better scholar.

Other teachers allowed me to finish this book. The staff at the JCC Early Childhood Center in Buffalo and Trinity Child Development Center in Oklahoma City have given me the time and peace of mind necessary to complete this book. Knowing my child was in good, caring hands made all the difference. A special thank you to Emily Malucci, Lourdes Peña, Irene Ngoma-Koutouma, Lisa Ottolia, Sarah Wickersham, and Robin Boyer.

Most importantly, I want to acknowledge my family. All of them have had boundless enthusiasm for this project and patience with my slow pace. Rosie has been my anchor in good and hard times. Ellen Malka, Bernard Malka, Jaclyn Connell, and Michael Connell gave me a home away from home in Atlanta. My sister, Diane Mateus, grounded me in turbulent times and offered unmitigated support in all other times. My mom, Amy Holland, constantly reminded me to keep body and mind together, and offered the comforts of home when both needed a break. Without my dad, Geoffrey Holland, this project would never have existed. His love of inquiry, debate, and history formed my youth and made it hard to envision doing anything else but this. Finally, I must thank my grandparents—Nancy, Paul, Louise, and Norval—and my great, great uncle Russell. Without them, this would not have been possible.

Last but never least, I want to thank Adam Malka and Isaac Holland-Malka. They are the two best things that have ever happened to me. For over ten years, Adam has supported me with humor, food, companionship, a lot of sports talk, and deep conversations about history. He has been a great editor, co-parent, and partner. He has made days that should have been hard, precious beyond words. Isaac was born in 2017; since then, he has brought a lot of chaos and an immeasurable amount of joy into my life. I wouldn't have it any other way. This book is for them.

Introduction

Trent Franks came of political age wearing a fetus on his lapel. The story of how the pin got there began in the shadow of the Cold War West, in a small uranium mining town in southwestern Colorado. Franks's 1950s hometown, Uravan, was a typical "yellowcake" town, complete with company dominance and high levels of cancer.[1] By the 1970s he was working in another classically western endeavor: oil drilling. But Franks began to chart a new career trajectory in Utah, where he took a course at the National Center for Constitutional Studies—formerly the Freemen Institute. The Freemen Institute was a religiously inspired right wing, free market group with links to the ultraconservative John Birch Society, and Franks named this one of his most important educational experiences. A short time later, he had his political epiphany. It came in the form of a pro-life film. "It showed a child in the throes of dying from a saline abortion," he recalled. It "made an indelible imprint on my heart forever." Franks soon became, according to the *National Review,* a "pro-life warrior."[2] One of the emblems of this war could be found on his jacket, near his heart, where he wore "a tie tack in the shape of the feet of a fetus, as a constant reminder of his anti-abortion-rights views."[3]

Franks' anti-abortion convictions drove his subsequent life choices. Once he moved to Arizona, he joined the local Right to Life group, picketed clinics, and helped found a Tempe crisis pregnancy center.[4] Elected to the Arizona legislature in 1984, Franks made abortion his singular focus while in office. He lost his seat in the 1986 election, but he continued to work on socially conservative issues. In 1992, he led an effort to put a constitutional amendment banning most abortions on Arizona's ballot (the amendment lost).[5] Once he was elected to the U.S. House of Representatives in 2003, he made national news for suggesting that African Americans were better off

1

under slavery than in twenty-first-century America. "Half of all black children are aborted," Franks claimed. "Far more of the African-American community is being devastated by the policies of today than were being devastated by policies of slavery." He argued the anti-abortion movement was "the civil rights struggle that will define our generation."[6] In fact, 50 percent of *unintended* pregnancies for black women ended in abortion, yet unintended pregnancies were only 7.9 percent of all of black women's pregnancies.[7] Such statements led many members of the press to label Franks an ultra-conservative crackpot, akin to a "nutty relative who lives in the attic." Dismissing Franks as an anomaly, however, obscures the very real ways that he was a product—and a vaunted spokesperson—of a powerful movement that arose in the final decades of the twentieth century.[8]

Trent Franks came from a movement that aimed to meet people in the intimate spaces of their ordinary lives. He, like so many others, was touched by the pro-life movement's cultural campaign to change hearts and minds. Franks's own political awakening was owed to a film, which he probably viewed in his evangelical church. Like many pro-life films, that one surely spoke in the language of biology—heartbeats, chromosomes, and brainwaves—but the setting reassured viewers abortion was a religious issue too. In spaces like these and with tools like these, anti-abortion activists politicized a host of white people, who then in turn committed themselves to end legal abortion. The white pro-life activists who surrounded Franks regularly compared abortion to slavery and genocide, often with graphic photos hovering in the background as evidence. They passed around pins of fetal feet and asked Americans to think of their relationship to fetuses, humanity, life, and murder. In these political and cultural conversions, pro-life activists changed the way people thought not only about abortion but also about themselves. Trent Franks told the Eagle Forum in 2014, "If I die and *Roe v. Wade* still stands . . . I will die a failure."[9]

This book argues that anti-abortion activists made the political personal to many white Americans like Trent Franks. Activists brought fetal imagery and its attendant politics into crisis pregnancy centers, onto public thoroughfares, and to schools, churches, and homes. They inserted fetal politics into profoundly intimate relationships: between husband and wife, child and parent, people and their God, to name a few. Those politics invited white people to think of themselves as abolitionists and the nation's saviors. In the process, activists developed and fostered a constituency of white Americans for whom anti-abortion politics became essential to their sense of self. Turning a core feminist principle on its head, activists made a political abstraction—fetal life—into a facet of everyday life. Yet unlike second-wave feminists, pro-life activists usually did not take personal experiences and give them political meaning.[10] Because so few of these activists had themselves had an abortion, their work became not to make the personal political, but to make the political personal.[11] They transformed their political beliefs—that fetuses were babies and abortion was murder—into a lived reality for many Americans who had never been touched by abortion. When these personal politics were successful, activists helped their audience identify with and see themselves in the fetus. They helped many individuals think of a fetus as a "tiny you."[12]

Anti-abortion political activism was cultural work, and its effects infiltrated the seemingly apolitical spaces of Americans' lives. When activists took gory photos of aborted fetuses, fetus dolls, embalmed fetuses, videos of abortions, and symbolic funerals and cemeteries into private and public spaces, they waged a war for hearts and minds.[13] The ongoing legislative battles that dominated many state governments were predicated on this more intimate activism. They were built upon ecumenical organizing in religious communities, where the devout recited prayers against abortion, heard pro-life sermons, read about local anti-abortion efforts, and watched anti-abortion films. They were built upon the activism done in crisis pregnancy centers, which beckoned pregnant women to their doors, implicitly offering abortion referrals but only providing pro-life counseling. They were built upon the "educational activism" anti-abortion activists did with young people in schools, churches, and homes. And they built upon a "family values" politics that activists employed in arenas large and small, from self-help groups to statehouses. This work ultimately trickled up into the halls of power and flowed onto the sidewalks outside of abortion clinics.

These cultural politics are a part of national story but, like Trent Franks, they are also a part of a regional one. The work of anti-abortion activists touched all parts of the United States but they affected some regions more than others. In places with large populations of white conservative Catholics, evangelicals, and Mormons, the movement made its largest impression, reshaping both everyday life and formal partisan politics. This book's dramas play out in one of those regions: the Mountain West. *Tiny You* examines the movement in Arizona, New Mexico, Colorado, and Utah, or the Four Corners states. There, anti-abortion activism was a product of Cold War migrations and transformations. Both new migrants and longstanding residents eventually remade the region's conservatism, from the New Right libertarian focus of the 1960s to a religious, social conservatism by the 1980s. This book tells the story of this everyday activism that transformed a region and a nation.

THE RIGHTS OF FETUSES

It was not just feminists from whom conservatives borrowed. In rhetoric as well as strategy, anti-abortion activists appropriated liberal tools writ large. Pro-life activists developed a discourse that envisioned abortion as evidence of the perversion of modern science, a genocide akin to the Holocaust, and a product of racist or otherwise hierarchical thinking that privileged some lives over others. In other words, they made the fetus into the victim of modern society and their campaign into a social justice movement by claiming that only through the protection of the fetus could Americans successfully protect the rights of all oppressed people. Conservative activists thus borrowed the rhetoric of civil rights—an ideology forged in the crucible of southern segregation and extended in campaigns for the rights of women, Latinx, Native Americans, LGBTQ people, and many others. Anti-abortion activists put that elastic but liberal rhetoric to conservative ends. While other social conservatives used the language of liberty, the pro-life movement wagered on the power of civil rights.[14] Because of this, abortion was able to outlast other socially conservative issues that drifted in and out of focus over the years.

The activists who repurposed the language of civil rights in this movement were almost all white. They were drawn from similar demographics as other mid- to late-twentieth-century conservatives. But white conservatives of the late 1960s and 1970s faced new challenges. When in the 1970s Americans began to recast the civil rights movement as righteous, not riotous, southerners who resisted desegregation were left outside of history's moral arc. This transformation had repercussions beyond the South; it had the potential to damage the Republican Party of Barry Goldwater and states' rights, even in the minds of an increasing number of white Americans. The embrace of rights discourse was partially a response to the moral rupture of massive resistance. White conservatives had to rethink the moral and ideological basis of whiteness in the aftermath of a civil rights movement which made the defense of segregation and white supremacy publicly untenable.

Anti-abortion activists offered one way out of this conundrum by building a civil rights movement for fetuses. They constructed a narrative in which white elites—from doctors to university professors, mainstream Democrats to radical feminists—were indoctrinating the American populace, leading them away from basic truths about humanity, gender, and life. Additionally, they suggested that many people of color—a group that activists fit into the old category of "the undeserving poor"—were destabilizing society from below. Because of the machinations of these two groups, abortion had become and stayed legal. Activists argued abortion threatened not just fetal lives but also Christianity, womanhood, the haven of childhood, and the "traditional family." When white activists tied their own identities to fetal victimhood, white conservatives too became victims. Regular white Americans, meanwhile, became the "moral middle" under threat from both the top and the bottom.[15]

Through this civil rights movement for fetuses, regular white people could be both the victims of modernity and potential saviors. When social conservatives borrowed the new social currency of civil rights and put it to socially conservative ends, white religious people—southerners, northerners, and westerners alike—were able to represent themselves as abolitionists, not segregationists. This was no small task, not least because anti-abortion activists usually figured fetal victims as white. But they often implied they would rescue people of color as well. In this way people of color, especially black people, were implicated in the pro-life movement, as one-dimensional victims of a liberal, feminist, or "anti-life" society in need of a white conservative savior. They came on stage, so to speak, largely to prove the morality of the white protagonist.

These proliferating victimhoods redeemed the Right at the expense of those from whom white conservative activists borrowed. Victimhood was always a hierarchy in the pro-life worldview, with the innocent fetus sitting at its apex. All others were tarnished by their potential corruption by liberal forces or by the fact that they were born. Born humans, after all, had a certain amount of personal responsibility for their circumstances in a way that fetuses could not have. Fetuses, and only fetuses, could be truly innocent. In a post–civil-rights era, white social conservatives asked that people of color and other marginalized groups fall into line with a civil rights movement for white people. This was one reason white anti-abortion activists never strayed into "other" civil rights issues; it was also why people of color, even conservative religious ones, rarely strayed into anti-abortion activism.

The pro-life rhetoric of fetal civil rights was supposed to distract from another group who could make a claim to "rights": women. The anti-abortion movement worked hard to hide the abortion-seeking woman, her civil rights, and her reasons for abortion. By focusing on the fetus, pro-life activists could sidestep the fraught issue of women's rights in an era when feminist values were infusing popular culture and politics. Pro-life activists were always deeply concerned with changing sexual mores and the status of women in society, but in the movement's infancy, activists realized that an anti–woman's rights platform would not help them win the day. Facing the rising tide of feminism, anti-abortion activists chose not to attack women directly but instead focus attention on the rights of the "unborn."

Although women who sought abortions might have been hidden, they were never fully gone. Recently, a handful of scholars have focused on the liberal origins of the anti-abortion movement, arguing that it was human rights, anti-poverty, or proto-feminist beliefs that motivated many early pro-life activists.[16] There is some truth in this reassessment, but pro-lifers' beliefs in human rights or the power of the state to better people's lives were almost always paired with an overriding concern about the insidious power of women's excessive sexuality. Unplanned pregnancy was the physical manifestation of that sexuality, and abortion was its murderous cover-up. Indeed, errant sex and the women who enjoyed it continued to crop up in anti-abortion politics, despite many activists' best efforts. When these women did appear, activists figured them as irresponsible elite white women, dangerously sexual women of color, or simple dupes of a corrupt system.

While many anti-abortion activists, like Trent Franks, were white men, white women had an important role to play too in this "civil rights movement." They were essential to the claim that this movement was not "anti-woman." This book, however, is not a history of women in the anti-abortion movement. Others have written that story, and written it well.[17] *Tiny You* is, rather, a history of the gendered political culture of an anti-feminist movement. In this book, women's activism is not much different from men's. Both men and women all used roughly the same arguments in defense of fetal lives, and took those arguments into intimate spaces. Let me be clear: These similarities should not suggest that the women of the movement were incidental to the direction and shape of pro-life political culture. In fact, they were likely responsible for it. Anti-abortion activists went to churches, homes, and schools; they politicized religious people, women, children, and families. These places and these groups of people, historically, were the province of women. The broad contours of this intimate activism were surely a product of a movement where white conservative women constituted the majority of activists. Pro-life action was not limited to these spaces—public streets and legislatures were obviously central—but it was in the domain of women where activists laid their movement's groundwork.

The white men and women of this movement claimed that theirs was a civil rights movement. Older visions of moral degradation transformed into more modern conceptions of rights abuses. Activists claimed that fetal rights derived from the Declaration of Independence. which secured Americans' right to life; but they were really riding a much more modern political wave. They borrowed much more from the black civil rights movement and the international human rights movement when framing their story. But make no mistake: This language was always in service of denying others their rights. Women seeking abortions were a perpetual thorn in the side of the movement. Were they murderers, jezebels, dupes, or trauma survivors? The movement easily named the victims, but the transgressors were harder to pin down.

ON BARRY GOLDWATER'S DOORSTEP

By the 1980s, the pro-life movement had reshaped conservatism and the Republican Party, even in the home of one of the most famous and influential New Right conservatives: Barry Goldwater. Goldwater, Arizona senator and 1964 Republican presidential nominee, embodied the libertarian, anti-tax, anti-federal government conservatism of the 1960s, a kind of politics that seemed quintessentially "western" both to his supporters in the 1960s and to historians ever since.[18] Goldwater, however, did not oppose legal abortion. In fact, his wife Peggy Goldwater was a longtime and vocal supporter of Planned Parenthood in Arizona, and Barry Goldwater had helped his daughter secure an illegal abortion in 1956. Goldwater was struggling to retain his Senate seat in 1980. By then, Mr. Conservative needed social conservatives to win. So he assured Arizona Right to Life that he would tow the pro-life line and support the Human Life Amendment, proposed by Arizona's other senator, Dennis DeConcini, the son of an early anti-abortion activist in the state. Because of this promise, Goldwater received the endorsement of Arizona Right to Life and other family values groups. Their support was critical. He won that election by only 9,000 votes.[19] Live-and-let-live, anti-government conservatism could no longer secure an election in Arizona without anti-abortion support—even for Barry Goldwater.

Goldwater has loomed large in histories of modern conservatism, but his region—the Mountain West—generally has not. The Sunbelt has been the most important landscape for studies of the New Right, but these have most often focused on California or the South. The geography of anti-abortion histories has been slightly different. "Place" has played a minor role in case studies of early movements in California or New York, and in work on radicalism and the places Operation Rescue besieged in the late 1980s and 1990s. In both Sunbelt and anti-abortion historiographies, scholars have been drawn to origin stories, firsts, and moments of political explosion. Adding a place like the Mountain West to our stories of social conservatism changes how we think of the conservative revolution. It shows how the pro-life movement remade most of America but most especially the middle regions. It shows how widespread, fundamental, and intimate those transformations were.

This book's events take place in the vibrant heart of the Mountain West, the Four Corners states—Arizona, New Mexico, Colorado, and Utah. Home to rapidly expanding suburban metropolises, these four states were each part of the massive political and economic realignment that created the Sunbelt in the second half of the twentieth century.[20] Military contractors as well as an assortment of other industries moved to the region during these years, all looking for cheap land, low taxes, and open spaces. Because of the resulting economic explosion, the Four Corners states subsequently drew scores of new migrants from the U.S. North, South, and Midwest in the 1950s and 1960s. This growth only accelerated as the century wore on. By the 1990s and 2000s, the population of these states was growing three times faster than the rest of the country.[21] Sunbelt urbanization unified these states, which until then had only been linked by their interconnected landscapes and histories of settler colonialism. Arizona, New Mexico, Colorado, and Utah all soon had heavily urbanized, multiracial populations, diverse economies, and strong residual rural identities.

This study does not claim that the pro-life movement was born in this region, nor that it was bigger, stronger, or more innovative there. It did, however, have a handful of "firsts," perhaps most importantly that Colorado passed the country's first abortion reform law in 1967, which mobilized one of the nation's earliest grassroots anti-abortion groups. The pro-life movements in the Mountain West birthed national leaders—like Carolyn Gerster (president of National Right to Life from 1978 to 1980), John Jakubczyk (lawyer to the national group Pro-Life Action League), and Norman Weslin (founder of radical rescue group Lambs of Christ). But any region of the country was home to some "firsts," not to mention a handful of prominent activists. Like every other place, the movement in the Mountain West was staffed and maintained by hundreds of people who had little to do with national leadership. And like every other region, its activists innovated some political strategies but mostly mimicked others from around the country.

And yet, this study of anti-abortion activism in the Four Corner states helps us see a national movement through new eyes. It reveals how race worked for a largely white movement in a multiracial—as opposed to a biracial or monoracial—environment. It uncovers how religious coalitions operated in societies with large populations of Catholics, evangelicals, Mormons, and non-believers. It shows how a movement claiming the mantle of tradition operated in a very modern landscape, in states made over by postwar economic transformations, Sunbelt migrations, and racial justice movements. In the end, the Mountain West allows for a study of political culture on multiracial, religiously diverse ground. It illuminates why and for whom fetal politics mattered.

Religious people of all stripes made their home in the Mountain states, alongside nonbelievers and people dedicated to New Age spiritualities. Religious historians Mark Silk and Andrew Walsh describe this region as "sacred landscapes in tension." New Mexico and Arizona were the "Catholic heartland," Utah was a part of the "Mormon corridor," an area culturally and politically dominated by the Church of Jesus Christ of Latter-day Saints (LDS), and Colorado had no dominant religious community but was home to people of Catholic, Protestant, Mormon, Jewish, and a variety of American Indian faiths.[22] In the postwar period, Colorado and Arizona, especially, developed large southern evangelical populations. Thus, the region as a whole had a large number of the type of white Christians who supported and joined the pro-life movement in the waning decades of the twentieth century.

Anglos, white ethnic people, African Americans, Asian Americans, Indigenous people, and Latinx all found homes in this mountainous landscape. In New Mexico, Anglos were one part of a polyglot society of Navajo, Apache, and Pueblo peoples, *hispanos,* and *mestizos.* While most *nuevomexicanos* struggled to preserve the lands and economies upon which they depended in the face of Anglo migration, some people of color—especially elite *hispanos*—maintained a modicum of power in the state.[23] Unlike New Mexico, Arizona was quickly dominated by Anglo Americans, though it too had a racially diverse population—including white Protestants and Mormons, Apache and the Akimel and Tohono O'odham peoples,

Mexican Americans, Mexican immigrants, and a small number of African Americans.[24] In Utah, white Mormons made up the overwhelming majority—LDS people did see the state as their promised land after all—but they lived alongside small numbers of Utes, Paiutes, and Shoshones, as well as small Greek, Italian, Japanese, and Chinese immigrant populations.[25] Colorado became a regional hub in the twentieth century, drawing laborers of many stripes, health seekers, and tourists to the state, leading to a diverse population of Native peoples, ethnic Mexicans, African Americans, Anglo Americans, Japanese Americans, and European immigrants.[26] The character of the region's population was a product of specific colonial histories, producing unique and complicated social hierarchies. In the late twentieth century, that population was also a cross section of America. This was a multiracial region in an increasingly multiracial nation.

Because the Four Corners states and the American West as a whole contained such a wide array of people—and such a large number of people of color—they were home to longstanding, intense disagreements about appropriate forms of reproduction. Women of color had long borne the brunt of public scrutiny about supposedly errant reproduction and its effects on the composition of the nation. This scrutiny took many forms in the late nineteenth and early twentieth centuries—from promoting white reproduction through better-baby contests to permanently ending women of color's reproductive capabilities through coercive sterilization. Western state governments enshrined their ideas about appropriate reproduction in both sterilization laws and anti-miscegenation laws that banned intermarriage between white people and others.[27] This meant that by the mid twentieth century, western people of color had already been implicated in national conversations about appropriate bodies, sexuality, pregnancy, and birth. Late twentieth-century social conservatives did not duplicate those older eugenicist conversations. They did, however, implicitly draw from and build upon these prior histories to make claims about the "right kind" of reproduction and its effects on the national body.

Social conservatives in the Four Corners states worked in a region that prided itself on being at the forefront of women's rights campaigns. Western states—and particularly those in the Mountain West—were the first to secure women's right to vote in the nineteenth century. Because of this, Margaret Sanger, the famous leader of the birth control movement, believed that the Mountain West states would be more hospitable to her movement in the 1920s and 1930s. She was mostly right. Colorado opened its first clinic in 1926, and Arizona and New Mexico followed within a decade.[28] Utah, the second state to give women the right to vote, did not however welcome the movement to free women from their reproductive constraints; the LDS Church called the use of birth control "one of the most heinous crimes" and banned it until the mid-1990s.[29] At least rhetorically, the Mormon Church joined the Catholic Church in opposing efforts to increase women's access to birth control. Half a century later, as women joined the feminist movement in the region and returned to the issue of reproductive rights, some of the same religious institutions would link arms to oppose them. Thus, at the end of the twentieth century, the Mountain West was home to a host of social conservatives and women's rights activists, both with extensive roots in the region.

The demographics that made this region unique offer important insights about the pro-life movement. In a region with a large population of Mormons, LDS people played the same role as they did elsewhere. They joined Catholics and evangelicals in the movement but participated only in subsidiary ways. In a region with many Latinx and Native American Catholics, the anti-abortion movement was still mostly white, drawing largely on white Catholic traditions and culture. In a region with relatively few black people and Jews, the movement relied heavily on historical comparisons of African American slavery, the civil rights movement, and the Jewish Holocaust, as it did everywhere else in the nation. Place did not change the movement's ideology, tactics, or reception. The unique demography of the Mountain West shows how uniform the movement was.

In the Mountain West and elsewhere, this relatively uniform anti-abortion movement remade the party of Barry Goldwater. According to much of the literature on the New Right, it was in the suburbs, especially those outside of Los Angeles, where white people ignored their own government handouts, made "meritocracy" and "free markets" into articles of faith, and began the conservative revolution.[30] If we look to the churches, schools, homes, and clinics in a region like the Mountain West, we can see why those conservative seeds bloomed at the end of the twentieth century. "Moral" conservatives altered many white Americans' everyday lives and eventually their subjectivities. It was not "liberty" that motivated their particular political revolution, but "life." Social conservatives did not simply extend a conservative revolution, they remade it.

In the 1980s, social conservatives took Goldwater's place in representing the western and conservative wing of the Republican Party; one was Trent Franks. Franks was one part of the Republican ascendency—with social conservatism at its heart—that transformed the region and the nation. By the late 1970s, the Mountain West had become a Republican stronghold, with Republican majorities at all levels of government, which only grew as the century progressed. When political scientists Theresa Marchant-Shapiro and Kelly D. Patterson analyzed the motivations for the Republican wave in the Mountain West in the 1980s, they found that two issues compelled the region's voters: distrust of the federal government and abortion. They argued that in the 1980s "the region became much more pro-life" and this "account[ed] for the increased Republicanism in the region."[31] Social conservatives—most especially pro-life activists and voters—are absolutely essential for understanding the region's and the nation's conservative turn in the last three decades of the century. Looking beyond movement pioneers, headline-grabbing personalities, or national organizations to the local activism in one region, we can learn how a relatively homogenized movement reshaped many Americans' sense of self, their definitions of conservatism, and ultimately the nation's politics.

THE SINGULARITY OF ABORTION

This book is the first history to truly reckon with the pro-life campaign for American hearts and minds. Because abortion stood as the pinnacle issue of social conservativism at the end of the twentieth century and the beginning of the twenty-first, it is an essential story to American political history as a whole. In the 1970s, the Equal Rights Amendment and the employment of gay teachers were socially conservative hobbyhorses; in the 1980s, the issues were AIDS, welfare, pornography, and anti-discrimination laws; in the 1990s, affirmative action, arts funding, popular music, and public funding for religious schools took center stage; and in the first decade of the new century gay marriage animated the cause. Each of these issues drew the ire of social conservatives for a period of time. None had the longevity of abortion. Recently a number of historians have surveyed the broad terrain of socially conservative activism at the end of the twentieth century, but few have taken account of legal abortion's singularity in the socially conservative movement. Perhaps most importantly, historian Andrew Hartmann has argued that the conservative culture wars ultimately failed. But did they? Perhaps some socially conservative causes floundered, but the fight against abortion did not and has not.[32] As of 2019 anti-abortion activists have not overturned *Roe v. Wade,* but by all other metrics, they have won their war.

Tiny You joins a bevy of work done by historians, sociologists, anthropologists, journalists, and public intellectuals who have attempted to parse out and explain this divisive issue.[33] This book depends on the story these scholars have told, but adds a critical element that has been left under-explored: how abortion became the singular issue for so many conservative Americans.

The broad outline of the abortion story offered by various scholars typically culminates—and descends—into radicalism. Usually the story begins in the late 1960s, with provincial Catholic activists and officials who by 1973 had begun to turn the tide against abortion reform at the state level.[34] As the story goes, *Roe v. Wade* reversed pro-life gains, but also stalled the momentum of the pro-choice movement as many feminist activists believed their work was done. In the 1970s, anti-abortion groups focused much of their efforts on state and national legislatures, especially upon passing an amendment to the U.S. Constitution (the Human Life Amendment) that would ban abortion. In the years that followed, activists debated among themselves whether to promote laws that would limit abortion or only those that would ban it outright. In the late 1970s and early 1980s, evangelicals joined pro-life coalitions. In the late 1980s and early 1990s, some of these new activists redirected the movement away from legislative change toward civil disobedience, especially clinic blockades. Certain elements of this radical movement went still further, embracing vandalism, arson, assault, and even the murder of abortion providers. Between the early 1980s and 2009, there were 153 assaults, 383 death threats, 3 kidnappings, 18 attempted murders, and 9 murders related to abortion providers. Eight of the murders happened between 1993 and 1998.[35] These acts were a part of a campaign of terror that touched every abortion provider in America.

Some scholars argue that specific individuals led the movement into increasingly radical action; national leaders Juli Loesch, Joan Andrews, John Kavenaugh O'Keefe, and Randall Terry have all been credited with directing the movement toward "by-any-means necessary" activism.[36] Others claim that apocalyptic narratives had dominated pro-life politics since the mid-1960s, inspiring activists to see themselves as God's messengers and motivating more radical and violent action.[37] Whatever the case—as historians tell it—this tidal wave of radical action began to slow when, in the early 1990s, courts began to uphold Racketeer Influenced and Corrupt Organizations Act (RICO) convictions against activists, and when Congress passed in 1994 the Freedom of Access to Clinic Entrances (FACE) Act, which imposed stiffer criminal and civil penalties on those blocking access to abortion clinics. RICO convictions and FACE did not stop anti-abortion protest, but they largely ended the massive civil disobedience that was the most public and contentious expression of the movement at the end of the century.[38]

I do not take issue with this narrative. In fact, its contours anchor my own story in the pages that follow. But the spectacle of a national rescue movement has obscured the importance of quiet, everyday activism that sustained the movement from its beginnings to the present day. This book argues that anti-abortion sermons, viewings of pro-life films in schools, or a casual glance at a fetal pin were more transformative than seeing radical activists block clinic doors. Through such everyday activism, the movement changed almost every urban area (and many rural areas to boot) in the United States, not just Pensacola, Florida, or Wichita, Kansas, cities most known for radical anti-abortion violence.[39] It was this kind of intimate activism, not the movement's more divisive civil disobedience, that produced the uprising of many white Americans around the protection of all fetuses. Moving away from the radical action that looks deceptively like the national story, this book attends to political culture in order to understand the development of a broad, national pro-life public.

In this endeavor, *Tiny You* joins a group of interdisciplinary feminist studies that have assessed the ways in which obstetrical, embryological, legal, and cultural knowledge has produced the fetus as a human subject.[40] These scholars have shown how central it was to the anti-abortion movement to get people to see the fetus as separate from the pregnant woman. Recent historians, most especially Sara Dubow and Johanna Schoen, have shown how social constructions of fetuses shaped legal statutes and the provision of abortion in America.[41] This book adds to this body of work by revealing how fetal politics remade conservative identities and how "life" became the primary political and moral concern for so many, over so many years. It shows how the fetus became essential to many, and why abortion became more important than tax policy to a host of conservatives, working-class and middle-class alike. Anti-abortion activists, I argue, not only made abortion a "bread and butter" issue; they made it *the* bread and butter issue.

Abortion, more so than any other issue, was social conservatism's political buoy. When other issues died—either at the polls, in the courts, or in the court of public opinion—social conservatives could cling to legal abortion as the unwavering evidence of moral decay. This issue continued to galvanize the broader movement, drawing new young activists and generating new political strategies. In a pinch, a conservative politician could always use the dog whistle of "life" to clarify a basic, moral difference between the two major parties. In fact, the "immorality" of abortion allowed (and continues to allow) the Republican Party to paper over a host of other sins. For a good number of conservatives, no weakness—political, familial, or even sexual—could outweigh the importance of a candidate's pro-life stance.

Some of the most passionate voices in this book come from twenty-eight oral histories I did with anti-abortion activists.[42] They generously gave their time to this project, even just an hour or two, telling me about their personal and political life stories. Most did not think their actions were historically important. This book, above all things, should put that misconception to rest. They may disagree with some of the interpretations I offer here, but I hope they see that their stories, their political savvy, and their cultural power have been accurately recorded. While I disagree with them about most political issues, this book would not be what it is without them.

This book is divided into two halves. Part One traces the personal and organizational origins of the movement and early activism. Chapter 1 centers on the 1960s, when both white, longstanding residents and new migrants formed religious and political social worlds that would serve as the basis for their pro-life activism. Other socially conservative movements—anti-birth control and anti-pornography campaigns especially—offered political tools for these future activists. One of the most important lessons pro-life activists took from their forebears was the power of an object of disgust closely held. When reformers passed the first abortion reform law in Colorado in 1967, anti-abortion activism began in earnest. In the next decade, which is the subject of chapter 2, activists linked their evolving rights rhetoric to fetal imagery and ephemera that activists could take into every part of their lives. In this decade, anti-abortion activists set the ideological groundwork for the movement while developing a new type of white identity—one based on their claims to morality and common sense. Chapter 3 follows these activists into American churches, the first important places where this ideology and its objects took root. In the 1970s, activists integrated pro-life politics in rituals of faith for many white Americans. They politicized religious spaces and made the preservation of fetuses central to how many white people thought about being a Christian in these years.

The second half of the book focuses largely on the 1980s and 1990s, when white anti-abortion activists decided that fetuses—and Christians—were not victims enough. In these years, they used pro-life politics to remake the identities of women, children, and families. Chapter 4 assesses the growth of crisis pregnancy centers, where activists tried to stop women from terminating pregnancies. In the 1980s, activists tried to "save" both fetuses and women; they hoped that women "damaged" by abortion and feminism would become the new faces of the movement. As chapter 5 shows, anti-abortion activists also sought to turn children into "survivors" of abortion. They remade a host of youth spaces to do this cultural work, integrating pro-life arguments and objects into schools, homes, and churches. Finally, chapter 6 examines how abortion opponents placed fetuses at the center of the late-twentieth-century family values movement. Pro-life activists took their fetus-focused family into a host of intimate and political spaces, trying to get the state to protect this family—what they called the traditional family—above all others. In so doing, they often shouted down or overshadowed the familial concerns of feminists, poor people, people of color, lesbian and gay people, and others.

In each of these chapters, white pro-life activists politicize a host of Americans—but those new political participants were almost always white. Even if anti-abortion activists believed their movement would benefit all Americans, people of color dissented, often silently, by refusing to join this new "civil rights movement." But that was no matter. By linking fetal preservation to many people's sense of self, anti-abortion activists had developed an unshakeable political coalition of white people who spoke in the language of racial justice all the same.

By the end of the century, activists had successfully integrated anti-abortion politics into the heart of American conservatism and, by extension, American politics. From the late 1960s onward, pro-life activists built a political culture that changed the meanings of life, reproduction, and abortion, but also what it meant to be a Christian, a woman, a child, or a member of a family. A history of pro-life activists producing knowledge in their homes and in their churches, in crisis pregnancy centers and on sidewalks, in wealthy white suburbs, working-class barrios, and sovereign Indigenous nations, is more than a single case study of postwar activism. It is, rather, the story of some of the most pressing cultural and political questions of American life in the late twentieth century.

NOTE ON TERMINOLOGY

Throughout this book, I use the terms "pro-life" and "anti-abortion" to refer to those opposed to legal abortion, and the terms "pro-choice," "abortion rights activists" or—if I am speaking of activists in the late 1960s—"abortion reformers" to refer to those who supported legal abortion. I use the more neutral descriptions but also the highly politicized titles activists used for themselves. "Pro-life" and "pro-choice," while both charged political claims, have become part of everyday speech. My use of them here is not a political endorsement but rather an acknowledgement of their ubiquity and a desire to call people what they wish to be called.

PART ONE

ONE

Rolling across Party Lines

Margaret Sebesta remembered the early 1960s version of herself as a simple, fun-loving young mother who "wanted to dance. That's all." In 1946, she had moved west, following in the footsteps of so many health migrants before her. Colorado's dry air helped cure the terrible asthma that plagued her in the Midwest. Sebesta had grown up in a small town on the Illinois prairie, with German and Irish Catholic parents who were dedicated to their church and the Democratic Party. As a child, she often had a hard time breathing but that rarely kept her from talking; her father told her regularly that her "tongue was tied in the middle and loose on both ends." Once in Colorado, Margaret took advantage not only of the state's environmental opportunities but also its social ones. She relished her independence and she loved dancing the jitterbug whenever possible. But she remembered a political thunderbolt interrupting her easy life in 1967. When a newspaper notice announced the possibility of abortion reform in the state, she remembered asking herself, "They weren't going to pass a bill that would kill innocent human beings in the womb? No." Years later, long after abortion was made legal throughout the United States, she looked back at her life and hypothesized, "I don't think I was put here [in Colorado] to cure my asthma. I was put here for something else. Probably tied to the tongue."[1] That thunderbolt in 1967 had motivated her to use her "gift of gab" for political ends.[2] She would become one of the most important pro-life activists in the state.

Sebesta's obituary explained her activism a different way. On her way out to Colorado, she was confronted with racial segregation for the first time. Because she had been "taught that everyone [was] created in God's image and likeness," she defied Jim Crow and "took a long drink" from a "Colored" water fountain. Her obituary explained that she refused to "obey an unjust law" and would continue her civil disobedience for the rest of her life. Of course, the rest of her life's activism centered on ending legal abortion.[3] The pro-life movement as a whole echoed Sebesta's narration of political awakening. Throughout the end of the century, anti-abortion activists recalled the beginning of their activism as either a political thunderbolt or an extension of their commitments to civil or human rights campaigns.[4]

Recently, historians have echoed these claims, especially the one about liberal origins. The pro-life movement "originated not among political conservatives, but rather among people who supported New Deal liberalism and government aid to the poor," according to historian Daniel K. Williams. In his narration, human rights and anti-poverty politics, not sexual moralism, were the intellectual predecessors of the anti-abortion movement.[5] Legal scholar Mary Ziegler largely agrees, though she suggests the movement had mixed liberal and conservative origins.[6] Both conclude that the movement only became conservative in the late 1970s when evangelicals and New Right conservatives wooed anti-abortion activists to join their anti-feminist movement and the Republican Party. These scholars are correct that many anti-abortion activists were Democrats and might have even considered themselves liberals. Some sexual moralists may have felt at home in the Democratic Party of the 1960s, but this did not make the early anti-abortion movement "liberal" when it came to women. Sexual moralism was never ancillary to this movement, nor was anti-feminism an afterthought. Beginning in the late 1960s, feminism and anti-feminism reshaped the definitions of liberal and conservative, making the word "liberal" synonymous with a commitment to women's rights *and* the welfare state. When the Democratic Party joined in this political shift, they slowly stopped centering their politics around the protection of the male breadwinner and his nuclear family. Social conservatives increasingly began to associate the Democratic Party less with the New Deal and more with civil rights, gay rights, women's rights, and most especially "abortion-on-demand." Ultimately the story of the anti-abortion movement is not one of activists who lost their liberalism, but rather one of sexual moralists who found their party.

The lives of Margaret Sebesta and the many others who staffed the first pro-life groups in the Four Corners states tell this story. Even if they recalled their conservative outrage rupturing their calm lives like a storm coming over the fields, they were socially, culturally, and politically prepared to answer that call. They came from certain demographics, religions, organizations, and professions that primed them for activism. Through these social institutions, future pro-life activists were influenced by sexually conservative movements like the anti-birth control and anti-pornography movements, much more than anti-poverty or civil rights movements. They may have been interested in the poor and the disenfranchised but those interests were not what motivated their anti-abortion activism. It was in the anti-porn and anti-birth control movements where they formed the intellectual frameworks that would later translate into anti-abortion politics. Even if some activists had been New Deal Democrats, they were always sexually conservative ones. Sexual moralism was in the movement's political blood from the very beginning.

In these moments, months, and years before the pro-life movement swelled, future anti-abortion activists were developing the primary elements of a politicized white identity. In the 1960s, conservative white religious people, most especially Catholics, experienced massive upheaval within their denominations and within American society at large. Those future activists began to stake out their political terrain, claiming to represent "the middle" and "the moral." White social conservatives separated themselves from both white elites and "dangerous" people of color. At the same time, early social conservatives claimed to be protecting people of color from a coercive state. From the 1960s onward, white conservatives fit themselves into both sides of America's racial story. They named themselves as the protectors of America from corrupting people of color, while also being the protectors of people of color from a corrupting America. Through such rhetorical moves, social conservatives began to use liberal and conservative tools to recreate a special place for white people in the era of civil rights.

White moralistic activists, in places like Tucson, Denver, and Albuquerque, were more representative of the movement as a whole, not Catholic officials in Rome who talked of human rights or a handful of anti-war or feminist pro-life activists. Examining the activities of social conservatives at the local and grassroots levels reveals the rhetoric and tactics that resonated with most activists, and how their tools evolved in context. Some of these activists only participated in pro-life groups for a few years, while others committed their entire lives to the cause. No matter the duration of their activism, these activists—the type that started and staffed early organizations—molded the institutions that would carry the movement through the end of the century.

This chapter examines the lives and politics of those activists in the 1960s and early 1970s.[7] The first half focuses on the social worlds they inhabited before legal abortion. A majority were relatively recent arrivals to Arizona, Colorado, New Mexico, or Utah, coming either in the early twentieth century or in the immediate postwar period from the Midwest, the Plains, or the South. They were often drawn by health or work opportunities in the region. Once there, they found homes in exploding urban areas, often in new, upwardly mobile neighborhoods. A large number of these future activists were of Irish Catholic descent and quickly enmeshed themselves in Catholic social networks. An important breed of future activist—the pro-life doctor or nurse—found their social homes in Catholic or secular medical societies. The new migrants built communities with long-standing residents in medical and religious spaces, which would become the organizational basis for their later activism.

The second half of the chapter focuses on the political cultures in which these future activists were already involved. These were the social environments and political causes that prepared activists to respond to the "thunderbolt" of legal abortion when it happened. Through Catholic organizations, many witnessed the inner workings of anti-pornography or anti-birth control campaigns, and took part either as activists or sympathetic observers. They also learned how to fight sexual modernity with conservative experts and arguments about civil rights, human rights, and the poor. Perhaps most importantly, they learned the power of a well-placed image (or item) of outrage to motivate social action. By the time abortion reform arrived in the region, the majority of anti-abortion activists were already concerned with the issues that would become the basis for social conservatism: cultural immorality, social relativism, the power of liberal elites, and, most importantly, changing mores around women's sexuality.

These nascent social conservatives did not have a single partisan home; some were Democrats like Sebesta while others were avowed Republicans. Socially conservative activists had not yet housed "morality" within the party of Lincoln. Neither Democratic affiliation nor use of liberal rhetoric, like that of human rights, can stand in for an interest in bettering the lives of women or for promoting gender equity. Pro-life Democrats and Republicans were always concerned about sexual morality. This social conservatism did not preclude some civil rights and women's rights activists from imagining affinity with the anti-abortion movement. But when they did, they had to ignore the strong tides of gendered and racial conservatism that already swirled around the question of legal abortion.

The women and men who built the pro-life movement were movers, living in a region shaped by exiles, migrations, and manifest destinies. Most had a migration story of their own, while a select few could claim longer roots in the West. But the majority arrived in the postwar period, staffing the area's military bases and middle-class professions. These future activists were one small stream in a flood of people in those years, when the region shifted from colonial backwater to booming Sunbelt. But these future activists stood apart from their fellow nomads moving into the Mountain West. Unlike so many others, they were drawn to social action. Their identities, their communities, and their interest in prior political causes primed them for socially conservative activism, and they in turn made the movement that would define social conservativism at the end of the century. These migrants did more than just arrive in the West. Through their migration and their political efforts, they transformed the region.

Not all were new to the region. Many had classic western migration stories. Ora DeConcini (née Webster) descended from nineteenth-century Mormon pioneers called by Brigham Young to settle Arizona. The Webster family had come to the upper Gila River Valley in the 1880s to create an "oasis in the desert," but this oasis was grown in the ruins of war. The Websters settled within miles of the San Carlos Reservation, a homeland and a place of exile for its recently defeated Apache residents. Ora herself embodied older stories of Anglo western progress: she was the first child in her family to be born with the help of a physician, a teen who sought new horizons in Los Angeles, and a young woman who went to college in both Utah and Arizona, receiving degrees in education, finance, and accounting. Eventually Ora married outside of her faith and into a rising political family, becoming the wife of a future Arizona attorney general and state supreme court judge and mother of a U.S. senator.[8]

Others came to the region as economic refugees. Libby Ruiz's father immigrated from Mexico in 1900, fleeing the policies of Mexican president Porfirio Díaz, who pushed thousands of rural people to the brink of starvation. Many of her father's fellow travelers were disappointed with their new homes across the border, but he was not one of them. Ruiz's father named his daughter "Librada" (Liberty) in honor of the United States.[9] Carolyn Gerster's migration to the Mountain West was born out of homegrown economic depression. She came to Arizona as a child in the early 1930s with her newly divorced mother, who left San Francisco hoping for work and a cure for Carolyn's respiratory problems.[10] These women, and others like them, would be important allies for postwar migrants.

The Mountain West was a different kind of oasis after World War II. No longer just an escape for those fleeing poverty or religious persecution, the Four Corners region drew the upwardly mobile to its exploding urban areas in the postwar period. Denver's population tripled between 1940 and 1970, Phoenix's increased five times in the same period, and Albuquerque's grew sevenfold. Outside urban areas, smaller cities like Los Alamos and Colorado Springs drew new migrants, often rising professionals seeking success in the Sunbelt's booming economy.[11] Future pro-life activists were no different in this respect from their co-migrants. John Gillette came to Tucson to build his medical practice, though he was the son of a successful Iowa state legislator.[12] Muriel James got a bachelor's degree at the University of Michigan and a graduate degree in public health nursing in Missouri before arriving in Albuquerque in 1953.[13] Gillette and James, along with a host of other postwar migrants, populated the region's white-collar professions as doctors, nurses, lawyers, ministers, and social workers.

Of these professionals, it was health care workers who were most likely to join the movement. Medical professionals—both new migrants and those from older generations—staffed many early anti-abortion organizations. This was true in every one of the four states but especially so in Phoenix, Arizona. There, the first pro-life groups included nurses and family physicians, alongside prominent thoracic and pediatric surgeons, cardiologists, and oncologists. Virginia (Ginny) Clements explained the reasons she joined the movement: "My father is a doctor, I married a doctor, I'm a nurse and I've taught nursing."[14] To her, opposition to abortion was the natural outcome of a medical background.

These doctors and nurses extended a long history of medical opposition to abortion, dating back to the American Medical Association (AMA)'s nineteenth-century campaign to outlaw abortion. Doctors pushed for these laws because they claimed that doctors alone—not midwives and certainly not women themselves—had the knowledge to determine when life began. Twentieth-century medical advances broadened doctors' interest in fetal life. After World War II, new technologies allowed doctors to view and treat fetuses in new ways, allowing some to look to fetal bodies for cures to persistent human problems. This process ultimately personified and individualized

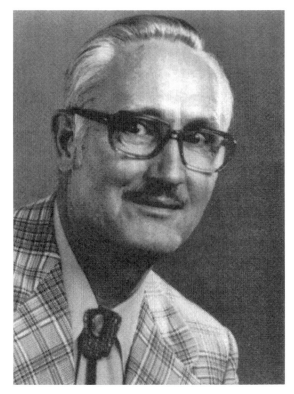

FIGURE 1. Wallace McWhirter, one of the founders of Arizona Right to Life, 1979. (Courtesy of Dr. Robert Allman; *Journal of Radiology*)

the fetus.[15] It is not surprising that activists like Arizona radiologist Wallace McWhirter believed his pro-life commitments began in medical school where he learned that abortions were "wrong and illegal."[16]

Postwar medical practice and politics, though, were not as clear-cut as the McWhirters of the world would have liked. In the 1940s and 1950s, many doctors quietly provided abortions to women in need and others, like New York gynecologist Alan Guttmacher, advocated for abortion reform. While McWhirter often implied there was medical consensus on when life began, his own biography suggested otherwise. McWhirter remembered seeing both Guttmacher and a pro-life doctor speak, and siding firmly with the latter.[17] This anti-abortion speaker might have been one of the vocal postwar physicians, usually Catholic, who argued that abortion laws should become more strict, not less. They believed that the legal loopholes that allowed abortion in very select instances should be closed. Such doctors continued to oppose any legal abortion, even when the AMA changed their stance and supported abortion reform in 1967.[18] By the late 1960s, doctors and nurses staffed the emerging movements on both sides of this issue, a debate that became an essential question of medical ethics.

Even more than the medical and health professions, it was the U.S. military and its related industries that built the postwar Sunbelt economy and drew new migrants. The Mountain West offered the military-industrial complex relatively cheap land, open spaces, sunshine, and temperate climates, all elements aggressively promoted by western boosters.[19] Between 1946 and 1965, the federal government spent 62 percent of its budget on defense, making the military-industrial complex the nation's largest business.[20] Such largesse attracted hordes of Americans to the region, some of whom would eventually join the ranks of the anti-abortion movement. William Riordan and Jack Arnold served as bombardiers during World War II, while William Reese joined the Air Force after the war. Eventually they would enter the private labor force and the pro-life movement, but all three first came to southern Arizona because of the Davis-Monahan Air Force Base.[21] Others were drawn to the region by industries linked to the U.S. military. Leo Dunn was an engineer who came to work for New Mexico's Sandia Corporation, an off-shoot of the Los Alamos laboratory and eventually the largest private employer in the state.[22]

The region's booming metropolises, and their wealth of high-paying jobs, were an attraction for Americans living in the U.S. South and Plains. Wallace McWhirter, for example, was the eighth of nine children born to a farming family in Roff, Oklahoma. A Protestant doctor, he found his way to southern Arizona and helped found Arizona Right to Life.[23] Some historians have credited migrants, like McWhirter, with the "southernization" of the U.S. West and the "southernization" of U.S. politics. Southern evangelicals brought with them commitments to unregulated capitalism, local governance, and the sanctity of the individual all "wrapped in a package of Christian, plain-folk Americanism," according to historian Darren Dochuk.[24] McWhirter, however, should not be held up as evidence of evangelical institutions' support for anti-abortion conservatism. Importantly, McWhirter was at odds with the religious institutions of his Protestant faith. In fact, he resigned from his congregation at some point in the late 1960s when he learned the minister and the denomination supported abortion reform.[25]

In the 1960s and early 1970s, evangelical denominations, in the West and elsewhere, were not institutional breeding grounds for pro-life politics.

Evangelical leaders most often supported abortion reform. In 1968, preeminent evangelical scholars, pastors, and physicians issued a statement saying that although they could not agree on the sinful nature of abortion, "about the necessity of it and permissibility for it under certain circumstances we are in accord."[26] In 1971, the Southern Baptist Convention passed a resolution supporting abortion reform and urged members to work for legislation that would allow abortions in cases of rape, incest, fetal deformity, and when it was likely the pregnancy would cause "damage to the emotional, mental, and physical health of the mother."[27] The convention reiterated this position in resolutions after *Roe v. Wade,* in 1974 and 1976.[28] Many evangelicals simply felt that the Bible did not provide a clear answer on the morality of abortion. Thus it was not southern evangelicalism that made the socially conservative revolution, at least not in this corner of the country, and not in the context of this movement.

Catholics generated the ideological basis for pro-life conservatism and staffed the movement's early ranks. Catholics had long believed that any act to limit the possibility of reproduction in sex was contrary to God's purpose. Pope Pius XI made the church's stance abundantly clear in his 1930 *Casti Connubii* encyclical, which, according to historian Leslie Woodcock Tentler, "summoned all priests to the frontline stations in a veritable war against birth control."[29] While contraception and abortion were both violations of natural law, contraception received most of the attention for most of the twentieth century. This was not because Catholics thought abortion was a lesser sin (they did not), but rather because, after the 1930s, the Catholic Church often felt alone in condemning birth control. Many Protestant and Jewish denominations had loosened their restrictions. Even as Catholic leaders and priests focused on the more common crime of contraception, they regularly reminded the laity that abortion was the murder of an unborn and unbaptized child and a profoundly immoral act. Some Catholics fed a steady diet of "moral law" were eager to join the fray in the late 1960s.

Catholic dominance of the early anti-abortion movement went beyond states with deep Catholic roots, like Arizona and New Mexico, into states with small Catholic populations like Utah. Many of Utah's Catholics migrated to Zion in the nineteenth century to help work in the state's mines and build the transcontinental railroad.[30] Perhaps unsurprisingly, it was a handful of Catholic laity, some priests, and the diocese's bishop who staffed the state's first pro-life organization, the Utah Right to Life League, in the late 1960s.[31] Emanuel Floor, who headed the movement in 1969, hailed from the state's Greek community and had converted from Greek Orthodox to Roman Catholicism in the mid-1960s. He explained, "I simply felt a little more complete in the Catholic Church." Floor was a rising star in the state's advertising world, tasked as the director of Utah's Travel Council with drawing outsiders to the state's tourist destinations. As an important public figure, Floor took no public political positions except on abortion.[32] Catholicism was so interlaced with this issue that, when Mormons began to join the movement in the early 1970s, they formed their own separate organization, the Utah Anti-Abortion League.[33] Thus, even in one of the most religiously unique states in the country, the religious contours of the early anti-abortion movement were the same. Catholics led and a small number of other religious people participated, usually in marginal ways.

Before their involvement in the anti-abortion movement began, future activists inhabited a Catholic world fraught with debates about modernization and reform, the purpose of traditions and unchanging religious dictums, and the importance of social justice. The Catholic Church experienced incredible theological and structural change in the 1960s. For most American Catholics, this process of reform began with the Second Vatican Council, which one historian calls "the most important event in the history of Roman Catholicism since the Reformation."[34] Between 1962 and 1965, three thousand theologians, bishops, and cardinals discussed how to move the Catholic Church into the modern world.[35] They covered a wide array of issues, from anti-Semitism to the way Catholics took communion, and they instituted sweeping reforms. The council empowered laity to become more involved in parish ministries, arguing that they were the theological core of the church. The Vatican Council confessed to past mistakes, advocating dialogues between denominations and tolerance of all faiths. They changed the language of mass from Latin to the vernacular language of the individual parish. Many rituals of mass changed as well. For example, congregations were encouraged to recite new prayers and to read the scriptures, and the priest now faced the congregation during most of the mass.[36]

At turns disorienting and empowering, these reforms touched every believer in this allegedly unchanging church. For many Catholic conservatives—those future pro-life activists—these changes were more than disorienting, they were "unbridled lunacy," according to sociologist Michael Cuneo.[37] When the Pope reaffirmed the church's opposition to birth control in the 1968 *Humanae Vitae* encyclical, many conservatives rejoiced, seeing much desired evidence of Catholic continuity. In the 1960s and beyond, conservatives, both men and women, latched onto reproductive issues to defend their church and their country against social change. They would put the church's resources and organizations to their use in this fight.

Future anti-abortion activists, more than simply being Catholic, regularly participated in Catholic organizations; they took part in local and statewide chapters of the Knights of Columbus, the Catholic Lawyers Guild, the Catholic Council of Nurses, the Christian Family Movement, and Catholic social groups. Anti-abortion activists in other parts of the country came from such organizations as well.[38] The most important incubator for pro-life activism, however, was the Council of Catholic Women (CCW), which had groups at deanery, diocesan, or archdiocesan levels.[39] The Council of Catholic Women, a federation of laywomen's organizations, was founded in 1920 in order to combat feminism and the "moral gangrene" it allegedly spread.[40] Since then, the group had created space for Catholic women to organize as political actors while also opposing the "unnatural" social forces that took women out of the home. The council adopted some progressive stances throughout the twentieth century—on issues ranging from child welfare to equal pay to nuclear disarmament—but it never let go of its concerns about the erosion of women's special status in society. Because Vatican II empowered lay organizations, the council provided an inspirational setting for modern Catholic women in the 1960s; Catholic women could become leaders, change their communities, and reconceive their place in the church.[41] This inspirational social action, however, always occurred within the frame of religious sexual moralism. For example, at a 1958 CCW meeting in New Mexico, a local priest warned his audience about excessive "sex in advertising" and the corrupting "pagan climate" in America today; he said the women should be "alert in [their] reading." One woman in that audience was future pro-life activist Muriel James.[42]

Even as CCW leaders embraced at least part of the church's reforms, especially Vatican II's empowerment of lay groups, the council maintained a fervent opposition to birth control, divorce, and abortion.[43] For example, in 1968, future anti-abortion activist Shirley Hellwig called on New Mexico's archdiocesan Council of Catholic Women to get involved in the campaign to oppose abortion, and she reassured members that the leadership knew how to lead them into the political fray. She said they "brought back the know-how" from the recent National Council of Catholic Women conference.[44] That CCW "know how" became the political bedrock of the nascent pro-life movement.[45]

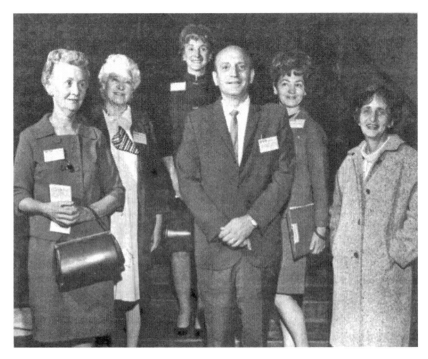

FIGURE 2. Two of the women in this New Mexico delegation to the 1968 National Council of Catholic Women conference went on to found the anti-abortion movement in the state: Shirley Hellwig (second from right) and Mrs. Leo Dunn (far right). (Courtesy of the Archdiocese of Santa Fe; *New Mexico Catholic Renewal*, Center for Southwest Research, University of New Mexico)

Importantly, white women dominated Councils of Catholic Women, even in the Southwest where ethnic Mexicans made up a large percentage of the region's Catholics. The leadership of Arizona's Councils of Catholic Women sheds light on the demographics of these organizations. Out of eighty-two Arizona women identified by newspapers as CCW leaders in the 1960s, only eight had Spanish-surnames (9.7 percent).[46] These eight women occupied low levels in the council leadership, such as heading a deanery-level committee or being the point person for a special mass. The marginalization of ethnic Mexican women in Arizona's CCW built on a longer history of racial discrimination in the state's Catholic community. In the early twentieth century, for example, Phoenix's ethnic Mexicans had to worship in a church basement. The Anglo priest insisted that the services remain segregated because Mexican immigrants were "untid[y] ... peons."[47] Though the church had improved since that nadir, many of their organizations still remained highly segregated by 1960. Thus, while Catholicism did organize the lives of many ethnic Mexicans, they were often cut out of the institutions that motivated pro-life activism. All over the region, it was white Catholic newcomers, not the Mexican Catholics with centuries-long roots in the region, who were most likely to take their concerns over changing sexual mores and turn them into social action.

In Catholic social settings like the CCW, white Catholic women developed ideas about white religious people's relationship to societal morality. Whiteness was a central, if unacknowledged, part of their worldview and their politics. These Catholics occupied racially exclusive or, at best, racially hierarchical spaces. There, CCW women focused on birth control and abortion, and sometimes on America's racial strife. But that strife was usually a southern problem, not a western one, and certainly not a problem of which they were a part.[48] CCW women in the Four Corners states were able to envision the white women that surrounded them as society's moralists, in both racial and gendered matters. In 1963 the *New Mexico Register* explained Catholic women's mission in the world this way: they were "the salvation of men, of the family, [and] of the nation."[49] White religious people, and most especially women, became protectors of womanhood, the keepers of decency, and sometimes the saviors of people of color. Such constructions built on older notions of the moral superiority of white women. After the Civil War, white southerners re-envisioned white womanhood as fundamentally moral, chaste, and pure—a status that united women across class. This was an adaptation of the separate-spheres ideology that was common in nineteenth-century America. Northern and western white women reformers turned some parts of this racial construction to their political benefit. In turn-of-the-century reform politics, for example, white religious women gained "moral authority" by protecting women and "rescuing" the poor and people of color, according to historian Peggy Pascoe.[50] In the postwar period, white women in the CCW repackaged older notions of moral and racial uplift for a modern moment.

Many of these Catholics, who would go on to start the anti-abortion movement, came from the Midwest. They were often from rural and urban areas in states like Iowa, Illinois, Indiana, Michigan, and Missouri.[51] Perhaps midwestern migrants were fleeing the declining industries in the much-maligned Rust Belt or they were simply looking for sunnier shores in the rapidly expanding metropolitan West. Norman Weslin, for example, left his home in the Upper Peninsula of Michigan for Colorado twice, once following his fiancé who sought work in Denver and then again when he retired from the Army in 1968.[52] Colorado exerted a strong pull on Weslin, who would go on to found Colorado Springs Right to Life and later the radical group Lambs of Christ. Locals noticed the arrival of midwesterners like Weslin and worried about their effect on their state's party politics. In the 1950s, for example, political observers in Arizona claimed that midwesterners were to blame for their state's conservative turn.[53] While midwesterners cannot be solely credited with such large political transformations, many surely brought a certain type of conservatism with them to the Mountain West. What was often called "midwestern conservatism" exemplified what many Americans considered "small-town values": a concern over fairness and decency, skepticism of corporate and eastern establishments, and a provisional, not absolute, belief in small government.[54] The type of midwesterner that moved west to work in the Cold War defense industry might have been especially likely to bring along this very specific constellation of political commitments. That conservatism masqueraded as "common sense" for many of its adherents—a common sense born from and carried by white (often midwestern) Americans.

Even though these soon-to-be activists proclaimed their dedication to "tradition" and "old-fashioned values," their lives were more a hodge-podge of old and new, and the women of the movement highlight this fact. A majority of early women activists had large families. For example, Shirley Hellwig of Albuquerque had five children plus a number of foster children; Helen Seader of Tucson had eight; and Helen Onofrio of Denver had ten.[55] Margaret Sebesta remembered that her early pro-life group in Denver was made up of a handful of women but the meetings felt much bigger. They included "something like 30, 35 children."[56] Many of these women, however, were also educated professionals, with jobs in medicine, social work, and politics. Carolyn Gerster, who helped found Arizona Right to Life and eventually became president of National Right to Life, was an accomplished internist and cardiologist. In the 1960s, she regularly turned up in Arizona newspapers, combatting tuberculosis and Valley Fever and starting a much heralded medical practice with her husband.[57] In the media coverage of this new breed of career woman, Gerster portrayed herself as a traditional mother who also happened to have an important job. She told Arizona newspapers that she stayed home in the mornings because it was "important [that] children see their mother in the morning" and showed off her culinary skills with a published cheesecake recipe.[58] When she was asked to address Arizona State University's female students on Women's Day, she delivered a somewhat complicated message. She said that women doctors bore a great responsibility to continue their careers because they had taken a man's seat in medical school.[59] The labor market was and should be a male world, she implied, but women could prove they had a reason to be there. Gerster and other women in the pro-life movement embodied postwar contradictions around womanhood. They embraced the idea that motherhood and the home were still a woman's highest calling while also meeting Cold War expectations of educational success. Future feminists called out the hypocrisy of these contradictory expectations. Many conservative women, however, seemed to balance their lives precariously at their intersection.[60] They strove to excel professionally and change American political life, all while doing so in the name of motherhood.

The racial demographics and rhetoric of this movement highlight the ways that anti-abortion activists incorporated "modern" ideologies into older social frameworks. Joan Sebesta Weber, one of Margaret Sebesta's children who grew up in the movement, remembered it as racially diverse, if unconsciously so. "We look back on it now [and] we realize that we were part of this group that knew no political boundaries, no ethnic boundaries, no religious boundaries. But we didn't know that at the time. [We] were just friends. We took them for who they were; we didn't look at them and like oh you're Black or Hispanic or whatever." According to her, this was a racially diverse movement, or even a postracial one. But the person she pointed to as evidence of this diversity was Chuck Onofrio, who was, according to Weber, "Mexican or Spanish."[61] In fact, Chuck Onofrio was an Italian immigrant who married a Mexican-American woman (Elena, who anglicized her name to Helen).[62] Perhaps his wife's race rubbed off on Chuck Onofrio in Weber's memory. Or perhaps an Italian, misremembered as Spanish, felt a little exotic to the movement's members. Either way, the pro-life movement was far from the postracial, multiracial utopia that Weber remembered from her childhood. From the late 1960s onward, the movement was almost entirely white, as members found it hard to recruit any significant number of people of color, even ethnic Mexican Catholics or black evangelicals.

Two women in the Southwest bucked this trend: Emma Gomez in Albuquerque and Libby Ruiz in Tucson. Gomez came to the movement like so many of her white counterparts. Before her politicization, she was enmeshed in her parish's alter society, her state's Council of Catholic Women, and the Christian Family Movement, a group dedicated to bringing spirituality to every part of the family and translating that into social action.[63] She was a nurse, like many other early activists, and her husband worked for the military industrial complex through the Sandia Lab.[64] Though she was a woman of color, she was incorporated in largely white Catholic and medical spaces, which helped shape her and so many others' activism.

Libby Ruiz was more of an outlier, if a fascinating one. Ruiz, the daughter of a Mexican immigrant who loved America, was a strident anti-communist and a voice for working-class, Mexican-American conservatism. Unlike Gomez and her white counterparts, Ruiz was not solidly middle class. She was the daughter of a plasterer and the wife of a railroad worker. She became a housewife with four children, and in middle age she committed herself to conservative politics. Initially, she was involved in the John Birch Society's Movement to Restore Decency, which formed in 1969 to attack sex education in schools "on the ground that Communists are behind the programs."[65] Over the next ten years, Ruiz blended radical anti-communism, assimilationist ideology, and social conservatism. In letters to the editor and public forums, she contended that big government made "leeches out of people" and that social "permissiveness" motivated poor people to break the law. The Chicano movement, according to her, had done ethnic Mexicans no favors by representing them "as poor, oppressed, deprived, and sometimes stupid" in order to access public funds. Ruiz turned to the individual, free enterprise, conservative morality, and the nation as the solutions to her city's and her community's problems. She translated these commitments into action through the anti-abortion movement, a Mexican-American anti-busing group, a city council election, and eventually a bilingual talk show on Tucson politics. The Tucson press treated her as an oddity, condescendingly describing her as "a well-meaning homemaker" and a political "novice." Her public speeches often drew "bemused looks" from the audience.[66] And truly, Ruiz was unusual in many ways. Unlike most other pro-life activists, radical anti-communism and assimilationist Mexican-American politics inflected her social conservatism, giving her denunciations of "moral decay" a different tenor.

Libby Ruiz was not unusual in all ways though. Every activist, including Ruiz, was trying to build a conservatism that rolled across party lines. Coloradoan Margaret Sebesta remembered that everybody was a Democrat because "being a Democrat meant you cared for people, you took care of your neighbors, you treated people right." She was right about the region's politics in part. Electoral maps of the Mountain West in the postwar period were solidly blue.[67] Future anti-abortion activists were just as much a part of this political trend, perhaps more so. Catholics—social liberals and conservatives alike—had longstanding commitments to the Democratic Party in this region as well as others. If anything, the Democratic Party of the 1960s had a greater claim to "protecting the family" than Republicans did, as historian Robert Self has argued. Since the 1930s, Democrats had made the protection of the male breadwinner—the male citizen worker with a family of dependents—the centerpiece of their social and economic policy. In the 1960s, the broader goals of President Lyndon Johnson's Great Society were to rehabilitate and support poor men, so they in turn could support their families.[68] Before the mid-1960s, among Democrats and Republicans, the assumption that the nuclear family was the ideal unit for individual fulfillment, for societal stability, and for social protection went largely unquestioned. It is not surprising then, that budding anti-feminists would have been completely comfortable in either political party of that era.

But the 1960s was also a time of partisan flux. Some staunch Democrats aired their growing discontent with their party and especially its younger, more radical contingent. Jack Arnold was deeply involved in Arizona's Democratic Party, running as the party's candidate for the state Supreme Court and later becoming the chairman of the Pima County Democratic Central Committee. However even this committed partisan complained about the direction of his party and the young people "who insist[ed] on their own terms."[69] His complaint was likely about younger activists who were demanding that the party commit itself to progressive stances on issues of race and gender. In the 1960s, Democratic pro-life activists, like Jack Arnold, and their state legislators could still reasonably hope that their party would join them when they opposed abortion reform.

Not all activists were Democrats. Some activists came to the movement from right-wing movements that fell outside the two-party system. Bruce Bangerter of Utah ran for Congress in 1972 under the American Independence Party on "freedom, constitutionality, and the right to life of the unborn child."[70] Many more were standard Republicans. Bernadine Haag of Tucson was a GOP loyalist who worried about the influence of drugs on young people, rising crime rates, government spending, and the erosion of constitutional liberty. She also warned her opponents—"good and loyal Democrats"—to be wary of radicals, like "SDS, WEB DuBois Clubs, Black Panthers, and SNCC," who were going to start "new left communiversities."[71] Perhaps Democrat Jack Arnold would have been receptive to such an admonition, even though Haag and Arnold occupied opposite ends of the political spectrum. In general though, party affiliation was not a good indicator of conservatism when it came to issues of gender and sexuality during this period. Libby Ruiz embodied the diverse political affiliations of this movement; she was a John Birch Society member who ran as a Democrat in Tucson city elections. Only in the 1980s would she become a Republican.[72] The movement as a whole would follow her partisan trajectory.

In the postwar period, before they joined "the cause," future pro-life activists were both a part of trends that shaped their region and also stood apart from them. These white midwestern professionals joined a stream of Americans pouring into the postwar West. Like so many migrants, they joined existing social institutions in the region, like medical societies, Catholic groups, and political parties, and subtly changed those institutions. Future anti-abortion activists infused a midwestern conservatism—a belief in an implicitly white, Middle American common sense—into spaces already laced with medical and religious conservatism. Those activists often participated in party politics in the 1960s, with both Democrats and Republicans envisioning their party as a possible home for moral conservatism. When these future activists stood apart from their fellow travelers and started a movement, they might have felt alone at first, but they should have known that there were already many institutions in the region quietly protecting their backs.

SOCIAL EXPERIMENTATION AND SMUT

Some might have been inclined toward pro-life social action because of their religious, professional, and regional identities, but it was other socially conservative movements that helped shape what form that action would take. In the Four Corners states, and elsewhere, movements against birth control and pornography animated activists' political imaginations. Some joined these campaigns while many others were a part of organizations where these movements flourished. When the possibility of legal abortion arrived in the late 1960s, anti-abortion activists borrowed and remade many of the tools, tactics, and arguments deployed in 1960s socially conservative movements.

Both anti-pornography and anti-birth control movements had roots dating back to the nineteenth century, but they had new import in an era of "sexual revolution." In the 1960s, many Americans worried that young people were abandoning old sexual mores for new, radical types of sexual and social groupings. There was massive change afoot but, as historian Beth

Bailey has argued, that change was not all led by radicals on the East and West coasts. Both in America's heartland and on its coasts, single and married women sought to separate sex from reproduction, especially when they enthusiastically embraced the Pill. Others sought more individual autonomy by rejecting some of the sexual controls, like curfew, that their communities had imposed on them.[73] By the late 1960s, activists from women's liberation movements and gay liberation movements asked for more radical change; they demanded sexual freedom, the decriminalization of homosexuality, and the right to control one's body. As importantly, these activists demanded that the citizenry rethink the place of sex and sexual moralism in American life.[74] It was because the call for sexual change reached so many in the 1960s—from co-eds in Lawrence, Kansas, to gay communities in Greenwich Village—that it was so threatening to social conservatives. In this era, birth control and pornography were about more than just obscenity, they were a part of a broader revolution in American sexuality.

One of the anti-abortion movement's most important precursors was the anti-birth control movement. This was especially true in Colorado which into the 1960s, still had some of the most restrictive birth control laws in the country. Its "little Comstock laws" prohibited the discussion of birth control or abortion and the possession of instructions for preventing conception.[75] Over the course of the decade, these restrictions would gradually be rescinded.[76] In 1965, legislators proposed a bill that would allow state employees to offer birth control information to people on state aid if they requested it. The bill did not force welfare recipients to use birth control or require state employees to discuss family planning if it conflicted with their religious beliefs, but despite these protections, social conservatives opposed the bill and tried to kill it.[77]

In the early 1960s, the Catholic Church organized much of the opposition to birth control reform in Colorado; their primary concern was about promiscuity. Archbishop Urban J. Vehr told a Senate committee that the bill "will lead to promiscuity and adultery which are against the laws of Colorado."[78] A Knights of Columbus chapter called it "state sanctioned adultery."[79] Other opponents contended that contraceptives would be given to young, unmarried girls, and thus encourage prostitution.[80] In the minds of these activists, fear of pregnancy was the only thing standing between a young girl and her john, an adulteress and her paramour. Once women were untethered from their reproductive restraints, their desires would become uncontrollable. Physical lust and desire for money would drive women away from the marriage bed, undermining "the sanctity of the home."[81] Local Catholic journalist Paul Hallett got to the heart of the matter: "Contraception itself is always an act of irresponsibility, because it seeks to elude the responsibility that nature has attached to the reproductive act."[82] This situation would affect more than just an individual here or there. The "contraceptive mind" was a contagious condition, leading society to demonize children and accept abortion, leading eventually to "moral chaos."[83] Ultimately, this relatively narrow bill sparked deep anxieties about women's sexuality and its role in stabilizing both heterosexual marriage and American society.

Conservatives coupled their panic about the prospect of loose women with arguments about poverty. Some contended that the poor were being targeted by the state and would be potentially coerced into limiting their families. According to opponents, the bill's premise was that poor women's reproduction was a social problem that needed to be fixed, and that fix amounted to "social experimentation."[84] These concerns were relayed to Catholic parishioners through their clergy across the state.[85] There was some truth to the claim that many who worried about overpopulation saw limiting poor women's reproduction as the solution.[86] But birth control advocates— and the subset that worried about overpopulation—were a varied lot, who offered a range of solutions from simple access to more coercive practices. Their opponents believed that all birth control activists had the same motivations and no amount of language protecting women from government pressure would be enough.

Opponents of the bill worried not only about the oppression of the poor, they also worried about the poor becoming a greater social burden through their excessive sexuality. The Catholic bishop of Pueblo paired his concern about social experimentation on the poor with a belief that the bill would be "costly."[87] Others argued the bill would increase tax burdens.[88] Catholic journalist Paul Hallett agreed. He forecasted a massive increase in venereal disease, which the state would have to pay to cure.[89] Another anti–birth control activist criticized the poor for relying on the state at all. "If indigent mothers can afford cigarettes, they can afford contraceptives," the opponent contended.[90] In this classic argument against state aid, the speaker imagined a woman who consumed irresponsibly, had sex irresponsibly, and then relied on the public to pay for her indulgences.

The conservative response to the 1965 Colorado birth control bill was part of a cultural re-envisioning of who the people were who were seeking to benefit from "scamming" the government. Beginning in the 1960s, social critics no longer pointed to errant white men or poor migrants, but rather to black people—and black women in particular—as the primary culprits.[91] In the mid-1960s, the media increasingly put images of black people alongside the most critical and unsympathetic portrayals of poor people.[92] Black women drew special attention, from liberals and conservatives, in this decade as they were blamed for poverty itself.[93] In the comments on the 1965 birth control bill, conservative white Coloradoans renewed the link between women and irresponsible public assistance. While conservatives named the sex of the "undeserving poor" in their comments, many surely had a race in mind as well.

Activists also levied broader critiques of government action. They argued that the government would be "invad[ing] the 'free conscience' of the individual" and "invad[ing] the sanctity of the home."[94] This language of invasions pitted citizens against the government in a war over women, sexuality, and the home. This was not a war of arms, but a war of culture. Lydia Bushenko wrote to the *Denver Catholic Register* that bills like the birth control law were facilitating a general moral decline. "Our government has litter baskets all along the highways to 'Keep America Beautiful,' yet she lets the soul and heart of our youth in America decay by allowing laws to protect . . . foulness," she argued.[95] Once the government intervened with issues of "family life," individuals lost their initiative and their morality.[96] Many of these activists were New Deal Democrats and yet, their belief in the power of the state to better people's lives did not extend to the realm of women and their reproduction.[97]

Critiques of government led Catholic journalists in Colorado—later the heralds of the state's pro-life movement—to make some tortured leaps into the southern past and present. Paul Hallett held up black civil rights activists as emblems of "moral resolution" but he also argued they should redirect their energy toward other "moral needs, every bit as imperious as those of civil rights." With more than a hint of resentment, he said that President Johnson had used the force of government to protect black rights, but would not do the same to oppose "immorality."[98] In a single editorial, Hallett imagined civil rights and social conservatism as twin movements, while also posing them as competitors for state resources. *Denver Catholic Register* journalist Frank Morriss looked a little further back for an analogy to the birth control debate, to the moment when the North "invad[ed]" and defeated the South by "force of arms," making much of the Constitution "dead letter." This was a cautionary tale for "Catholics who have thought you could have a little bit of welfarism . . . without too much regard for the Constitution."

Twentieth-century Catholics, according to Morriss, would learn what nineteenth-century southerners had: that "there is no realm of life the government will not eventually invade."[99] His rendition of the Civil War, where embattled white southerners and not African Americans were the heroes, dredged up Lost Cause mythologies in order to condemn government action.

While disagreeing about who were the analogous moral crusaders in the U.S. South, Hallett and Morriss did agree on a couple of key points. First, they saw in the South—and its struggles over states' rights and human rights—a parable for a nation at risk. They also both articulated an ambivalent-at-best relationship to the African American struggle. Morriss erased it entirely while Hallett used it for moral gravitas, quickly cast it aside, and then re-centered his own political concerns. Neither of these journalists, and almost none of the future pro-life activists who read their paper, would join racial justice movements in the region. Insofar as black history mattered, it was deployed in ideological service of modern social conservatism.

Hallett and Morriss were a part of a larger debate about race in the Catholic Church. It was not until the late 1950s that Catholic leadership named racism and segregation immoral. In the 1960s, American bishops lent support to the civil rights movement and demanded that Catholic institutions integrate.[100] This advocacy alongside open condemnation of abortion might seem to suggest that anti-abortion activism was born from socially liberal circles, that in fact a defense of people of color did translate into a defense of fetuses. There is no doubt that some activists certainly mixed racial liberalism and sexual conservatism. But more often racial and sexual conservatism went hand in hand in local Catholic papers and among the laity.

In the era of Vatican II, the white Catholics who enthusiastically embraced change were often the most outspoken about racial injustice and the most restrained when it came to the church's sexual politics. The reverse was often also true. For example, in the late 1960s, Fred McCaffrey, a liberal, was the editor of Santa Fe's archdiocesan newspaper, the *New Mexico Catholic Renewal*. Under McCaffrey's leadership, the newspaper published strong critiques of American racism, the war in Vietnam, and what he considered outdated church traditions. Equally important, the newspaper questioned the 1968 *Humanae Vitae* encyclical and even the burgeoning anti-abortion movement. "Many old-fashioned members of the Church," McCaffrey wrote, want laws "which enforce our particular beliefs" on the general public. He hoped "anti-abortion-bill arguers will be a little hesitant this session in telling people they 'represent' the Catholic Church."[101] Conservative readers boycotted *Renewal* because of its liberal politics, and the *Denver Catholic Register* tried to capitalize on this exodus by encouraging *Renewal* subscribers to come over to a "real Catholic newspaper."[102] In the same years, the *Arizona Register,* the newspaper of the Diocese of Tucson, rarely wrote about racial discrimination and frequently agonized over sexual change. Even if many in the Catholic hierarchy mixed civil rights commitments with their denunciations of sexual immorality, most priests, members of the laity, and their newspapers committed to one movement or the other.

Ultimately the 1965 birth control bill did pass in Colorado. Socially conservative activists lost this battle in the war against "state-sanctioned promiscuity." Even more importantly, later that year in its *Griswold v. Connecticut* decision, the U.S. Supreme Court ruled that laws limiting married couples' access to birth control information violated their right to privacy. After that ruling, social conservatives could no longer count on the state as an ally in their fight against birth control. But anti-birth control movements—in places like Colorado—proved an important testing ground for future pro-life activism. Activists extended old connections between women's reproduction and the health of the nation, all while envisioning "the contraceptive mind" as a contagion ready to afflict all Americans. They imagined the poor both as victims of government interference and as promiscuous leeches on the body politic. Government efforts to secure women's ability to control their own reproduction amounted to a campaign to undermine the sanctity of the individual and "invade" the private sphere. Finally, activists dabbled in southern allegories and the history of black people to authenticate their own moral crusade. In this debate, and many others like it, activists tried and tested socially conservative ideas, many of which would prove useful a few years later when they approached the threat of legal abortion.[103]

The other movement that proved an important testing ground was the anti-pornography movement. Moralists "rediscovered" pornography in the 1950s. Even in the midst of its rebirth, many critics viewed the anti-porn movement as a religious movement bent on censorship. In order to escape the stereotype of the backward Catholic book burner, anti-porn activists, especially the group Citizens for Decent Literature (CDL), modernized their movement.[104] When they did, they developed new tools used in the fight against secularism and liberalized sexuality. Pro-life activists would borrow from that toolbox only a few years later.

In the Four Corners states, Citizens for Decent Literature formed individual groups while also organizing drives through the Knights of Columbus, the Council of Catholic Women, and other Catholic groups. In 1957 in New Mexico, the Knights of Columbus organized a rally that included more than 1,100 men from seventeen parishes condemning the "dirt being poured out" into their communities.[105] Catholic organizations remained the backbone of the anti-pornography movement throughout the 1960s and yet, the movement's rhetoric downplayed their role. Activists emphasized that their righteous indignation had no single religious source. Protestants, Jews, and Catholics all were a part of the movement, one advocate insisted. He explained, "We all find our meeting ground in morality. The principles that guide us emanate from the divine law."[106] CDL projected an aura of religious pluralism and "sexually healthy Americanism [that] distance[d it] from its dubious and unpopular 'humorless puritan' forebears," argues historian Whitney Strub.[107] In the late 1950s and 1960s, anti-porn activists tried to make religious activism more palatable to an American public that was growing skeptical of Catholic movements that infringed on individual rights.

Another key innovation of the anti-pornography movement was the use of the conservative expert. Activists used their own social authorities to wage war against liberal and academic "elites."[108] The anti-porn movement used a whole host of experts—from psychiatrists, to social scientists, to police officers—to prove that pornography negatively affected society. One such expert was journalist James L. Kilpatrick, editor of the *Richmond Daily Leader,* who worked tirelessly to incite massive resistance to desegregation. In his 1960 book *The Smut Peddlers,* Kilpatrick turned his attention to pornography, condemning it through a history of obscenity law. The *Denver Catholic Register* hailed the book as a blend of common sense and expert opinion. The reviewer suggested that Kilpatrick was a new breed of thinker who could combat "the ivory towers of a fact-ignoring liberalism." He was "a representative of that new surge of thought that rolls across party lines called Conservatism." This conservatism, according to the reviewer, could stand up to modernity because it used liberal tools: "It adheres to tradition and the common standards of our civilization, while being prepared to meet liberalism or relativism on its own ground."[109] Together, Kilpatrick and his sympathetic reviewer helped develop conservative expertise as legitimate truth-telling, while painting liberal expertise as "fact-ignoring" obfuscation. This provided a way to undermine major social institutions like universities, media outlets, and government commissions while using similarly formal knowledge production to buttress moral claims.

In these years and beyond, conservative activists imagined both "fact-ignoring" liberal experts and "common sense" conservative experts as white.

Yet in these contexts, the whiteness of liberals and conservatives did not bind them together. Rather, conservative activists used the production of "truth" and the politics of social issues to differentiate types of whiteness. "Ivory Tower" intellectuals were white elites disconnected from "moral" Middle America. Those elites supposedly used their social authority to change society in unnatural ways. Class, education, and most importantly politics marked theirs as a threatening, betraying whiteness. Even as conservatives used more formal expertise to support their political claims, their experts avoided being grouped with elite intellectuals. The truth of conservative expertise lay not with the evidence but rather the "common sense" or "tradition" of ordinary (white) Americans. Their formal knowledge did not produce truth, it simply reflected truth already established by moral Middle America.

One primary way that anti-pornography activists gave their arguments both the aura of truth and the lure of titillation was through film. Citizens for Decent Literature made a number of short films about the effect of pornography on society. For example, in 1965, a Catholic school in Denver showed parents "a true-life film, that depicts the slaughter of an innocent youngster by a 16-year-old boy" who had read "obscene magazines."[110] These films amounted to a "sexual safari, exposing various sexual kinks to [their] audiences," according to historian Whitney Strub.[111] Such films were often the highlight of CDL meetings and anti-porn campaigns in sympathetic organizations, like the Knights of Columbus.[112] Benedict Urbish, Thomas Glennon, and Jack Arnold, who were Knights and future pro-life activists, likely viewed such films. In anti-porn campaigns, social conservatives learned the power of images and films to arouse, attract, and outrage viewers. The films—and the possibility of simultaneously stoking both offense and arousal—drew attention in ways that words could not.

A 1969 controversy over a sexually explicit poem highlights how the anti-pornography movement's rhetoric and tactics motivated socially conservative activists. At the University of New Mexico, Lionel Williams, an English graduate student, had assigned six poems by San Francisco poet Leonore Kandel. The class was well prepared to deal with the poetry, but the broader New Mexico community was not. One poem, "Love-Lust," caused the state to devolve into a broad, almost hysterical, debate over obscenity, sexuality, and the role of the university. The poem discussed oral and genital sex in frank, evocative prose.[113] Someone circulated the poem outside the classroom and the outcry mounted quickly. The governor received 1,500 telegrams about the issue in just two days.[114] The uproar led to the suspension of two graduate teaching assistants and the resignation of two English faculty members. Punishments rippled outside the university when a professor was fired at another university for openly supporting the UNM grad student, and a bookstore owner was arrested for selling Kandel's book.[115]

The debate became a referendum on the university itself.[116] Even though the president of the university took swift action, New Mexicans around the state condemned the state's flagship educational institution. The school, they argued, no longer represented the taxpayers. Robert P. Tinnin, an insurance executive and one-time director of the U.S. Chamber of Commerce, told a crowd that UNM educators were not representing the people and the university should be "completely fumigated."[117] Activists caricatured the "libertine" university and its "vermin" professors as being in opposition to the moral citizenry. One woman wrote to her local newspaper that the university fostered "pornography, subversion, alcoholism, sex orgies, hippies, yippies, drug addicts, degenerates, traitors and Communists."[118] Many within and outside the university pushed back on such defamations, arguing that it was a place for the exchange of ideas that produced upright, productive citizens. A school official maintained that the poem controversy was just a cover for people with a wide range of issues with the university from student dress to "manifestations of Black Power."[119] As it turned out, sexual hysteria was a useful organizing tool for UNM opponents. The state legislature quickly redirected $50 thousand of the university's budget toward an investigation of the school's role in the dispute. Activists argued that universities—like many other major societal institutions—had become a place of sexual and political indoctrination for the state's youth.

The phantom of sexually depraved blackness stood at the center of conservative condemnations of the university in 1969. Many argued that the only reason that "Love-Lust" became an issue was because a black man assigned the poem to a class that included white women.[120] Often the outraged used the language of lynching to convey their dismay. One person said they should cut the teacher's "tongue off," while another said if his daughter had been in the classroom, "we would not have to worry about Lionel Williams today." One New Mexican threw away all coding: "They ought to hang the ———."[121] Others called the reading of the poem a "sexual assault." White women were the innocent victims of the poem's obscene attack.[122] White elites at UNM—whether they were "hippies" or "Communists"—had allied themselves with "Black Power" activists and black grad students/metaphorical rapists. This alliance of "bad" people of color and white elites was the constituency against which white social conservatives launched their moral campaign.

Though social conservatives condemned the poem's presence in the classroom, they demanded copies for their own reading pleasure. A municipal judge said New Mexicans were eagerly passing the poem around—he ran "into it numerous times" in one day—even though, he cautioned, it might be illegal to do so under the state's obscenity law.[123] One state senator said that his constituents had demanded a mass meeting to distribute the poem "in order to know how bad it really was." One New Mexican suggested that the poem "be sent to every taxpayer in the state."[124] People wanted to read and keep the offending poem, desiring a more intimate relationship with the thing they reviled. Having the poem in their pockets helped perpetuate their outrage. It helped the reader understand himself or herself as upstanding, moral, and conservative. And of course, the sexually explicit poem had the potential to excite the reader in other ways. "Scandalized young matrons whipped copies of it out of their purses for the enlightenment of about-to-be-scandalized friends, while businessmen distributed it at the office, whispering the details to their innocent young secretaries," wrote one local reporter.[125] The poem motivated outrage, lust, and identity formation, a handy oar for social conservatives as they navigated political tides.

Those in possession of the poem however were hesitant to allow such intimacy. The state senator whose voters demanded the poem's distribution responded that he "would not be an instrument for circulating such filth."[126] Some local newspapers opened their doors so locals could read the poem in person, in the safety of a brightly lit, respectable newsroom. Of course, then the newspaper reported eagerly on visitors' reactions to the poem. One noted that more men than women came in but then, panting, recorded every woman's response to it.[127] There was titillation not just in reading the poem but watching other people read the poem—especially watching the women ostensibly being protected from smut by anti-porn advocates. Communal outrage could be an orgiastic affair. In the end, New Mexico's gatekeepers were not successful at keeping the offending poem from the offended masses. According to one journalist, "Love-Lust" "became the most read and discussed piece of poetry ever in the state."[128]

Women were not only the victims of pornography, but also the source of its moral contagion. "R.I.G." explained to *Denver Catholic Register* readers in 1960 that the only solution to the "cancer of pornography" was the reassertion of patriarchy—or as he put it—"the dignity of womanhood." That included "men tak[ing] back the authority that they have handed over to women," "women cast[ing] off their immodest and anti-feminine garments," employers denying married women work, and society putting all women "out of masculine roles in business and politics." If this did not happen, "there will be many, many effeminate men; and the streets will be full of rapings."[129] Without the harnessing power of traditional gender roles and marital sexuality, men would have both too much and too little masculine energy. The men most at risk, R.I.G. implied, were those white, middle-class men with familial and professional aspirations. Because of the influence of their liberated wives in "immodest" garments, those formerly respectable men would become consumers of pornography, rapists, homosexuals, and participants in contraceptive sex.

A number of future anti-abortion activists worked in anti-pornography movements and participated in Catholic organizations that heard anti-porn pleas.[130] Pro-life activists learned from their anti-porn brethren to hide their religious activism behind a veneer of a broader "moral" campaign. They learned "expertise" was a good weapon against modern knowledge production or "indoctrination" from educational institutions. They learned the utility of visual tools, like films, to compel viewers. Perhaps most importantly, future pro-life activists learned the power of having an object of outrage available in your pocket.[131]

Socially conservative activism—no matter how it was cloaked—was grounded in a deep concern over gendered, sexual, and often racial change. The liberation of women from compulsory housewifery, the threat of pregnancy from every sexual act, and even a rigidly "modest" uniform could spell social disaster. Men and women would spiral out of control, and into sexual aggression and homosexuality. It was moralists—those white Middle Americans—who would protect society from both white elites and black deviants. They would be protectors of "womanhood" and the "family" for the good of America.

The anti–birth control and anti-porn movements set the groundwork for the early anti-abortion movement in the Four Corners states and across the nation. John and Barbara Willke, two of the country's most prominent pro-life activists, said as much in their book on the history of the movement. The Willkes did not note New Deal programs or anti-poverty campaigns as precursors to their movement; instead, they focused intensely on birth control debates and concluded with the founding of the anti-pornography group Citizens for Decent Literature.[132] To them—activists who had been at the forefront of the anti-abortion movement since the 1960s—it was debates about contraception and pornography that were the necessary background for understanding the creation of their movement.

Even though abortion reform did not fully arrive in the United States until the late 1960s, some social conservatives were bracing for this change years earlier. They might be considered anti-abortion activists who did not yet have a movement. Before the formation of a grassroots movement, social conservatives often used the language of rights when they spoke about abortion: the right to life, rights of the "unborn," human rights. The National Catholic Welfare Conference asked the United Nations to include the right to life "from the moment of conception" in their 1948 Universal Declaration of Human Rights.[133] A handful of historians have used such rhetoric to suggest this group was truly liberal in the early years. The language of rights, however, rarely stood apart from a concern over gendered and sexual change. Pulling rights rhetoric out of its social conservative framework misunderstands 1960s pro-life activism and its foundational concerns.

One of the most important early abortion cases highlights the connection between rights rhetoric and concerns about the changing status of women. In 1962, Arizona TV personality Sherri Finkbine made national news when she sought an abortion of her severely deformed fetus. Finkbine had realized the sleeping pills her husband had brought home from Europe (thalidomide) were causing birth defects in Europe. She told a journalist friend about her ordeal in order to raise awareness of this problem in the United States. Soon after, Finkbine and her local hospital were flooded with letters and phone calls condemning her planned abortion. The hospital caved to the public pressure and Finkbine and her husband had to fly to Sweden for the procedure.[134] Finkbine garnered the sympathies of many in Arizona; media outlets represented her as a good mother making a difficult and tragic choice.[135] The Vatican, however, openly condemned her abortion using the language of life and murder. Referring to the fetus, Vatican Radio explained, "He was a man. He was alive. He was innocent. He has been killed."[136] The Diocese of Tucson clarified the Vatican's stance to its congregants: "The human fetus has the right to life."[137]

In the years surrounding the Finkbine case, a small number of activists connected abortion to the Jewish Holocaust, though this connection was still not very common in pro-life rhetoric. Knowledge of the Jewish Holocaust had been trickling out since 1945 with media coverage of the liberation of concentration camps and the Nuremberg Trials. By the early 1960s, comparisons to Nazi Germany and the Holocaust were relatively common—moving, according to historian Kirsten Fermaglich, from the "margins to the center stage of American public discourse." Intellectuals—from Betty Friedan to Stanley Milgram—used the Holocaust to explain some core aspect of the human condition or social governance.[138] The few anti-abortion activists who did make Holocaust comparisons were part of a growing national obsession with the Jewish genocide. In 1960, a Dallas priest wrote in his weekly column that abortion was "nothing less than a polite justification of Hitlerism."[139] According to him, Nazi Germany and its genocides were the necessary outcome when a government began limiting the fundamental rights of its citizens. The smattering of Nazi comparisons like this one may seem like a clear-cut use of liberal rhetoric, but the movement's "liberalness" never stood apart from its profound conservatism on gender and sexuality.

In the early 1960s, activists most often diagnosed the malady of abortion using the language of gender transgression, abandoning rights rhetoric altogether. Modern women were the symptom and source of society's problems. Mrs. W. Hughes of Arizona argued that women were increasingly "restless, . . . unhappy, [and] worn out" because of "social and moral" problems. The solution, she cautioned, was not "in clinics which teach men and women how to go to the dance without paying the fiddler."[140] Society was allowing women to abandon sexual responsibility, through birth control, divorce, and most importantly abortion.

Other pro-life activists placed their gendered concerns *alongside* arguments about Nazis. Mrs. Marceline Boyer of Kenosha, Wisconsin, wrote in a letter to the editor that while Hitler had been defeated, "the worst and most vicious war that can and will be fought" continued: a war against abortion. She then turned to the origin of the problem: "Vanity, so that women can adorn their body with fashion and beauty culture. . . . Now who is behind the scene encouraging this? Satan." This was a battle between good and evil where women's reproductive choices were all part of a broader, sinister plan. "Woman is [Satan's] chief concern because it is she who peoples the earth. So, to spite God, he is placing all devices and contraceptions for her use, to defy God's plans," she concluded.[141] Years later in a letter to the editor comparing abortion to the Holocaust, Doris Storms of Tucson put it even more succinctly: "Blame the mothers," she said.[142] For these activists, Hitler did not sit at the pinnacle of their visions of errant modernity, but rather he sat in a pantheon alongside bad mothers, narcissistic women, and Satan.

Activists were just as likely to look abroad to modern Japan and Sweden, rather than Nazi Germany, for their cautionary tales in the 1960s. When Sherri Finkbine was refused at her Phoenix hospital, many speculated that she would either go to Japan or Sweden where abortions were legal. (She settled on Sweden at the last minute.) In the context of the Finkbine case and after, social conservatives held up these two countries as examples of what happened when sexual modernism was enshrined into law, making divorce, sex education, birth control, pornography, and abortion legal. A *Las Cruces Sun Times* editorial bemoaned the "near-Scandinavian pornography level we have now" while a Denver journalist looked to Japan as evidence that birth control would be quickly thrown off for abortion because it was "100 percent successful."[143] Activists contended that it was in these two countries where "the contraceptive mind" had fully taken hold. Some conservatives explained this stance on sexuality through religion—"Japan is not even a Christian nation"—while others used the turn-of-the-century rhetoric of degeneration—Sweden is a "nation of degenerates leading the world in suicides, alcoholism, divorce, and venereal disease." These characterizations were so common that, in 1970, Dear Abby dedicated a whole column to misunderstandings about sex in Sweden.[144] The comparisons to Japan and Sweden eventually fell out of favor in the movement. In the 1970s, social conservatives gradually realized that these two countries were not good foils in their fight against legal abortion. Japan's and Sweden's sexual modernism did not cause them to slip down the slope to coercion and genocide, the outcome pro-life activists so frequently promised.

Concern over the changing status of women, which eventually transitioned into overt anti-feminism, was at the root of most early anti-abortion concerns. Pro-lifers in Tucson in the early 1970s offer a small glimpse into this sentiment. Bernadine Haag accused feminists of "trying to 'stick it down' American women's throats through fair means or foul—mostly foul!" William Reese criticized the "placard-carr[ying] . . . dissatisfied women" as do-nothings who simply liked to complain. Nancy Cousins grumbled that she was "sick of being represented by leftist libbers against baby's rights (for abortion)." Soon after the Equal Rights Amendment (ERA) was proposed, a whole group of Tucson pro-life activists vocally opposed this signature piece of feminist legislation.[145] Of all the activists covered in this chapter, only one articulated a pro-feminist stance: Dennis Deconcini, the son of Ora

Deconcini. In 1976, when he was running in a successful campaign for U.S. Senate, he supported the ERA but opposed abortion, though he hedged and told "women's lib groups" that he would not support all right-to-life bills. Ultimately, the only anti-abortion advocate who supported certain parts of feminism was more a sympathetic politician and less a full-fledged activist.[146]

Rights rhetoric was a part of 1960s pro-life sentiment, but the activists who used it were far from "liberal" in terms of gender and sexuality. The protection of the fetus could not be divorced from the condemnation of women. It was women who were leaving the home, taking jobs in the workforce, and engaging in politics. It was women who were allowing or promoting sex without "responsibility." It was women who were motivating the government to "invade the sanctity of the home." And it was women who were the faces of Satan in the battle for America's soul—a battle playing out over fetal bodies. "Murder" and sexual immorality were always intertwined.

. . .

When abortion reform arrived in the late 1960s, activists were primed with more salient rhetoric and political tools than they realized or acknowledged. Even in the story of Margaret Sebesta—that happy-go-lucky young mother struck by a political thunderbolt—there are clues about both the commitments and the organizations that grounded the early pro-life movement. Sebesta found out about Colorado's abortion reform bill from Marge Wilson, a member of the Young Democrats who got a copy of the legislation. The legislation was written by Susan Barnes, a student at Denver University—an institution which had already been "infiltrated" by supporters of Planned Parenthood, zero population growth, and communism, according to Margaret and her daughter. Marge Wilson then took the bill to her next-door neighbor, who was a nurse, who then went down the block to the head of the archdiocesean Council of Catholic Women.[147] Sebesta used this story as evidence that the movement was organic and spontaneous. Her story, however, reveals much more.

Far from "spontaneous" action, Sebesta's story shows the ways this movement was already building on existing socially conservative constituencies: Catholic activists and conservative medical practitioners. Organizations like local medical societies and the Council of Catholic Women helped shape members' socially conservative worldviews long before they joined the movement. These organizations welcomed new migrants to the Mountain West and gave them a platform to change the region. Through participation in such groups, these future activists witnessed or became involved in anti-birth control and anti-pornography movements. On that first day of the anti-abortion movement in the state, Marge Wilson, Margaret Sebesta, and their neighbors already knew who their allies were.

Sebesta's story also exposes how the pro-life movement built on existing ideologies that opposed sexual modernism. Through anti-pornography and anti-birth control movements, activists came to believe that sexual modernity was already embedded in schools, universities, and state governments. In these movements, activists began to craft essential tools that they would use in their war against legal abortion. It was these socially conservative movements, not New Deal or Great Society liberalism, that provided the basis for future anti-abortion work. In these years, activists, both Democrat and Republican, began to craft an ideology, a social conservatism, that would remake American political culture at the end of the century.

TWO

Imagining Life

In 1974 a seasoned conservative activist and staunch Catholic, Californian Virginia Evers, caught a glimpse of an anti-abortion ad in her local newspaper. It was a photograph of a Washington doctor holding the feet of a ten-to-twelve-week-old fetus. Evers already ran a small business, Heritage House, that sold nationalist paraphernalia for the U.S. bicentennial, but in the following years she began manufacturing and selling her most famous item: "Precious Feet," a metal pin of fetal feet inspired by the pro-life ad. Evers and her family moved to a small town in Arizona and began focusing almost exclusively on Precious Feet and other pro-life goods. Heritage House marketed Precious Feet as an item that "breaks the ice and helps you speak for those who cannot speak for themselves."[1] Activists were supposed to wear the pin to remind themselves and others of their dedication to "life." One satisfied pro-life customer wrote about the Precious Feet, "Clerks in stores, bank tellers, people in any crowd . . . inevitably ask what they are and it gives me a chance to impress a visual image on their minds that they will never forget."[2] Evers described the national and international response to her product: the tiny feet "were greeted with such tremendous enthusiasm that . . . during a meeting of worldwide pro-life leaders in Dublin, Ireland, they were officially proclaimed the 'International Pro-Life Symbol.'"[3] By the late 1970s and early 1980s, this replica of fetal feet was the right symbol for the movement. It condensed a number of central anti-abortion arguments—about fetal life, about rights, and about genocide—into a small metal pin. Pro-life activists had learned well from their anti-porn predecessors. An item of fascination that motivated moral outrage, if held closely, was a powerful thing.

In the late 1960s and 1970s, activists generated a host of fetal images and objects that were supposed to be transparent reflections of reality, but they were effectively so much more. Pro-life activists created a symbolic world of fetal imagery that became inextricably wed to their evolving ideology. Anti-abortion ephemera did not simply reflect a truth that was already there, but helped manufacture that truth. There was a creative and dynamic relationship between the political creators, the objects or images, and the society they sought to explain.[4] Catholics and their leaders had discussed the importance of fetal life and their opposition to abortion long before 1967. But with the advent of the movement, the shape and scale of anti-abortion sentiment changed radically. Through the movement's fetal imagery and ephemera, many came to see themselves as against abortion, and that political commitment became central to their subjectivities. Fetal images and objects helped constitute an anti-abortion identity for their recipients and shape pro-lifers' vision of the world.

In the 1970s, pro-life activists developed a repertoire of fetal imagery and arguments that represented their movement as a justice movement. As with earlier socially conservative movements, the anti-abortion movement sought to meet liberalism on its own ground. The first step was to humanize the fetus, in an attempt to secure for it the rights of a born human. This was at the heart of pro-life activism in 1967, as it would be well into the twenty-first century. Next, activists sought to convey the magnitude of the crime through historical analogy, latching onto slavery and the Holocaust as their primary comparisons. Finally, activists worked to convey that their politics were unifying and had the potential to join together the races, sexes, and religions which liberals had supposedly put asunder. In so doing, anti-abortion activists continued to develop a new type of white identity—one based on their claims to common sense and morality. They claimed white conservatives were the true inheritors of the black civil rights movement.

What activists built in these years was important, but just as important was what they erased: women who sought abortions. Despite the sexually moralistic politics that grounded this movement, many pro-lifers knew that women who sought abortions could never successfully be the movement's villain. Thus, in the late 1960s and 1970s, activists generally attempted, often unsuccessfully, to hide her and their sexually moralistic politics from view. The political culture activists built in these years did not resonate with all Americans, but for those primed to hear and see the pro-life pitch, it became a powerful way to re-envision the world and their place in it.

Colorado was an unlikely place for a reproductive rights revolution to begin. In the early to mid-1960s, activists in other parts of the country had begun calling for the reform of abortion laws, arguing that the law and public morality were at odds. At that point, all states in the United States had restrictive abortion laws dating back to the nineteenth century, most only allowing abortions when a woman's life was in danger.[5] Because of such laws, reformers contended doctors risked legal action, as many bent the law or broke it entirely to terminate women's pregnancies, and women risked death from self-induced abortions or back-alley abortionists. This group of abortion reformers was made up of doctors, nurses, legislators, ministers, and social workers, with a small handful of outspoken early feminists who called for women's liberation from "bodily slavery" and for "abortion on demand." These activists were motivated and sustained by an increasingly vociferous law-breaking public, who openly demanded contraception and detailed their experiences with illegal abortions. In the mid-1960s, there was a growing abortion reform/rights movement. California and New York were the hotbeds of reform activism, though there were individuals from Georgia to South Dakota lobbying their legislatures for change.[6] There was little conversation about abortion reform in Colorado before 1967, so what happened next took many by surprise.

In February of 1967, rookie state representative Richard Lamm brought an abortion liberalization bill to the Colorado legislature. The bill allowed abortion under certain conditions: if the woman's mental or physical health was endangered, if there was a high probability of a damaged or deformed fetus, or when the pregnancy was a result of rape or incest. The bill immediately gained forty-six recorded sponsors, nearly half of the Colorado legislature. The year before, Lamm had told a public audience that a liberalized abortion bill would not get even five. Within two months, the law passed easily, with sizeable majorities in both houses of Colorado's legislature, with support from Democrats and Republicans and from rural and urban legislators. The day had been won for liberalized abortion using less than one hundred dollars in promotion money.[7] Both supporters and opponents of abortion reform were shocked by the speed at which this monumental piece of legislation was passed.

A liberal Democrat and a lawyer, Representative Lamm had proposed the bill in order to address growing concern about overpopulation and women's oppression. He contended that the law would allow women to be more than "brood animals," forced to birth babies they did not want into an already overpopulated world. Overpopulation ravaged women's bodies and ruined children's lives, as "excessive reproduction" bred poverty, and abject poverty led to communism and authoritarianism, he claimed.[8] Lamm was a part of a growing group of Americans in the 1960s who saw impending doom in the world's increasing population and sought to limit reproduction both at home and in developing countries abroad.[9] Revising an old dictum, he suggested "be fruitful, but multiply cautiously." For him, the bill was both a state-centered approach to limit "excessive" reproduction and a path to loosen women's reproductive shackles. If the law passed, Lamm believed, "Colorado could become the nation's conscience center, where potential tragedy could end."[10] There would be no more back alleys, no more wire hangers or knitting needles, and no more legal shame.

In Colorado, as elsewhere, it was mainly Catholics—from archbishops down to laypeople—who were the first to oppose legal abortion. Catholic priests and bishops had been the most outspoken opponents of abortion reform every place it was raised in the 1960s. In 1970, the National Conference of Catholic Bishops organized National Right to Life. Even when the group transitioned into a lay organization three years later, it retained Catholic leaders, Catholic resources, and a largely Catholic membership.[11] In Colorado in 1967, the only organized opposition to legalized abortion was the Colorado Catholic Conference, a semi-official lobbying organization affiliated with the church.[12] Roused to action, the Colorado Catholic Conference sent appeals to all parishes in the area after the bill passed in the House. The Sunday before the Senate vote, all Catholics in Denver heard a plea from the pulpit to write their legislators to oppose the abortion bill. They also probably learned that there would be a public hearing where constituents could talk to legislators about the bill.[13]

Jolted by their priests and perhaps their consciences, hundreds came to the public hearing, packing the room and the hall outside. One reporter described the meeting that followed as "pugnacious, quarrelsome," and "ill-tempered."[14] The meeting was supposed to consist of five-minute speeches from supporters and opponents of the bill. The crowd, which largely opposed the bill, gradually got more and more unruly, eventually shouting at the legislators. One audience member remembered that many of the legislators did not seem to be listening to the speakers opposing the bill, but instead spent their time reading literature supporting abortion reform.[15] After one state senator shouted angrily at the crowd, the audience quieted a bit, enough to hear one of the more provocative speeches of the day.

Dr. Robert Stewart, a Denver gynecologist and former president of the Catholic Physicians Guild, approached the podium with a small suitcase in hand.[16] He spent five minutes discussing German measles, or rubella. The disease was relatively harmless to a healthy adult woman, but by the early 1960s, many Americans knew that if rubella was contracted during pregnancy it could cause miscarriages, infant deaths, and many serious birth defects, including severe mental disability. At the time of this public hearing, the United States was at the tail end of a full-blown rubella epidemic, the largest in recent memory. Many Americans were moved by the tragedy of children born without arms, legs, or fully working heart, unable to see, hear, sit up, walk, or touch. For the worst cases, many doctors saw death as "merciful."[17] During this outbreak in the 1960s, about 30,000 babies were born dead or quickly died after birth, and another 20,000 had major abnormalities.[18] The heartbreak of these families captured the imaginations and parental fears of many Americans—especially white, middle-class Americans. The power of rubella was that everyone interested in child-bearing, even the most privileged, felt susceptible as the disease seemed to have no economic or racial boundaries.[19]

In the heat of the early abortion debate in Colorado, Stewart took up this exact issue. He conceded that German measles could result in personal catastrophe. But he argued that of all the pregnant women with German measles, only one in six fetuses came out deformed. Why murder six for the sake of one tragic life, he suggested?[20] Here, he displayed a very different moral understanding of the disease than most Americans held at the time. Abortion reformers, and the birth control advocates who preceded them, argued that the promotion of "life" was not the highest goal but rather the "quality of life." Or, as one abortion liberalization advocate wrote to the *Denver Post,* the "state has no right to give aid to this ungodly promotion of quantity without regard to quality."[21] Stewart rejected this calculation. He rejected quality of life arguments (as would all pro-life activists after him) and he also disagreed that German measles threatened the American family. He said that the majority of pregnant women with German measles were not at risk. Of course, a few women would have babies with abnormalities, but these dangers should not be extrapolated to all. Stewart suggested that German measles hysteria was robbing five of six infected women of their healthy babies. The disease did not fundamentally undermine the dream of a middle-class white

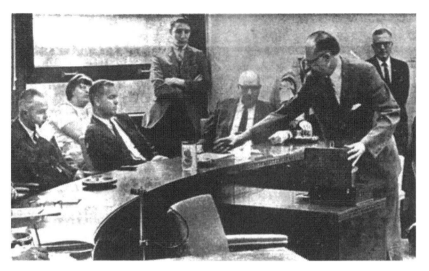

FIGURE 3. Dr. Robert Stewart removes a preserved fetus from the Senate committee table, April 1967. (Courtesy of Getty Images; *Denver Post*)

woman's easy reproduction and it did not undermine the white American family, he implied. Abortion, rather than disease, was the true tragedy.

Stewart spent his allotted five minutes on this issue and then asked the senators for more speaking time. When they refused, the doctor opened his briefcase and said, as one observer remembered, "Let's see what we're doing here." On the senators' desk, he placed two jars with preserved fetuses, supposedly at about ten weeks' gestation though the pictures suggest a much more developed fetus. The same audience member recalled that the whole room seemed stunned by the doctor's display and the chairman of the committee "came unglued." The observer at the public hearing—Margaret Sebesta, the young mother who just wanted to jitterbug—would go on to become one of the most influential pro-life activists in the state. She remembered this moment as a turning point in her activism, moving her to tears almost forty-five years later: "I was mad . . . because of . . . the reaction of the members of a legislative hearing committee over a real baby, a real human being. It affected me. I can see it to this day. God bless Robert Stewart."[22] For Sebesta, these fetuses were the perfect rebuttal to the day's hearings.

While the preserved fetuses caused quite a stir at the hearing that day, a good number of Americans were familiar with the sight of fetal bodies. Since the early twentieth century, preserved fetuses were common teaching tools in college science classrooms, medical schools, and scientific laboratories, used to demonstrate and examine the process of human development.[23] In these spaces, real fetuses (either miscarried or aborted) were examples of biological truths and human origins.[24] Beyond the classroom, there was another place in which Americans had become familiar with preserved fetuses: the sideshow. Part of an American obsession with the grotesque, fetuses populated exhibits of "the world's strangest babies," displays which titillated audiences with sensational congenital deformities. Sideshows connected these fetuses to bad behavior; abnormal fetuses were the physical punishments for premarital sex, drug use, and incest.[25] Such displays thrilled and scared viewers. Fetuses reassured audiences of their own normality while threatening them with gestational retribution for secret sins. Many Americans, in both educational and leisure settings, had sought "truth" in the fetal body. But there was much more instability in this truth than anti-abortion activists would concede. The "truth" in fetal bodies could be construed just as often to be about women's sin, personal weakness, and biological "monstrosities," as about beauty and "life."

Robert Stewart used preserved fetuses to make a very specific claim about abortion and about 1960s politics. He, like many anti-abortion activists after him, used fetal bodies to argue that modern politics and science ignored the truths that "old" science had proven long ago. Stewart, using his authority as a doctor and with his fetuses as evidence, made claims about biology, not religion. Many later pro-life activists would echo his claims, arguing that in the past, people had seen preserved fetuses in classrooms and elsewhere, where they learned that fetuses "were babies." These fetal bodies were the easy, self-evident teaching tools of biological truth, now hidden or cast aside. Modern white conservatives were the inheritors of that old common sense.

Anti-abortion activists would continue to use fetal bodies to tell biological stories. Within a few years, they began arguing that all people have their chromosomal "uniqueness" at conception, their heartbeats start between 18 to 25 days, their brain waves begin at 43 days, and all their "bodily functions" work at 11 weeks.[26] Such discussions were often paired with fetal imagery, either preserved fetuses or photos. As had Dr. Stewart, activists continued to use fetal remains and biological discussions in tandem, in an effort to make fetuses resemble born humans. A discussion of heartbeats and brainwaves confirmed the humanity of the fetuses pictured and the fetal bodies authenticated the biological similarities people could not otherwise see. This biological story would continue to be a preoccupation of the movement, as activists delved deeper into human biology to create an origin for human life through narratives of resemblance.

The public hearing and Dr. Stewart's display of two preserved fetuses were enough to motivate some opponents of the abortion reform bill to begin forming Colorado's first right to life group. The early members were mainly white Catholics, a majority of whom were women. Like the anti-pornography activists who preceded them, early anti-abortion activists denied that there was anything distinctly Catholic about their movement. This was not particularly easy because Richard Lamm repeatedly characterized the opposition to his bill as distinctly and provincially Catholic. During debates on the bill in the House, Representative Lamm argued that Colorado's legislators should not genuflect to the Catholic Church's moral stand against abortion. Rather than inerrant, he claimed the church had been inconsistent with its abortion prohibition. As evidence, he offered legislators this little history lesson: until the late sixteenth century, the church had allowed abortion within 40 days of conception for a male fetus and within 80 for a female one.[27] Then popes alternated between banning abortion altogether and outlawing it after "quickening," or the time when the woman felt the fetus move. Lamm intimated that even the popes of the past, the Vicars of Christ, disagreed on when life began. He concluded that Catholics played fast and loose with their own history, while trying to impose their modern-day morals on the rest of Colorado.

Activists could not escape this religious condemnation because reporters covering anti-abortion activities regularly asked attendees if they were Catholic. At one of the first anti-abortion protests, reporters claimed that most participants were Roman Catholic and asked at least one woman if this was a "Catholic movement"? Protestors pushed back against the characterization, carrying signs saying "Protestants against Abortion." Mary Ford, who was a member of the Council of Catholic Women, insisted that the movement was "primarily ... Protestant."[28] At a later protest, when reporters asked protestors' religious affiliation, almost all "refused to disclose their religion."[29] In these shifting claims to Protestant, ecumenical, or even secular identities, activists maintained that they represented a broader Colorado community or the mainstream, a status denied them if they were "just Catholics." During the 1967 protests, Reverend Frank Freeman of St. James Catholic Church asked rhetorically in a letter to the editor, "Could this bill have been enacted without the contrivance of religious bigotry?"[30] The persistent focus of reporters on the Catholic character of the movement was born of residual anti-Catholicism and also a growing belief (articulated by Richard Lamm and others) that religion should not influence public policy.

This posed an interesting problem for nascent anti-abortion activists: should they deny the role of religion in their movement or reinterpret the role of religion in society? In 1967, they emphasized the former. But over the course of the next decade, they expanded their vision to embrace the latter.

Pro-life activists in Colorado—from Dr. Stewart onward—emphasized medical, biological, and sociological arguments over religious ones, extending lessons learned in the anti-pornography movement. The name of the first anti-abortion organization reflected this: the Colorado Joint Council on Medical and Social Legislation. One of their first pamphlets contained a graph showing increasing abortions in Colorado alongside pledges to "preserv[e] and enhanc[e] the dignity of the individual person" and "to disseminate the most advanced scientific knowledge to help eliminate and treat the basic causes underlying the above problems."[31] The bulk of the group's members and constituency were women, though professional men occupied two of the three leadership positions. Margaret Sebesta had initially been president but she explained that she was "a housewife who kn[ew] how to make bread from scratch, but d[id]n't know how to conduct a meeting or an interview." So she called a lawyer she knew—John Archibold—to represent the group.[32] Having professional men at the helm helped give the group more social authority than if they had been "just" housewives or "just" Catholics. In the group's early promotional material and in their public presentations, the members of the Colorado Joint Council on Medical and Social Legislation tried to look more like sociologists or biologists than activists or moralists, in an effort to expose the "distortions" of modern medicine in a way people of faith could not. Within the next few years, pro-life activists would partially sideline the sociological and scientific formality of these early groups and re-engage with the question of religion in society.

Anti-abortion activists—throughout the rest of the century—retained the core argument pioneered by these activists in the movement's early years: modern doctors and social scientists had undermined "true science" out of a blind adherence to feminist, environmental, or simply liberal ideology. One of the most longstanding claims in this vein was that modern doctors—and specifically Alan Guttmacher, preeminent obstetrician and gynecologist and one-time president of Planned Parenthood—had changed the language of reproduction. They argued that Guttmacher (or an amorphous pro-choice intelligentsia) had created the word "fetus" to take the place of the "unborn" or just "baby." One Arizona pro-life activist, Phil Seader, saw the most nefarious of motivations in this linguistic shift: "you know, we're having a problem with abortion 'cause babies are cute, babies is a cute sound. So [Guttmacher] said, 'We're going to have to stop calling 'em babies if we want to kill 'em.' He said, 'We're going to call them fetuses.'"[33] According to anti-abortion activists, modern doctors and social scientists had pulled the linguistic wool over the eyes of the American public. Like the anti-porn movement, anti-abortion activists put the blame "on the shoulders of the sociologist and the liberals," all while marshaling expert knowledge in defense of their own cause.[34]

The modern elites whom anti-abortion activists were railing against were very clearly figured as white. Guttmacher and his cabal of obstetricians, social scientists, and physical scientists were viewed as the primary villains. These professions—in the American imagination and in reality—were overwhelming white and male in the 1960s. Conservative whiteness depended on differentiating itself from these white elites, often a more crucial divergence than with people of color. Anti-abortion activists relied on formal knowledge production to build their case, but the preserved fetuses proved that their acquired knowledge simply confirmed old-fashioned common sense. In so doing, white conservatives claimed to represent "moral" Middle America, while simultaneously claiming that opposition to abortion was about biology, not morality.

The early anti-abortion group in Colorado rarely discussed pregnant women in its literature. Pro-life pamphlets contained graphs, statistics, and discussions of law and public policy, but nothing on women seeking abortions.[35] The women of the movement tried to fill in for those absent women in public protests, even as they largely excused themselves from the group's leadership. A few days after the public hearing in Colorado, about fifty women "in their silk hose and high heels," along with babies and young children, marched around the capitol in protest. At this "Mother's March," conservative women made the argument that the women at stake in this debate were pro-life mothers, simply defending their children. Mary Ford noted, "We love our children."[36] Ford left her foil—the abortion-seeking woman who did not love her "children"—unspoken. By making this woman a phantom, early activists redirected the public gaze toward conservative women, and they implied what later activists would say explicitly: that women were hurt, not helped, by abortion.

Activists were not completely successful at erasing sexual judgment from their rhetoric. Condemnation of women's supposed sexual immorality came through most clearly when activists discussed the rape exception in the Colorado law. Leonard Carlin, of the Catholic Lawyer's Guild of Denver, suggested that statuary rape (which would have allowed a girl to get an abortion under the law) simply meant "she had intercourse and got pregnant." Additionally, Carlin said, in rape cases that involved adult women, the law was flawed because it did not require the victim to get "permission of the person who committed the rape."[37] For Carlin, even rape victims bore the responsibility for sex out of wedlock. In forums like the *Denver Catholic Register,* where activists did not have to worry about anti-Catholic backlash, pro-lifers continued to suggest, just as they had in debates about birth control and pornography, that abortion was an expression of sexual immorality, "compound[ing] ... the sin of fornication."[38] Such language reveals the persistence of sexual conservativism in anti-abortion circles. But the fledging pro-life movement in Colorado also acknowledged that vilifying the fornicating woman would not sell in a political world that was now talking about women's "bodily slavery" in earnest. Thus, the main proponents of the burgeoning pro-life movement sought to put at the heart of their campaign the image of the preserved fetus, with its attendant biological arguments, and omit the image of the illicit woman.

In 1967, the anti-abortion movement's arguments found little traction among Colorado's legislators. Many worried about Colorado becoming an abortion "mecca," while a smaller number contended that they were legalizing murder. But those concerns did not stop the legislature from passing the law or Governor John Love from signing it.[39] So as the law relaxed its strictures on abortion, Governor Love asked those doctors and psychologists helping women access legal abortions to remain vigilant not for attacks on the integrity of "life" but, in the words of one reporter, for the "flood of gals to the abortion mecca of the world."[40]

Coloradoans would never see that "flood of gals"—strict enforcement meant that few Coloradoans, let alone those from out of state, could get abortions there—but important seeds had been sown for the pro-life movement. Over the next forty years, many Americans in Colorado and elsewhere would encounter preserved fetuses outside abortion clinics, in crisis pregnancy centers, in churches, or in the news. Fetuses in jars would never be as available as Precious Feet pins, but nonetheless they became common, if grisly, trade in anti-abortion activism. By the late 1970s, pro-lifers were stripping fetal remains of their accessories, removing them from jars and presenting them in bare hands or blankets to grab the public's attention. As fetal remains appeared in places as varied as the Phil Donahue show and the Democratic National Convention, activists continued to try to convince

Americans of the "biological truth" of fetal life.[41] Even more common were the scientific arguments those fetuses represented. "True science" affirmed that life began at conception.

In the late 1960s and early 1970s, anti-abortion activists turned regularly to history—specifically American slavery and the Jewish Holocaust—to ground their arguments. They claimed that abortion was a type of mass violence and that, consequently, the pro-life movement was a justice movement. In these years, activists excised less useful comparisons, like those to modern Japan and Sweden, and focused more narrowly on the past. Activists attempted to place themselves within a historical genealogy that included heroic abolitionists and Nazi opposition. At the heart of these comparisons were the graphic photos activists used to create visual connections between abortion and historical violence. But even as the largely white anti-abortion movement claimed solidarity with justice campaigns of the past, the only true oppression, they argued, was that enacted on the fetus. Through such rhetorical work, activists created a moral whiteness, where conservative Americans assumed the role of freedom fighters and justice warriors. This political work occurred in pro-life movements across the country, even in one of the most irregular states: Utah.

Utah had been born out of an attempt to create a nation outside the boundaries of the United States. Relocating to the Great Basin in 1847, members of the Church of Jesus Christ of Latter-Day Saints soon found themselves back in the United States (after the end of the U.S.–Mexico War vastly expanded the nation's borders) and at war with the U.S. government over local sovereignty.[42] In the twentieth century, after disputes over federalism had been put to rest, the LDS Church continued to dominate the state's social and political life, leading one historian to call it a "democratic theocracy."[43] And yet, twentieth-century Mormons were different from their forebears; they still valued their identities as "peculiar people" and members of "the one true church," but they also sought admittance to the American mainstream.

Mormon assimilation took on political, economic, and even religious forms. Once strident opponents of federal power, twentieth-century Mormons embraced the welfare state through their support of the New Deal and voted for Democrats even after President Franklin Roosevelt's tenure.[44] By the postwar period, most Mormons considered themselves middle-class

American patriots who fully embraced capitalism, a radical change from their past commitment to economic communalism. In 1980, the church even added the designation "Another Testament of Jesus Christ" to the cover of the Book of Mormon, suggesting Mormons were akin to mainstream Christians.[45]

Claiming whiteness for themselves was another key step in the Mormons' path toward "Middle America." In the nineteenth century, Protestant Americans had considered Mormons not fully white, and compared them to Native peoples, African Americans, and Middle Easterners. These racialized comparisons signaled Mormons' ineligibility for full citizenship. In reaction, Mormons took a multipronged approach to prove their whiteness. Early in the twentieth century, they argued that Mormon families, with their numerous children, would help forestall the "race suicide" of white people. In the nineteenth century, Mormon fecundity was evidence to others of a "perverse" marriage system (polygamy), but in the twentieth, it became a commitment to white domination. Additionally, white Mormons contended that black Mormons were descendants of Cain, the cursed and murderous brother of Abel. In the first half of the twentieth century, Mormons used such arguments to exclude black men from the priesthood, the power given to worthy men to act in God's name. Thus, both white reproduction and black marginalization were central to Mormons' claim to racial privilege in the early twentieth century.

In the anti-abortion movement, Mormons made new claims for racial inclusion and privilege through another campaign for the "right kind" of reproduction. By the early 1960s, the times had begun to change for Mormons and the rest of white America. Church leaders supported, at least rhetorically, full civil rights for black people, while continuing to deny them full rights within the faith.[46] This created a conundrum for Mormons: How could they assert their belief in racial equality while also maintaining the racial hierarchies that structured their lives? The anti-abortion movement offered one solution. By defending uninterrupted reproduction and "life," Mormons helped make "moral" white people into the defenders of humanity, reasserting racial hierarchy by other means. Through the movement, Mormons helped create the fetus as the ultimate victim of modern society, an "innocent" (white) victim in a world of movements demanding the recognition of racial and gendered discrimination. Mormons got in line with their Catholic brethren on when "innocent" life began and what it looked like. To give their victim historical gravitas, Mormons used historical analogies to the Holocaust and slavery—the same ones used across the country. Such analogies borrowed from the victimhoods of black and Jewish people in order to make white conservatives into modern-day freedom fighters. Ultimately, pro-life culture offered Mormons a "moral" avenue for racial and political inclusion.

In 1973, Utah was still operating under its abortion statutes from the late nineteenth century, and there had been little effort towards abortion reform in the state. But in January of that year, the Supreme Court decided *Roe v. Wade,* ruling that state laws criminalizing abortion were unconstitutional. This forced Utah, along with forty-five other states, to revise its abortion law.[47] The court had decided that a woman in her first trimester of pregnancy (roughly to three months) had the right to terminate her pregnancy. In the second trimester (roughly three to six months), the state could regulate abortion in ways that were reasonable to maternal health. In the third trimester, the court considered the fetus viable, which meant that possibly it could live outside the womb. At this point in the pregnancy, the court said, states could prohibit abortion unless it was necessary to save the woman's life.

One of the first responses from Utahns was to rely on old ideas of Mormon moral difference, best protected by the state of Utah, rather than the federal government. The Utah Anti-Abortion League, the state's short-lived, largely Mormon pro-life group, pushed their legislators to use Article III, Section II of the Constitution, which allowed Congress to restrict the jurisdiction of the Supreme Court.[48] This was the most popular argument taken up by Utahns in the first year after the *Roe* decision. Many maintained that regulating morality was a state's right.[49] In a petition, the Utah Anti-Abortion League explained "other states may do as they please, [but] we insist that Utah should be free to protect all human life within this state."[50] Unlike most other anti-abortion activists, who wished for a federal law or court decision that would outlaw abortion across the country, the first instinct of many pro-life Mormons was to demand state sovereignty on social policy. The first knee-jerk reaction of many Utahns was to emphasize Mormon moral and political separateness.

Generally, however, Utahns borrowed heavily from Catholic pro-life culture, and thus argued their moral superiority was akin to that of other socially conservative white Americans. Anti-abortion groups in the state immediately used pictures, distributed by national activists, to convey their outrage and their arguments. In March 1973, the Utah Right to Life League bought a full-page ad in the *Salt Lake Tribune.* The main attraction in this ad was a large photograph of a fetus supposedly at twenty weeks' gestation.[51]

Imagery of this "victim" quickly became more graphic and more ubiquitous. The picture published in the *Salt Lake Tribune* had been relatively sterile; its origin is unclear, but it might have been a manipulation of an in-utero photograph. Though the fetus was separated from the woman, it bore no other visible signs of miscarriage or abortion. But very quickly, photos of aborted fetuses, bloody and dismembered, took center stage in Utah and around the country. Most of these came from one essential publication: John and Barbara Willke's *Handbook on Abortion*.[52] This 150-page book, first published in 1971, translated an assortment of pro-life arguments generated by activists all over the country into a single, easily consumable political tract. Some would come to call this the "bible of the anti-abortion movement."[53]

John and Barbara Willke were a couple from Cincinnati, Ohio; he was a family practice doctor and she, a nurse. Journalist Cynthia Gorney describes Barbara Willke as "caring," "small and vigorous," while John Willke had "an air of collected certainty" and a voice "that made some of his debate opponents feel as though they had been patted on the head and sent to their rooms."[54] By Barbara Willke's account, the two began offering marriage classes at their local Catholic church in the early 1960s, which expanded to lectures and books on sex education and, finally, abortion.[55] In the late 1960s and early 1970s, the Willkes became convinced that pictures were going to be their greatest tool in the fight against legalized abortion. They went about collecting images from sympathetic doctors and pathologists around the country.[56] At first they only put four pictures in the *Handbook*. They intended the book to be in the "pocket" or "purse" of "all who value human life." And in fact, as John Willke recounted, the book "went like wildfire because there was nothing out there."[57] Between the *Handbook* and the other anti-abortion material he distributed through his publishing company, John Willke generated some of the most important teaching aids of the pro-life movement. Or, as literary scholar Carol Stabile contends, Willke "put the fetus on the cultural map."[58] Though activists would go on to refine or even openly disagree with the arguments and tactics set out in the *Handbook,* the pictures remained a consistent, if not uncontested, presence in almost all corners of the movement.

In the early 1970s, the Willkes took their show on the road. In 1972 alone, they visited seventy cities trying to convince people that abortion was murder.[59] And they came repeatedly to Utah.[60] Their presentation included a slide show of graphic photos and a short video of an abortion. The video had been made for use in medical schools, but the Willkes silenced the original soundtrack and supplied their own pro-life voiceover. Once people viewed the film and their pictures, Barbara Willke said they made "a 180-turn" from "what" is being killed to "who."[61] The quick answer the Willkes wanted was, of course, "a baby." Such a response did not fully answer the question of "who" was being killed, in the anti-abortion worldview.

Most, if not all, of the photographs that the Willkes showed were of either white or racially ambiguous fetuses. In most pro-life paraphernalia, the fetus was a universal subject, supposedly a representation of all humanity. In the early editions of the *Handbook on Abortion,* the Willkes' public presentations, and in early pro-life literature in Utah, white bodies were supposed to act for all. Here again, as so many times before, efforts to represent all of humankind slipped into representations of the most privileged in society. This was a subtle reminder to conservative Americans that white people were victims of genocide and oppression too. In the early 1970s, activists sometimes supplemented their stock fetal images with the occasional photo of a black "victim" of abortion.[62] This addition served to accentuate the movement's claim that it was a "colorblind" justice movement. White conservatives then placed themselves as the saviors of people of color, and of humanity writ large.

Such images popped up across the United States, but their effect in Utah is especially instructive. In Utah, as elsewhere, the Willkes had an eager audience for their presentations. Based on the demography of the state, and on their presence at LDS Church events and at Brigham Young University, it is fair to assume that much of their audience was Mormon. They even met with the First Presidency of the LDS Church (the church's president and his top two counselors) in the fall of 1973 and received support for their talks and materials.[63] Margaret Fitzgerald wrote to her congressman that "after attending another Right to Life rally, I am more convinced than ever that the Supreme Court made a horrendous mistake.... Every judge, senator, and congressman ... should be compelled to view the films presented by Doctor Willke ... showing these aborted babies." Mr. and Mrs. Ralph E. Keller were also compelled by the Willkes' presentation: "I have just seen some appalling slides on abortions ... and I don't believe there was a dry eye in the audience." Margaret McGuire emphasized (in capital letters, no less) how much these photos had personally affected her: "UNTIL I SEEN THESE PICTURES AND READ WHAT HORRIBLE THINGS ARE BEING DONE I DIDN'T REALIZE WHAT SUFFERING IS CAUSED BY THIS LAW." Judy Prince was so moved that she invested in literature and her own slide show so she could lead anti-abortion seminars in her home.[64] People like Prince adapted the Willkes' presentation and turned a biannual speech by outsiders into an intimate presentation among friends, family, and neighbors. Whether through personal initiative or through the organizational channels of the fledging pro-life movement, the Willkes' pictures circulated quickly and often in Utah's abortion debate. Much like pornographic poems and films, these photos were both documentary evidence and sites of disgust, personal identification, and fascination for potential activists. For many, viewing these pictures marked an important political transformation, a moment when people became committed to the anti-abortion cause.

The charge that abortion was murder was somewhat at odds with Mormon theology. The First Presidency of the LDS Church issued a statement on abortion in 1972 calling abortion "one of the most revolting and sinful practices of the day," though permissible when the woman's health was at risk or in cases of rape. The sin of abortion was not, they clarified, on par with the unpardonable sin of murder of an innocent person. A pro-choice Utahn pointed this exact issue out to her congressman: "Are you familiar with . . . the Mormon practice of doing no temple work [sacraments done for the dead] for full term children . . . [who are] still-born? According to Mormonism, the spirit enters the body of the child *at birth*."[65] Core Mormon practices, she argued, demonstrated that those who died in the womb were to be treated differently, because they did not yet have a soul, than those who died after birth.[66] She pointed out that, according to the church, abortion was not same as murder.

When Mormon Utahns claimed that abortion was murder, they either willfully or naively disagreed with church teaching. A sociologist in the 1980s found that 61 percent of Mormons believed abortion was a form of murder and 53 percent believed the soul entered the body at conception.[67] This sociologist explained that the divergence between official doctrine and public opinion was a remnant of Mormon folk belief. It is just as likely, however, that many Mormons were compelled by non-Mormon anti-abortion activists. In the space between the church's condemnation and the Willkes' murder argument, many Mormons in Utah chose the more stringent "Catholic" stance on abortion. For Mormons, these religious and political maneuvers were a part a racial assimilation process, whereby they gave up (a little of) their distinctiveness for something that unified them with other socially conservative white Americans.

With graphic fetal imagery in hand, Utahns and other anti-abortion activists made the fetus into the ultimate victim and theirs into a movement for justice by borrowing from the history of oppression, slavery, and genocide. Comparisons to the Holocaust became the common refrain of pro-life Mormons, Protestants, and Catholics alike; by the 1970s, the Holocaust had become a central moral reference point for Americans.[68] Anti-abortion activists claimed that legal abortion, like Hitler's "final solution," was an example of state power run amok. While other conservatives in the 1970s worried about property rights and economic freedom, these social conservatives warned of a different, more insidious type of federal encroachment. They argued that with *Roe,* the government was not only infringing on individual state's rights to regulate morality, it was also infringing on people's right to life itself. They argued that once the government legalized what they saw as the murder of "the unborn," it was a slippery slope to killing the elderly, the disabled, and any people unwanted in society.[69] One Utahn wrote, "I am very much afraid that [*Roe*] will lead to further atrocities, such as the putting away of our elderly, and could eventually destroy man's love for man, the binding force which holds any nation together."[70] The Freemen Institute, a Utah-based right wing, free market group, placed this argument front and center when it covered abortion in its newsletter: "And let us look at recent world history, let us look at Nazi Germany. Where did they begin? They began with abortion."[71]

The slippery-slope-to-genocide rhetoric had much in common with the "contraceptive mind" of 1960s birth control debates. In both, personal "irresponsibility" masked a deeper moral violation. Each identified a contagious mindset, easily spreading to society at large, then escalating into grosser crimes. Activists argued that the very foundations of society were at risk if this social disease spread. Women's errant reproduction was the source of the problem in both, but the "contraceptive mind" of 1960s birth control debates named women as perpetrators, while the slippery slope rhetoric erased their presence.

If anyone questioned that abortion was murder, pro-lifers answered with graphic photos of aborted fetuses as evidence. One Utahn very clearly made the connection, referencing another of the Willkes' most famous photographs: "To view the pictures of the perfect body and member conformation of children no more than one to two months old . . . to view these little human beings, some still alive, unconcernedly thrown into hospital garbage cans like pieces of trash convinced me we are without a doubt a nation of degenerate butchers. . . . We have become Hitler. We are our enemy."[72] In subsequent years, pro-choice activists would cast doubt on the proclaimed gestational age of the fetuses in these photos, arguing that the truth of

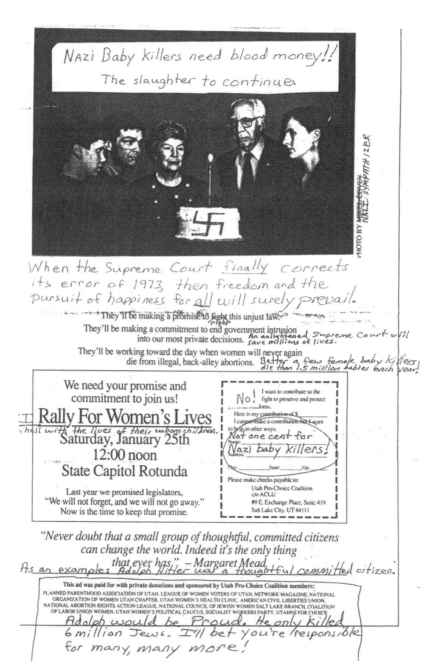

FIGURE 4. In 1991, the ACLU of Utah received this piece of hate mail with anti-abortion words written over their donation request letter. The author argued that campaigns for reproductive rights and Nazism were one and the same. (Courtesy of the ACLU of Utah; Special Collections, J. Willard Marriott Library, University of Utah)

pro-lifers' claims depended on whether these bodies were similar to ones legally aborted in the first or second trimester or to near-term fetuses protected by federal law. But for most anti-abortion activists, these pictures were evidence that Americans, and especially pro-choice Americans, were engaging in what came to be known in activist circles as "the Abortion Holocaust."

Utahns were among the many activists who employed these comparisons, and they did so with the help of the *Handbook*. The Willkes explicitly and implicitly linked abortion with Nazis. They argued there was no difference between the idea of "quality of life" and that of the "Master Race."[73] The Willkes' photos then seemed to prove the connection. Utahns took up this torch, discussing the "genocide" of abortion with fervor, often describing *Roe* as a break with a fundamentally good American past. The common question was: How could this freedom-loving, civilized, Christian country become like barbarous Nazi Germany? One Utahn wrote that legalized abortion "would turn our nation . . . into a sterilized concentration camp that would make Adolph Hitler envious."[74] In these dystopian visions, abortion led the United States toward fascism and genocide, bringing the future America closer and closer to the Nazism defeated only twenty-five years before. While most Americans of the time used Holocaust analogies "for the purposes of national self-congratulation," according to historian Peter Novick, anti-abortion activists did something very different.[75] They used Holocaust analogies to convey the magnitude of a national "crime," while casting white social conservatives as the resistance.

Early pro-life activists also argued that the same ideas underwrote the institution of slavery. Unlike comparisons to the southern past in the birth control debate, anti-abortion activists fashioned themselves as morally upstanding abolitionists, not Confederates subject to the whims of an oppressive North. In the *Handbook on Abortion,* the Willkes made the direct comparison between slavery and abortion, and more specifically the *Roe* decision and the 1857 *Dred Scott* decision, which ruled that black people—slave or free—were not citizens and thus not protected by the Constitution.[76] The Willkes argued that both cases made some groups "less than human" and both practices—slavery and abortion—degraded life. Frank Morris, the *Denver Catholic Register* editorialist who had in 1965 connected social conservatives with white Confederates, had reversed his analogy by the 1970s. Now he compared pro-lifers to the Americans who "mounted the bloodiest war in history to end slavery" and described one anti-abortion leader as "Lincolnesque."[77] The Civil War and southern chattel slavery became the key historical analogies for pro-life groups around the country.[78] Even in Utah, activists did not use local histories for comparison, turning neither to the history of Mormon persecution nor the history of nineteenth-century Mormons buying Indian children for purposes of conversion and labor.[79] Instead they followed the lead of pro-life groups across the country and used analogies that would deemphasize differences between white Mormons, Catholics, and Protestants. All used the argument that the Civil War was the last time good Americans had to defend against "anti-life" elements from within. In this historical comparison, black people were history's victims (analogous to modern-day fetuses) and white abolitionists and pro-life activists were history's heroes.

Were women then akin to slaveholders in this story? They were never named as such and the organs of the movement continued to try to hide them from view. Pro-life letter writers did not necessarily follow the party line of movement leaders and often explicitly or implicitly condemned the "irresponsible" women who sought abortions. One bemoaned a world where a woman could have an abortion "as casully as one might have a tooth pulled." Another looked back with fondness to older, more punishing days: "Perhaps if girls were made to pay for their mistakes like in the olden days there would be no need for legal abortions."[80] These activists believed modern women needed to be restrained from casually terminating pregnancies and avoiding their social and biological responsibility.

For the activists who used historical analogies to explain the problem of legal abortion, though, the practice was not just similar to slavery and the Holocaust; it was worse. It was worse because the fetus was innocent and helpless, and thus the ultimate victim. In February 1973, U.S. Representative Wayne Owens received the same pleading form letter from many of his constituents: "We now implore that you work to eradicate the killing of innocent and helpless humans."[81] One Utah couple concluded their letter to Owens, "As far as I [am] concerned this is far more tragic than anything Hitler ever did, at least his victims weren't completely helpless and could fight to a degree for themselves."[82] Born humans "could fight for themselves" and thus were less "helpless and innocent." Here conservative rhetoric about personal responsibility for one's own circumstances merged with religious arguments about sin. Only fetuses could be truly "innocent" in a social and existential way. Anti-abortion activists effectively created a hierarchy of oppression, where the (white) universal subject—the fetus—could sit at the top as the ultimate victim.

Many pro-lifers were even more outraged at the injustice of "killing" the innocent because, as of 1972, the Supreme Court would no longer let states execute the guilty. That year the court had ruled all existing capital punishment laws unconstitutional because they violated the Eighth and Fourteenth Amendments; the court opined that capital punishment was cruel and unusual because it was applied "capriciously" and disproportionately to people of color.[83] Utah pro-lifers were indignant. Mrs. John Lyman wrote her congressman, "What do you think of a country where we abolish capital punishment for convicted murderers and yet slaughter thousands of unborn babies each year?" Another contended that laws protected "coyotes and other predators" but not "the highest form of life, the little unborn human being."[84] In these letters, "coyotes," "predators," and "convicted murderers," while raceless terms, operated as racial code. As historian Michael Flamm has argued, urban crime and juvenile delinquency began to take on a racial cast beginning in the late 1950s, prompting a full-blown campaign by many white Americans for "law and order" in the 1960s. Anti-abortion activists combined the racialized politics of law and order with the right to life, but in so doing the "right to life" slipped from a right for all humanity to a right for the (universalized, white) "innocent." Here, white social conservatives extended their ambivalent relationship with people of color. As in the birth control debates, poor people of color were, at turns, in need of a white conservative savior or the source of society's problems.

In the pro-life worldview, abortion fit in a genealogy of oppressions and genocides even as it negated all others. The "abortion Holocaust" was the most brutal in its execution, the most numerous in its numbers of victims, and the most inhumane in its choice of targets. The fetus became a victim that no born human could be. Once born, individuals—especially those "coyotes and predators"—were partly or completely responsible for their own situation, not governments, institutions, racism, or sexism. Using the Holocaust and slavery, anti-abortion activists named white pro-life people as defenders of social justice and ultimately sustained the rhetoric of individual responsibility even in the most dastardly circumstances. In practice, pro-lifers in Utah and elsewhere used the Holocaust and slavery to argue that fetuses were the only real innocents, the truly helpless. Everyone else was potentially culpable for their own oppression and even, their own genocide. Anti-abortion activists claimed that their campaign was the embodiment of all campaigns for justice and equality, while undermining some of those campaigns' core assertions. They implied that if legal abortion could be stopped, it would be a victory for the political philosophy of "life," and all other rights would flow from there.

In Utah, where few white people joined movements for racial justice or openly opposed black men's exclusion from the priesthood, many joined or sympathized with the pro-life movement.[85] Mormons, however, were often only supporting actors in the anti-abortion movement, organizing often in exclusively LDS spaces.[86] Because they used movement tools—especially graphic photos—Mormons were as enmeshed in pro-life political culture as Catholics, however. These tools produced a relatively homogenized movement, which helped unite white Mormons with white conservative Catholics and Protestants. Anti-abortion activists had created a social justice movement with reference to the histories of slavery and the Holocaust, but without committing themselves to anti-racism or the elimination of anti-Semitism. For them, the main systemic problem with American society was a fifth column promoting anti-life policies around the country. Thus, the primary victim in this modern world was the fetus. In this movement, Mormons and others created a moral whiteness, where conservatives shored up their racial privilege by claiming to be racial saviors. The only way to combat the influences of this abortion (or previously, contraceptive) worldview, pro-lifers argued, was for good Americans to defend the fetus.

NEW MEXICO, 1976

In the mid-1970s, anti-abortion activists in New Mexico and across the country began developing imageries of racial reunion. Their campaign for the fetal victim, activists believed, had the possibility of uniting Americans across race. Pro-life activists drew on a re-purposed imagery of the civil rights movement to claim that social conservatism was where race was no longer important, where people could come together in support of a higher cause.[87] These arguments took many forms across the movement but in New Mexico, they played out most clearly in annual multiracial symbolic funerals to mark the anniversary of the *Roe v. Wade* decision. Here white activists enlisted people of color to prove theirs was a justice movement, and staged funerals of fetal subjects to convey the unifying potential of their civil rights campaign.

In many ways, the anti-abortion movement faced an uphill battle in New Mexico. The state had legal abortion before 1919 and after 1969. Until 1919, New Mexico accepted the quickening doctrine, the common law principle used across the United States that made abortion legal as long as it occurred before the time that a woman felt the fetus move.[88] After 1919, for the next fifty years, abortion was illegal in the state except when a woman's life was in danger. During that time, New Mexico's women broke the law to self-induce abortions or sought midwives and doctors to help them.[89] In 1969, New Mexico reformed its abortion laws, allowing a legal abortion in cases of rape or incest, if the fetus was likely significantly deformed, or if the woman's mental or physical health was in danger. But because New Mexican doctors interpreted this law more liberally than their counterparts in Colorado, abortion was much easier to access in New Mexico than in Colorado in the four years before the *Roe* decision.[90]

After *Roe,* New Mexico continued its relatively pro-choice policies, despite having some very strong pro-life politicians in state and federal office. Over the years, politicians repeatedly drafted anti-abortion bills in the state legislature. Despite their persistence, between 1973 and 2000, New Mexico's legislature passed no law requiring parental notification or consent for a minor's abortion; no "informed consent" law, requiring women to read pro-life-slanted medical information before an abortion; and no law requiring a waiting period or counseling before an abortion.[91] These types of laws, ruled constitutional by the U.S. Supreme Court, passed in many states around the country in the 1980s and 1990s. As in almost every other state in the union, New Mexico's legislature did pass a conscience exemption allowing health care providers to refuse to provide or aid in abortions.[92] In 1998, the New Mexico Supreme Court ruled that the state's Equal Rights Amendment, passed in 1972, protected the right of women on state assistance to access abortions using state funds.[93] This court decision led experts on abortion policy to conclude that "New Mexico's state constitution gives more protection than the federal constitution for a woman's right to choose."[94]

Facing a generally pro-choice New Mexican audience, New Mexico Right to Life relied heavily on the language and imagery of racial justice movements. The name of the group's newsletter, *Viva Life,* reflects how important race was to its narratives about abortion. The use of Spanish in the title suggested that the group had a multilingual and multiracial audience. The use of such rhetoric to appeal to people of color as well as white conservatives was a break from early pro-life politics. In other parts of the country, in the early 1970s, anti-abortion activists had banked more on the power of racial resentment than on racial reunion. Historian Gillian Frank has shown how, in 1972, white pro-life activists in Michigan sold their cause using racially targeted ads: pictures of white babies were sent to white voters to suggest abortion put white people in particular at risk.[95] Explicit racial resentment worked in Michigan in 1972, but in the following years, most anti-abortion activists would make a different political calculation. They put both racial resentment and hope of racial reunion to work. In New Mexico and elsewhere, activists hoped that in the right context, multiracial imagery and the promise of racial reunion would appeal to both whites and people of color. By 1976, white conservatives wished to look like the legitimate inheritors of the black civil rights movement, borrowing the emotional power of a movement that had recently been recast in American memory. However, racial resentment lay just under the surface of this co-option, and few people of color joined the movement. The movement sometimes secured the participation of people of color for a day or two, but it could rarely translate that participation into long-term activism. This was because the language and imagery of justice movements was always used to promote a conservative vision of racial harmony through fetal rights, rather than racial justice.

New Mexico anti-abortion activists were at the forefront of this shift because narratives of racial harmony and human unity were central to the state's vision of itself. After New Mexico achieved statehood in 1912, boosters drew tourists to their state using Anglo Americans' interest in racial and cultural differences. Many white people came to see the beautiful landscapes and the supposed harmony among "Indian," "Spanish," and "American" people.[96] In the 1960s and 1970s, when New Mexicans read about the deterioration of "racial harmony" around the country, the state's politicians assured the populace that their state was different.[97] In 1971, the attorney general contended that New Mexicans were "fortunate to have achieved a degree of racial harmony and understanding. Extremes of intolerance and injustice are not nearly so prevalent here as in some of the states."[98] Anglo Americans believed New Mexican communities had solved the "race problem" that was afflicting the rest of America.

This narrative of racial concord was more than wishful thinking on the part of New Mexico's politicians; it was a political counternarrative to the stories activists of color were telling. By the late 1960s, a variety of New Mexican activists were critiquing Anglo dominance in the state and working to reform its institutions. Younger ethnic Mexicans, who increasingly identified as Chicanos, and American Indian activists contended that U.S. conquest had been a cultural and physical dispossession. More than that, some argued that the United States had attempted genocide. Pro-life activists disregarded most aspects of this political critique while using some of its ideas to support their own arguments. In the midst of this racial uprising and the concurrent rising tide of feminism, anti-abortion activists attempted to harness the power of civil rights, human rights, and racial harmony toward anti-feminist ends. Protecting the fetus could be the multiracial work that galvanized races and religions to unite in the face of the social divisions that liberals and radicals had supposedly created.

This vision for racial reunion can be seen most clearly in New Mexico Right to Life's annual memorials for *Roe v. Wade.* Each January, from the late 1970s through the 1990s, New Mexico's anti-abortion activists marched up to the state capitol and gave red roses to legislators to symbolize the "beauty of the preborn child." This ritual was begun by the New York pro-life group Women for the Unborn in 1971 and expanded by the national March for Life, an annual march in Washington, DC, beginning in 1974.[99] But in the years after the *Roe* decision, New Mexico Right to Life created its own program. In 1974, the group marked the anniversary with what members called "a memorial service," which included a panel discussion and the screening of two films at a local Knights of Columbus hall.[100] If the group held some kind of commemoration in 1975, it did not make the news. But in 1976, the New Mexico Right to Life committee organized something a little more provocative, a little more sensational. The group decided to host an interdenominational, multiracial funeral service.[101]

This service was a part of a "pro-life week" with a variety of activities and multiple chances for activists to display their commitment or to recommit themselves to the cause. Organizers probably drew inspiration for their January Respect Life week from the Catholic Church, which held a Respect Life week in October of every year. Activists planned a conference with many speakers and held a "family life" hour at a local Lutheran church.[102] They asked pro-lifers to skip a meal to protest abortion—"Miss-A-Meal for Life"— and to donate the savings from that meal to their organization.[103] But the centerpiece that January was a mock funeral.

The ceremonial funeral service was to be held at the Metropolitan Temple Church of God in Christ in Albuquerque. This parish was a part of the Church of God in Christ denomination, a predominantly African American sect of Pentecostalism.[104] Though the denomination began at the turn of the twentieth century in the South, much of its inspiration came from the West. One of its founders had been motivated by a Pentecostal revival in Los Angeles. In the early twentieth century, this southern church expanded into the North and West, especially in urban areas.[105] Albuquerque's Metropolitan Temple had begun in 1957 in a living room and a beauty shop, near one of the well-established black neighborhoods of Albuquerque. Reverend W.C. Griffin, a black New-Mexico-born minister, led the church and participated in the funeral service, though his pro-life activism seems to have been limited to memorials in 1976 and 1977.[106]

The anti-abortion funeral was billed as a "symbolic interdenominational service" in memory of the "10,000 aborted babies killed in New Mexico during 1975."[107] The main focus of this service was a white casket used to symbolize all aborted fetuses; it was surely the subject of prayers and pleas from the pulpit, and it was visible to those sitting in the pews. This symbolic casket was transported by highly symbolic couriers: the pallbearers were "children representing various cultural backgrounds."[108] Mourners followed the casket with its child pallbearers throughout the day's events.

Once they left the multiracial funeral service in one of Albuquerque's few black churches, mourners moved along one mile of the Santa Barbara–Martineztown neighborhood en route to a symbolic burial and graveside service at Mount Calvary Cemetery, a largely Catholic burial ground. The Santa Barbara–Martineztown neighborhood had been a Hispano village established around 1850 and annexed by the city in the post-1945 period. By the mid-1970s, the neighborhood was an impoverished urban barrio, but with a "stable close-knit community" that included residential and commercial buildings.[109]

Jesuit priests had founded what would later become Mount Calvary Cemetery in the Santa Barbara neighborhood in 1869.[110] Since then, it had been the place where Santa Barbara–Martineztown residents put their relatives to rest and where they sent their children to play. Without a park in the neighborhood until the late 1970s, the cemetery had served as an informal playground.[111] So when pro-life activists made their funeral procession from Metropolitan Temple to Mount Calvary Cemetery, they did so through Albuquerque's segregated and impoverished urban landscape. They moved through the streets of the barrio toward the cemetery where there was a headstone to memorialize those killed by abortion.[112] Once there, in view of pro-life mourners and perhaps a handful of children at play, activists held "a symbolic burial of the hopes, ambitions—and life—of the 'unwanted' and unprotected."[113] Using the imagery of death and racial reunion, activists attempted to make abortion the origin of all oppression—all "unwantedness"—and the abandoned fetus the symbol for all injustice.

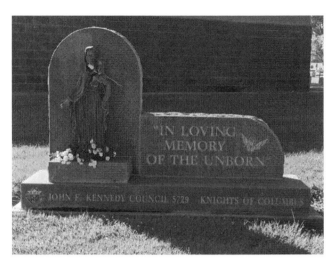

FIGURE 5. Anti-abortion memorial in Mount Calvary Cemetery, Albuquerque, site of the 1975 symbolic burial and gravesite service. (Author's photo)

Unlike preserved fetuses and graphic photos, the white casket was a symbolic representation of fetuses rather than a literal one. Anti-abortion funerals, memorials, and gravesites symbolized the death of many, in a manner similar to the various Tombs of the Unknown Soldier. Established after World War I, such tombs were where people could come to the resting place of one anonymous body in order to mourn all those who died in war, while also mourning a broader cultural loss. Literary scholar Laura Wittman argues that the Tombs of the Unknown Soldier were "at once a representation of the body of the nation and of the human body, both felt to be ruptured, perhaps permanently." It was "not so much about anonymous bodies," she continues, "as anonymous people," a condition of the modern world that cannot be reversed and must be confronted.[114] Pro-life activists used the gravesite for the unborn in similar ways but to different ends. The anti-abortion memorial endowed an anonymous body with public meaning; it was intended to bind a movement and prompt protest against what activists saw as a national genocide. Across the country in the next decades, pro-life activists regularly put up permanent memorials in Catholic cemeteries, like the one in Mount Calvary; they also built makeshift symbolic graveyards to remember those "lost" to abortion.[115] By 2017, there were fifty-one permanent gravesites of aborted fetuses and hundreds of memorials across the United States, where activists could go to mourn.

Another of the day's intended symbolisms was the multiracial commitment to "life." It was not happenstance that the funeral moved from a largely white Lutheran church for "Family Hour" to a largely black Pentecostal church for the funeral to a Catholic, largely ethnic-Mexican cemetery. The choice of pallbearers also betrayed this symbolic purpose; they were a group of children from "various cultural backgrounds" (probably a euphemism for different races). If the spaces through which the casket traveled were racially distinct, the casket's primary witnesses, the pallbearers, were racially diverse. The tragedy of abortion and the mourning of those aborted was intended to join people across race and across religion. In that day's theater of racial harmony, black, white, and ethnic Mexican, Lutheran, Pentecostal, and Catholic religious practitioners were unified as "humanity protecting humanity."

With a few exceptions, New Mexico's African Americans and ethnic Mexicans did not join the movement. Like Rev. W. C. Griffin, some may have participated in a pro-life event now and then, but not regularly. As in Utah, Arizona, and Colorado, anti-abortion groups in New Mexico were made up largely of white religious people.[116] People of color may have prayed at memorial services or said the rosary in private or at a public event, but they were almost never the activists on whom pro-life groups could depend. Many years after the funeral processions, an Anglo New Mexican activist suggested there were no African Americans in New Mexico to recruit. When asked whether the pro-life movement in the state included other people of color, the same activist replied that New Mexico's Native American and ethnic Mexican populations were personally pro-life but did not "vote it."[117] Her response, while not directly answering the question, made the larger point: she did not see people of color in her state taking public stands against abortion. Even if there were substantial numbers of Native American, ethnic Mexican, and black pro-life people, they did not join New Mexico's pro-life groups. If this was a civil rights movement, it was largely a white one.

At the same time, Chicano and American Indian activists also demanded that the public pay attention to reproductive politics, attacks on the family, and, what one activist publication termed, "the theft of life."[118] The theft they spoke of was not abortion, however, but sterilization. In the mid-1970s, Chicano groups in New Mexico, aware of the forced sterilization of ethnic Mexican women in Los Angeles, held meetings to warn locals and prepare them for interactions with medical professionals.[119] American Indian activists and a government investigation exposed that the Indian Health Service had also been sterilizing huge numbers of Native women without their consent. Activists said that at least 25 percent of all Native women in the United States in the 1970s had been sterilized.[120] Some activists saw such abuse as a part of a broader campaign against the family, but their critique was very different than the one leveled by white social conservatives. For the American Indian Movement at least, it was sterilization abuse, the removal of Native children to foster care, and the removal of the elderly to old-age homes that undermined the Indian family.[121] For many in these two movements, colonialism and racism were at the root of their families' problems, not secularism, sexual modernity, or abortion.

The majority of American Indian and Chicano activists who were concerned about reproductive politics, racist coercion, and genocide in their communities in the late 1970s and early 1980s disassociated those concerns from the issue of abortion. Most simply did not discuss abortion when they spoke of "the theft of life." But those who did discuss abortion usually said it was very different than sterilization. According to them, the problem of abortion was not that it was legalized genocide, but rather that it was too hard to access for poor women of color. In 1978, the National Indian Health Board said that "while abortion and sterilization on the surface seem like related issues," sterilizations were being forced on Indian women, whereas laws banning the use of federal funds for abortion made the procedure virtually impossible to get for all but the wealthiest Native women. The National Indian Youth Council added that anti-abortion laws were not a curb on state reproductive coercion, but rather part of it. Without access to legal, publicly funded abortion, and "with little hope of a decent standard of living for the babies they bear, more and more poor women will be forced to choose sterilization as one of their few remaining options."[122] According to them, anti-abortion laws gave Native women, and poor women more generally, less control over their lives and less support for their families, not more.

While ignoring Native and Chicano concerns over sterilization, white pro-life activists regularly co-opted the struggles of people of color. In the 1970s and 1980s, New Mexico anti-abortion activists repeatedly invoked the black civil rights movement, and especially Martin Luther King, Jr. New Mexico Right to Life newsletters used King's words—"I fear the silence of the churches more than the shouts of the angry multitudes"—as rallying cries. At a Right to Life rally in Las Cruces in the 1980s, a pro-life leader told his audience, "If [King] were here today, he would say, 'Let freedom and justice ring for the born and the unborn.'" When describing the gestalt of her movement, New Mexico activist Dauneen Dolce said succinctly: "It's civil rights."[123] The national movement made similar claims in these years. Early on, they relied on the face of Mildred Jefferson, a black woman and president of National Right to Life between 1975 and 1978, to do this work.[124] They also relied heavily on black activists like Jesse Jackson, who, in the early 1970s, saw birth control and legal abortion as a part of a long history of efforts to limit the reproduction of people of color.[125] Later, in the 1980s and 1990s, activists used King's niece Alveda King to authenticate the political connection between anti-abortion work and civil rights. Speaking on behalf of Priests for Life, Silent No More Awareness Campaign, Heartbeat International, Georgia Right to Life, and the National Black Pro-Life Coalition, King regularly argued that her famous uncle was pro-life.[126] Having people of color of the past and present represent the anti-abortion cause, even if only for a day, was an essential way of authenticating their movement as a "civil rights movement."

One goal of this strategy was to erase women seeking abortions. In 2000, a pro-life publication in Arizona explained the purpose of the strategy succinctly: "We must frame the issue so as to attract civil rights supporters because we will lose if the public concludes that abortion is a civil right."[127] The person for whom abortion might be a civil right loomed large and yet went unaddressed. From the beginning, many abortion rights advocates had argued that legal abortion was a prerequisite for a woman's full citizenship. She had to be able to control her own reproduction to control the conditions of her existence. In order to deny abortion as a right, and deny feminists the cultural inheritance of Selma, pro-life activists claimed theirs was the civil rights movement. Activists relied heavily on token people of color and multiracial imagery to authenticate this claim in the 1970s and onward.

This civil rights movement, though, had very clear boundaries. When people of color or Jews linked social justice to reproductive rights, anti-abortion activists claimed that those people betrayed the broader justice movement. For example, in 1989, pro-life activists in New Mexico picketed an Albuquerque synagogue during Yom Kippur, one of the High Holy Days in the Jewish year, with signs equating Jews to Hitler. The synagogue's rabbi, Paul Citrin, had been vocally pro-choice, and Jews in New Mexico, more generally, supported abortion rights.[128] For the picketers, who represented no particular organization, the Holocaust was a result of an "abortion-mentality," an antagonism to "life," rather than anti-Semitism or fascism. Jewish New Mexicans, then, were culpable for a modern Holocaust, and philosophically complicit in the Nazi Holocaust of the past. These anti-abortion activists attempted to make their point about abortion as a human rights issue by openly opposing those most closely associated with genocide in recent historical memory.[129]

Anti-abortion activists' interest in racial reconciliation also had its limits. No pro-life activists in the Four Corners states joined in coalition with Chicano, black, or American Indian civil rights groups in the region. They did not engage in or even discuss the many civil rights issues on which their few allies of color worked. Even as anti-abortion activists foregrounded racial reunion, racial ambivalence and resentment continued to crop up within this white civil rights movement. One example came from Colorado activist Margaret Sebesta. She recalled an encounter with a reporter at an early pro-life protest: "[He asked] what would I do if my daughter were raped by a big black nigger? This was of course much before politically correct speech was imposed upon us and he said it the way he thought about it. And I was so mad. I was banging my hand on the hood of a car. . . . I wouldn't kill anybody."[130] Sebesta placed racism at the heart of the abortion liberalization movement. She envisioned herself and her pro-life compatriots as anti-racists, unwilling to kill. But she also aligned herself with this racist white reporter by mourning the time before "politically correct speech was imposed upon us." Even in the whitewash of memory, this was clearly an anti-racism made for white conservatives. Activists borrowed the language of racial justice movements and sometimes their criticisms of eugenics to discredit the pro-choice movement, rather than seriously wrestle with modern racism.

· · ·

Throughout the late 1960s and 1970s, white anti-abortion activists developed rhetorical tools—focusing on biological arguments, comparisons to slavery and the Holocaust, and civil rights genealogies. To make their point, they relied on conservative sociological and medical expertise rather than religious arguments. They borrowed the tools of leftist movements to extend a conservative, moralistic agenda. Activists, like Dr. Robert Stewart, pushed the conversation toward questions of biological origins: bodies, chromosomes, heartbeats, toes, and fingers. With preserved fetuses and grisly pictures, activists worked to make conception into the baseline for humanity and the fetus into the ultimate victim of modernity. To do so, activists co-opted the historical narratives of slavery and the Holocaust and argued that abortion was the worst genocide of all time. Finally, activists used token people of color to claim the movement was a civil rights movement. Primarily white activists used the emotional power of the civil rights movement, while imagining the fetus as an entity that would unify all Americans. In so doing, they made "regular" white Americans into abolitionists, saviors of people of color and the nation as a whole. All together, these activists used liberal tools to dismantle sexual liberalism.

These arguments were not just voiced but seen. Preserved fetuses carried around in bottles were the first objects the movement used to convey anti-abortion arguments, but they could not be the items of fascination that would compel a daily commitment to "life." They were too rare. Other, more common objects and images quickly filled the void. Graphic photos of aborted fetuses could be in anyone's pocket. Makeshift graveyards outside of abortion clinics or permanent ones in Catholic cemeteries could catch the attention of any passersby. These were just the tip of the cultural iceberg: fetal models, fetus dolls, bumper stickers, license plates, children's books, T-shirts, and, of course, Precious Feet pins all became common pro-life tools. Each brought anti-abortion politics deeper into the everyday lives of Americans. Anti-abortion activists argued these were simply evidence that fetuses were babies, but they were much more. They were the carriers of the pro-life story.

———

THREE

Claiming Religion

In 1971, Coloradoan Ruth Dolan realized she was in the midst of a religious revolution. That year Colorado legislators had proposed a bill that would repeal all abortion restrictions in the state, claiming the 1967 reform bill had not done enough for the state's women. Dolan remembered calling Denver churches to find out what they were doing to oppose the bill; she found out "most of them didn't know or didn't care" and a few were openly supporting repeal in the state. "That astonished me," she recalled.[1] Until the early 1960s, all major religious traditions—Jewish, Catholic and Protestant—had been unanimous, at least in their official pronouncements, in their opposition to abortion.[2] By the late 1960s, however, this unanimity had splintered and many began to advocate for abortion access. Across the nation, religious leaders called for the reform and repeal of restrictive abortion laws from their pulpits—the "healing of body and soul in the name of human compassion" in the words of one New Mexico minister.[3] Others did much more. In Colorado, the Clergy Consultation Service (CCS), a group of forty local priests, ministers, and rabbis, counseled women who wanted abortions and then helped them skirt the law to get them. In so doing, the clergy of CCS placed moral decision-making with the pregnant woman, and confessed their own inability to determine whether the fetus was a life.[4] By 1970, CCS clergymen in twenty-six states were counseling 150,000 women a year.[5] Many national religious leaders joined their reform-minded clergy to advocate for change. In 1963 Unitarian Universalists became the first Protestant denomination to support abortion reform, and many Christian and Jewish dominations soon followed. Even Protestant churches that would later oppose liberalized abortion laws, like the United Methodists and the Southern Baptists, cautiously supported abortion reform in these years.[6]

Many conservative Americans, like Ruth Dolan, were shocked to realize that the sexual revolution had gone to church.

A decade later, this evolution had largely been erased from public memory as conservative activists convinced many Americans that the pro-life perspective was "the religious perspective." In the intervening years, activists politicized religious spaces across the country, integrating fetal politics into rituals of faith and convincing their co-religionists to join the cause. In those years and after, houses of worship became sites of political transformation. In fact, it was for religious white Americans that activists first made pro-life politics personal. Many began to experience opposition to abortion as central to their identities as Christians. Through this work, activists expanded their base of activists from middle-class professionals to all classes and occupations. Any (white) Americans who considered themselves conservative and Christian were asked to take a stand against abortion. This work was often done within the confines of the parish, congregation, or ward, but gradually activists built bridges across denominations. Activists motivated many to overcome their theological differences to stand under the same political tent.

By the 1980s, white anti-abortion activists had reclaimed the authority of "religion" from liberals and placed it squarely in the domain of the Right. White conservatives used abortion politics to both narrow the definition of religion and reconnect religion with a certain version of political whiteness. When white activists politicized their religious spaces, they made abortion central to many white people's relationship with their faith. When they sacralized anti-abortion political space, white conservatives brought their fusion of religion and politics into the public square and asked passersby to see that space through their eyes. And finally when white activists worked across denominational lines with other white conservatives, they were able to use claims of religious pluralism as evidence of their universal "morality." As white conservatives claimed to speak for "religious people," they denied religious authority to pro-choice people, who anti-abortion activists believed to be a part of the white elite manipulating society. They also ignored or marginalized religious people of color who did not fit into activists' politicized worldview.

Much of this political work was done in pews and from pulpits, in Catholic parishes and LDS meetinghouses, in intimate and holy places. This kind of religious activism was often overshadowed by the movement's legislative work at the state and national level. In the 1970s, anti-abortion activists in the Four Corners states and around the country directed much of their

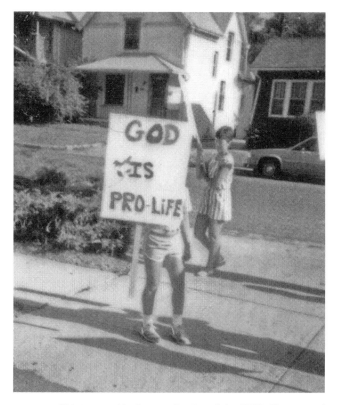

FIGURE 6. Picketer outside Denver abortion clinic, 1986. (Courtesy of Planned Parenthood of the Rocky Mountains; Western History and Genealogy Department, Denver Public Library)

legislative energy at the federal government. They supported the Hyde Amendment (which prohibited federal funding of abortions through Medicaid) as well as a constitutional amendment banning abortion. The constitutional amendment debate was riven with debates over strategy; should the movement push for an outright ban or just an amendment that would return the issue to the states? While the Hyde Amendment passed in 1976, no pro-life amendment received enough support to pass in either the House or the Senate or to trigger a constitutional convention. Through the lens of these legislative drives, the pro-life movement of the 1970s looks divided and largely unsuccessful.[7]

If we direct our gaze at the parish rather than the statehouse, however, the movement looks wholly different. There, the movement was dynamic, developing cohesive political ideas and ecumenical bridges. Religious people laid the organizational and theoretical groundwork for the movement for years to come. A cadre of energized activists compelled their religious institutions to remake themselves into bulwarks against abortion. Through their work, anti-abortion activists motivated many religious people to join their cause and changed the political tenor of many congregations. By the end of the decade, pro-life activists had claimed "religion" as their own.

WE COULD HAVE SHUT THE COUNTRY DOWN

In pews all over Arizona, in January 1975, Catholics heard about the problem of abortion.[8] If priests in the Diocese of Phoenix followed their bishop's suggestions, they planned a regularly scheduled mass or a special evening mass on the "Christian concern for life" in order to "sensitize the congregation to the importance of the issue." The week before, church bulletins told parishioners that *Roe v. Wade* gave "parents and their doctor the legal right to take the life of innocent unborn children at will" and that together Catholics could "arouse a consciousness in our country of the evil of abortion." Many churchgoers certainly recited the suggested prayer that week: "That people of all faiths and religious convictions may join in the effort to obtain Constitutional protection for all human life, let us pray to the Lord." The following Sunday, on the anniversary of *Roe,* many parishes rang their church bells for fifteen minutes, as the bishop suggested. Others flew their flags at half-staff in "memory of thousands of innocent lives taken by abortion." The bishop suggested that priests draw from the liturgy for other religious occasions, especially the funeral mass for unbaptized children and the Feast of the Holy Innocents, the December holiday commemorating King Herod's killing, after Jesus's birth, of all Bethlehem boys under the age of two. In writing their sermons, some priests probably drew from the bishop's statement on abortion, which he attached with his other suggestions. Priests might have quoted rising abortion statistics and a growing "climate of social permissiveness," as the bishop's statement did. Priests might have mentioned women aborting out of "convenience," cited allegedly scientific proof that life begins at conception, or made comparisons to the gas chambers of World War II. They might have argued that civil law was based on "divine law," and worried aloud that the two were now in conflict. They might have asked their flock for a "renew[ed] determination to reverse the Supreme Court's abortion on demand decisions." Or priests might have written their pro-life sermon from scratch. Whatever the case, few parishioners would have left their services without some interaction with anti-abortion arguments and imagery. Few would have missed that January 22 was now "a day of mourning."[9] Of course many Catholics would have previously known about their church's opposition to abortion, but in the 1970s this belief took up much more space in church. It became integral to many Catholics' experiences of their faith.

From the late 1960s onward, white Catholics, Protestants, and Mormons witnessed some form of pro-life politics enter their rituals of faith. Sometimes church leaders took the lead in promoting anti-abortion politics, but more often white activist laity had to prod their religious leaders to prioritize abortion throughout the year. After the Catholic Church and its organizations primed their flock for pro-life activism, the hierarchy hesitated when it came to anti-abortion advocacy in the early 1970s. Thus, it was often lay activists who pushed their priests and ministers to give fetal politics a place in church and tried to convince their co-religionists to join the movement. In the Catholic Church, but also Mormon and Protestant churches, pro-life activists had to work to reassert their politically and theologically conservative vision within religious institutions. Lay activists, with the help of sympathetic clergy, brought fetal imagery and anti-abortion politics into religious spaces, thus changing the ways in which many experienced the moral and political facets of their identities as religious people.

While much of the country, especially in the 1970s, thought of abortion as a "Catholic issue," Catholic activists, priests, and bishops did not always agree on how to approach their opposition to abortion. Some Catholic leaders worried that outright advocacy would encourage more anti-Catholic sentiment in the public at large or that it would jeopardize the church's tax-exempt status. But questions about pro-life advocacy also touched a nerve in an already divided church. In the aftermath of Vatican II, the contest between liberal and traditionalist Catholics played out most intensely on issues of gender and sexuality: priests' celibacy, contraception, women in the priesthood, divorce, homosexuality, and abortion. Many of these debates filtered into local parishes, where liberal and traditionalist Catholics often co-existed.[10] The traditionalists accepted and even promoted the church's steadfast dictums. The liberals, however—a group that included laity, priests, men and women religious— broke the church's rules, sometimes openly, and demanded change. Some of the most public dissenters were excommunicated or removed from their posts.

Some liberal priests dissented simply by not prioritizing pro-life politics. Mike Berger, the Family Life Director for the Diocese of Tucson, noted, "I think some of the pastors did not give [abortion] the kind of importance that some of the people who were more active in the movement wanted it to be."[11] His observations were echoed on a national level as well. In 1976, Robert N. Lynch, the head of the church's committee for the pro-life constitutional amendment, offered this explanation for pastoral reticence: "Parish priests," he explained, "are turned off by the abortion issue" because pro-life activists were the same people who had opposed even basic sex education in Catholic schools.[12] A 1972 survey in New York found that 40 percent of Catholic priests disagreed or had concerns about the church's stance on abortion.[13] Only from the outside did the Catholic community appear unified on the issue; pro-life activists knew they pushed their cause within a politically fractured church.

Many white anti-abortion activists testified that they had to motivate Catholic priests and bishops in the late 1960s and early 1970s. Margaret Sebesta remembered that, in 1970, Catholic bishops in Colorado reached out to her group because they wanted "to have contact with the resistance." The bishops sent a young priest to meet with the activists and, at some point in the meeting, the two parties disagreed about politics or strategy. Sebesta, adept at turning a phrase, remembered telling the priest: "if he kept riding the fence like that he'd get splinters in his britches."[14] Even in a meeting created for political alliance and aid, the Catholic hierarchy did not want to commit in the ways activists like Sebesta wanted. While it is unclear whether Sebesta got the priest to stop riding the fence, it is clear that she and Colorado's nascent pro-life movement were pushing the local Catholic hierarchy, rather than the other way around. One Catholic author complained in 1971 that clergy and the church hierarchy had not sufficiently supported the anti-abortion movement and thus "failed as moral leaders."[15] In these early years especially, lay activists and many church leaders disagreed not on the immorality of abortion but on how active the church should be in the movement against it.

And yet, many priests did give activists religious space for their political work. An Arizona poll in 1967 found that when a reform bill was facing the state's legislature, 82 percent of the diocese's priests said they had offered some pro-life "commentary" to their congregations, 86 percent encouraged their congregants to write to their legislators about the bill, 63 percent gave their congregations the names of their legislators, 47 percent suggested that the church's auxiliary groups work on the issue, 42 percent delivered a sermon on abortion, and 37 percent put some mention of the bill in their parish bulletin.[16] Priestly efforts were probably lessened because parishes were supposed to be talking about the yearly diocesan financial drive that week. Priestly participation in anti-abortion politics only grew in subsequent years.

From 1967 onward, pro-life activists integrated fetal politics into the daily rhythms of faith on a parish-by-parish basis. Arizona anti-abortion activist John Jakubczyk remembered his early activism: "We'd have pro-life masses where we talked the priest into letting the pro-life group of singers play. . . . And then I would talk the priest into giving a homily on the subject and ask him to pass the basket to raise money so we could buy materials."[17] Activist Laurie Futch echoed Jakubczyk's memories of church-based activism. At the end of mass, she said, "we [would] give a short talk about what we do and then we would offer the Rose for Life or the Precious Feet lapel pins. And then we'd always say we need volunteers."[18] Catholic churches, especially those with white congregations, became so synonymous with anti-abortion advocacy that church employees often acted as surrogate activists. One woman called her Catholic church with concerns about legal abortion and the office put her in contact with a local pro-life activist from another Catholic church.[19]

When activists came to church, they brought with them their potent fetal imagery. In 1973, the Diocese of Phoenix began showing a fifteen-minute slide show "of unborn children," narrated by members of Arizona Right to Life, after Sunday mass.[20] Activists like Laurie Futch brought Precious Feet pins to the churches she visited. Later, activists showed films like *The Silent Scream* to religious audiences, even to children in Sunday school. In such moments, the boundaries between social conservative political work and religious observance disappeared, as Catholics were asked to defend fetuses and their faith to a secular world.

With Precious Feet pins in hand or with images of abortion before their eyes, congregants were asked to sign petitions and vote for pro-life candidates. One Utah man wrote his congressman in 1974: "Yesterday at Mass we were urged to sign a prolife petition to be presented to you. Father stated you had not made a public statement against abortion."[21] Anti-abortion activists appealed to churchgoers to write letters to their elected officials. For example, in 1979 in New Mexico, Governor Bruce King received hundreds of letters against abortion with the same four pro-life talking points. These letters were a part of a campaign organized by New Mexico Right to Life and promoted in the state's churches. The prompt gave religious audiences directions for their letters and demanded they get involved because "GOD NEVER INTENDED US TO KILL OUR CHILDREN." One woman sent the form to the governor with the explanation, "This letter was given to me in the Church. I think it's time we do something about abortion."[22] By 1978, one California legislator complained, "We're tired of being inundated with pulpit-initiated letter campaigns."[23]

When those "inundated" elected officials were Catholics themselves, they got a special brand of pro-life pressure. When, in 1969, the governor of New Mexico, David Cargo, had an abortion liberalization bill on his desk to sign, his fellow Catholics pleaded with him to veto it.[24] One New Mexican sent him a relic from Pope Pius XII so that the dead pope could offer the governor guidance. Another wrote, "I truly believe that God has placed you in the position of Governor principally in order that you would be able to veto abortion legislation."[25] Once Cargo allowed the legislation to pass, Catholic New Mexicans invoked their common faith to chastise him. One activist beseeched: "As governor and as a Catholic you could have born true witness to the Church by vetoing the bill, but you neglected to do so; Why?"[26] Years later, in 1977, a New Mexico pro-life activist wrote another governor with a similar condemnation: "How can you reconcile your conscience to permitting the slaughter of countless innocent unborn children in this State? How can you go to Mass? How can you go to the Sacraments? How can you sleep nights?"[27] These activists invoked Catholic officials as members of a common faith who were subject to strict church laws on abortion, murder, and sin. The founder of Colorado Springs Right to Life and later the radical Lambs of Christ, Norman Weslin, put it more bluntly: he said if a Catholic says they support legal abortion, "you must tell them: 'You are no longer a Catholic.'"[28] Activists pushed against those liberal Catholics, who, using their own moral compass, supported or did not openly oppose liberalized abortion laws. Not only did lay pro-life activists work to make anti-abortion politics integral to religious spaces, they also punished their co-religionists who disagreed.

By the mid-1970s, lay white activists had compelled the church hierarchy to take more public action against legal abortion. In 1975, the National Conference of Catholic Bishops announced a plan of action called the "Pastoral Plan for Pro-Life Activities." They called on all church-sponsored or "identifiably Catholic" organizations to pursue a three-point plan of action. They suggested an educational campaign directed at the general public and, more intensively, at the Catholic community. "The primary purpose of the intensive educational program," their statement read, "is the development of pro-life attitudes and the determined avoidance of abortion by each person." The second goal was a broader effort directed at women seeking abortion and those who had had abortions. They asked that this pastoral work provide moral guidance showing "that abortion is a violation of God's law" and providing services to pregnant women, "special understanding" for rape victims, and, finally, potential reconciliation for women who had abortions. The third goal of the Pastoral Plan was the development of an extensive legislative and public policy campaign. Finally, they asked that states, dioceses, and parishes organize committees to put the plan into action.[29]

The Catholic hierarchy took more action for the pro-life cause after 1975, but in the minds of many anti-abortion Catholic lay activists, it was too little, too late. Despite the Pastoral Plan, many activists remember this early period as a failure of moral leadership. Arizona activist John Jakubczyk argued, "I look back and say gosh they were still so respectful of the system instead of just screaming, No! Can you imagine in 1973 if the Catholic Church had said any legislator who supports abortion is automatically excommunicated? . . . And . . . we are going to have the entire Catholic population sit down and not go to work until you think this thing through. We could have shut the country down. Could have woken everybody up. . . . We should have been bolder in the earlier days."[30] Catholic leaders had failed both Catholic activists and the country as a whole, Jakubczyk suggested. They had overestimated the power of the opposition and underestimated their own power to motivate American Catholics and change American politics. Because of this failure to politicize Catholic people, Jakubczyk believed, abortion remained legal and the pro-life movement had to continue working for incremental change in parishes, at state capitols, and outside abortion clinics.

MORMONS AND PROTESTANTS JOIN THE "CATHOLIC" MOVEMENT

When reflecting on where most anti-abortion picketers were from, a Tucson anti-abortion activist said "mostly churches, mostly churches" and those churches were not just Catholic.[31] Early pro-life groups often included Mormons and people from a variety of mainstream and evangelical Protestant denominations. In the Northeast, they even had the occasional Orthodox Jew. The religious nature of this movement was not by accident; nor was it because religious people were naturally pro-life. The politicization of Protestants and Mormons was a product of institutional and grassroots activism within those faiths. Over the course of the 1970s, white conservatives across many faiths began to feel that abortion was central to their religious identities. As they did, they were able to envision alliance with those with whom they had profound, and irreconcilable, theological disagreements. White conservative Catholics, evangelicals, and Mormons could, together, be a part of the "moral middle."

The scale of this activism ranged from the monumental to the minute. A Tucson activist remembered that church bulletins were the first forum where her group warned the public about the growing availability of abortion.[32] Later bulletins followed up with nuts-and-bolts updates on the movement, pro-life meetings, current threats, and suggested donations. Norman Weslin, founder of Colorado Springs Right to Life, first heard about legal abortion this way. In 1969, his church bulletin notified the congregation that a pro-life doctor was giving a lecture on how to stop legal abortion. The notice and subsequent lecture motivated Weslin to join the movement—a movement that would become his passion.[33] While others in Weslin's congregation probably ignored the same notification, a select few like Weslin responded with enthusiasm.

Some types of religious activism could not be ignored. Rev. James Mote led a conservative revolt in his Denver Episcopal parish. When the Women's Council of the Episcopal Church passed a resolution calling for repeal of all restrictive abortion laws in 1970, Mote grumbled that that he knew "of no women competent to make such a decision." Years later, he got his parish to secede from the Episcopal Church because of the church hierarchy's support of divorce, women's ordination, and legal abortion.[34] Socially conservative activism caused an epic rupture for this congregation, motivating its members to abandon their denomination. But everyday and monumental activism were related. Surely there were many political bulletins and sexually conservative sermons in Mote's parish before his parishioners voted to leave. Those small, and seemingly inconsequential, political acts built a socially conservative consciousness for many, allowing for congregation-wide activism. These intimate and grand politicizations occurred in both Mormon and Protestant faiths, though they often took denomination-specific shapes.

Mormons were common allies even in the early days of the movement. This was partly because LDS opposition to abortion was not new, even if Mormons were conflicted over when ensoulment occurred. Nineteenth-century Mormon leaders opposed abortion, but with a view firmly toward eastern Protestant power. Throughout the second half of the nineteenth century, Mormons and non-Mormons engaged in a pitched battle over polygamy—and by extension, sexual norms, families, and Christianity.[35] Beginning in the late 1860s, Mormon leaders used abortion as an example of eastern excess and immorality, an argument for why Protestant American leaders had no right to impose monogamy on Utah. As the U.S. government ramped up its judicial and legal attacks on polygamy, President of the Church John Taylor wrote of easterners' Protestantism: "Their god is overlaid with gilt and tinsel, but inside it is pregnant with its twin adjuncts foetecide and infanticide."[36] In 1884, Taylor argued that easterners had actually brought abortion with them to Utah, infecting good Mormons with their immorality.[37] Critiques of the aborting East were criticisms of the failures of monogamous marriage, the hypocrisy of easterners' moral outrage at polygamy, and the excesses of federal power that eastern monogamists levied against Mormons. It was in this period that punishments for abortion were most severe in the church; President Taylor threatened that any woman who had an abortion would be "sever[ed] from the church" and never "inherit the Kingdom of God."[38] For LDS leaders in this moment, abortion was a symbol of eastern political and moral degradation and thus a betrayal worthy of excommunication.[39] In the twentieth century, the penalties lessened.

If the nineteenth-century LDS Church was fraught with debates about gender, so too was the church of the 1970s. In this decade, the church was transitioning toward a global, modern church but not without some growing pains, especially around issues of black men's access to the priesthood and the role of women in the church. The church had become increasingly interested in international conversion, a movement that had begun in the 1950s but grew exponentially in the 1970s. In 1951, the church's members numbered only a little more than one million and were concentrated in the American West; by the early 1980s, the international church alone numbered 1.5 million.[40] Though the church eventually solved its priesthood problem in a 1978 revelation by the church's prophet allowing black men the privileges of LDS manhood, the church doubled down on the place of women. In 1972, when the proposed Equal Rights Amendment (ERA) to the U.S. Constitution was sent to the states for consideration, Mormons began a decade-long, acrimonious debate over whether the Mormon tradition sanctioned equality for women or a special, different place for women in families and in society.[41] The church eventually openly opposed the ERA, helping secure its national defeat. Throughout the 1970s, the church hierarchy and regular conservative Mormons pressed the idea that motherhood was a woman's sacred role in society and feminism threatened that holy pedestal.

One important piece of this conservative turn was a more explicit opposition to legal abortion. Though most twentieth-century Mormons disapproved of abortion in most cases, their opposition was largely unspoken until the early 1970s. Between 1919 and 1971, the General Authorities of the church (which included members of the three highest governing bodies) did not address the practice in their public talks. In the 1970s that changed as opposition to abortion became a regular part of Mormon leaders' speeches and testimonies. Between 1971 and 1973, leaders of the church discussed abortion 12 times in their public addresses, and between 1973 and 1980, 43 times.[42]

The LDS General Conference was perhaps the most important forum for these talks. The General Conference was a biannual series of meetings and lectures about Mormon interests and theology—what one scholar described as the "cement that held together the Mormon" community since the nineteenth century.[43] At every general conference in the 1970s, Mormons heard about abortion from their leaders at the General Conference. For example, at the May 1975 conference, James E. Faust, an assistant to the Quorum of Twelve apostles, gave an entire talk about "the sanctity of life." Directing his comments to women because "only they can honor the holy calling of motherhood," he combined quotes from church authorities and talking points from non-Mormon pro-life leaders. He called abortion "evil" and "abhorrent," arguing that reproduction in marriage was the only thing keeping people from "becoming mere addicts of lust," even as he remained vague about the precise moment of ensoulment.[44] More importantly, President of the Church Spencer W. Kimball included condemnations of abortion in the conference's opening talks almost every year during the 1970s.[45] Because Mormons consider their president to be a prophet and modern-day revelator, his comments carried the power of official church doctrine.

These talks reached an incredible number of Mormons. The conference began to be broadcast on the radio in 1924 and on television in 1949.[46] By 1970, the conference was carried by 100 radio and 200 television stations and had a worldwide audience of "millions."[47] Additionally these talks were distributed in print version through church periodicals and incorporated into lesson manuals for children and adult Sunday school classes, male priesthood quorums, and functions for the Relief Society, the primary LDS women's group.[48]

With the president's blessing, many Mormon pro-lifers brought their activism into religious forums. As early as 1973, some leaders of the Relief Society asked Mormon women to oppose abortion.[49] In 1977, Barbara Smith, head of the Relief Society, used her platform to oppose abortion because "eternal progression [toward godhood] is dependent on mortality." She added that "it should be no surprise then to find [Mormons] standing against abortion, actively working against it, and urging our members to support and join the battle to preserve life."[50] At the church's flagship academic institution, Brigham Young University, the associated student group worked on anti-abortion letter campaigns and other pro-life activities.[51] Certain wards financially supported anti-abortion organizations through donations and fund-raising activities.[52] This was all in addition to pro-life ideas that circulated around the weekly LDS education classes attended by good Mormons of all ages. For most Mormons, the church structured every day of their lives in one way or another and thus, in the 1970s, pro-life politics became a part of Mormons' daily expression of their devotion.

For Sandra Allen, a Mormon woman living in Las Vegas but with familial ties to Arizona, Utah, and New Mexico, social conservatism shaped relationships with her friends and family and her liberal, non-Mormon neighbors. In the late 1970s, Allen was an overworked housewife in her mid-twenties, writing daily in her diary. Her primary solace in a chaotic life was her friendship with other Mormon women. "Sitting with [godly Mormon women] and talking about truths was like sitting in on a meeting with the 'great and noble.' . . . Heaven would not be heaven if I was ever denied the right to work with them in the eternities," she wrote.[53] Another day she envisioned a "pure power in the bond that binds me with these women."[54] Allen and her friends had intensely intimate relationships, where they gave each other blessings, shared energies, fasted and prayed together. The women who Allen loved struggled to perfect their relationships to God and pushed Allen to be a better mother, wife, and Mormon.

When Allen had to enter sexually liberal spaces she often felt physically cold, subsumed by a "spirit of darkness." She described many of the liberal non-Mormon women she encountered as "cold and hard," and others as potential prostitutes.[55] Sexual moralism was imprinted on Allen's senses. Shades of darkness and light, sensations of cold and warmth differentiated the upright from the unprincipled. It was not uncommon for Mormons to feel separate from their "gentile" neighbors—Mormons were, after all, a "peculiar people"—but in 1978 Allen experienced her own difference as much through the lens of politics as religion.

Sandra Allen felt no darkness or cold when she interacted with pro-life non-Mormons, only exhilaration. Around the anniversary of the *Roe* decision in 1978, she joined a big anti-abortion march where she was delighted by the large crowd of "concerned Christians" protesting together. She noted that Mormons were in the majority that day, but "the Catholics gave us a run for our money." "We all left pleased and excited," she recorded.[56] Church meetings promoted political understandings of members' moral, not just religious, identities. A week before the march, Allen attended a church event where members discussed the threat of feminists who advocated for the ERA and legal abortion. From that meeting, Allen got the sense that "there is so very much evil going on about us—I feel angry and helpless. I want to know what I can do to change things."[57] This political excitement moved her to action when an activist friend asked Allen to get involved and join the battle lines of American politics.

Once she did, Allen continued to rely on feelings of cold and darkness— plus the "God Nod," or divine guidance through prayer—to prove that the Divine sanctioned her politics.[58] When NOW (the National Organization for Women) organized in Las Vegas—or as she put it "when the enemy was in town"—Allen "went cold in the realization of the reality of this battle."[59] In Allen's world, politics was not separate from her sense of self or even from her bodily reactions. Moral politics infused her relationships with other women, with her church, and with her God. For Allen and many other Mormons, pro-life politicization seamlessly blended into a world already wrapped around family, conservative gender roles, and church allegiance.[60] Anti-abortion politics also stimulated Mormons like Allen to expand their ideas of "the moral" to include some Catholics and Protestants.

Even as Mormons jumped into anti-feminist politics, few became reliable movement activists. LDS people usually played supporting rather than main roles in the theatre of abortion politics.[61] New Mexico pro-life activist Dauneen Dolce explained why Mormons had such a small presence in the movement: they "have a way of kind of working their own maybe from history of how things happened. . . . [Even now,] I don't get the Mormons in to speak." Dolce also argued that "trust" was a problem for LDS people within pro-life coalitions made up of Catholics and Protestants who, Mormons worried, harbored anti-Mormon feelings.[62] According to National Right to Life officials, LDS leadership told them in 1973 that Mormons preferred to pursue anti-abortion initiatives within the confines of their own church.[63]

Another explanation for the marginal participation of Mormons in the movement is that LDS leaders treated abortion differently than they treated murder in the twentieth century. If a member of the church committed murder, that person was immediately excommunicated. A member who terminated a pregnancy, on the other hand, was "disciplined by Church councils, as necessary." Abortion, unlike murder, was for Mormons "amenable to the laws of repentance and forgiveness."[64] Specifically, in cases of rape, incest, when the fetus was extremely deformed, or when the life or health of the mother was in danger, the practice of abortion was morally sanctioned by the church, as long as the woman had discussed the issue with both her husband and her bishop. Thus when non-Mormon activists proposed laws that would ban abortion in all cases, Mormon pro-lifers could not support them.[65]

This difference between the Mormon stance and the movement's stance meant that the church usually offered rhetorical support for the pro-life cause, but they did not use their extensive church apparatus to aid the movement the way they did for other conservative causes. In their campaign against the Equal Rights Amendment during the 1970s and 1980s, and later, their campaign against gay marriage, the LDS Church pushed its members to political action. Many have credited the LDS Church, at least partially, for the defeat of the Equal Rights Amendment in 1982, the success of an anti-gay marriage bill in California in 2000, and the passage of an amendment to the California constitution banning gay marriage in 2008.[66] On the issue of abortion, however, church leaders often left overt anti-abortion activism to the individual activists.

By the late 1970s and early 1980s, the pro-life movement began to attract members of another faith community in large numbers: white evangelical Christians. Evangelical activists came from a variety of denominations and independent Christian churches, entering pro-life coalitions across the country, and especially in Arizona and Colorado. Beginning in 1952, Southern Baptists and other evangelical groups helped reinvent evangelicalism as open, flexible, and compatible with modernity. They also began missionizing in the West. By the late 1990s, the region was home to some of the largest evangelical congregations in the United States, including Phoenix's First Assembly of God with 9,500 members and Denver's Heritage Christian Center with 3,500 members.[67] Colorado in particular became a vibrant hub for evangelicalism, home to a variety of evangelical industries and nonprofits, including James Dobson's Focus on the Family.

For evangelicals, especially the white ones, pro-life belief became central to their religious identities. Initially, evangelical dominations were ambivalent about or even supportive of abortion reform.[68] But even as many evangelicals equivocated about the morality of abortion, there were a handful of ministers and laypeople who were outspokenly pro-life, pushing their congregations and dominations toward activism.[69] A Texas pastor, Robert Holbrook, had been outraged by the *Roe* decision and immediately formed Baptists for Life. Holbrook worked with pro-life groups in the region and lobbied the Southern Baptist convention to change its stance on abortion.[70] Ultimately, people like Rev. Holbrook won the day, motivating many to equate pro-life sentiment with evangelical Protestant belief.

By 1980, grassroots activists had pushed fetal imagery and pro-life politics into white evangelical spaces. Many historians have identified Francis Schaeffer's four-hour documentary called *What Ever Happened to the Human Race?* as the instigator of evangelical pro-life action.[71] In 1979, Schaeffer, a respected speaker and documentarian, released the film, which combined extended anti-abortion arguments with powerful imagery of abortions and abortion's supposed victims. The most remembered scene of the movie was of Schaeffer in front of the Dead Sea, which was filled with plastic dolls representing those "killed" by abortion. The film came to churches and meeting halls all over the country, and was, according to two scholars of the pro-life movement, "mobbed like rock concerts."[72] This film, however, was a match that ignited conservative drybrush. In the 1970s, fundamentalists were pushing evangelicalism into more rigid theological and more conservative political territory.[73] This theological rigidity combined with sexual change in evangelical circles. White evangelicals began embracing the sensual joys of marital sex, while more vehemently condemning all practices outside its boundaries.[74] When Schaeffer's film came into white evangelical religious spaces, it made pro-life politics personal and relevant to communities in the midst of a conservative sea change.

This type of politicization was less common in black evangelical churches. African American leaders were less likely than their white counterparts to advocate for particular social issues. Black congregations were politically active, but their activism usually focused on issues most of their congregants could agree upon, like community outreach programs or voter registration drives. Moreover, white social conservatives often ignored communities of color. In a roundtable on the Religious Right and people of color in 1994, one participant explained: "They're not organizing, building constituencies or pulling people of color into their groups—that would require accountability."[75] As a result, white evangelicals became more uniformly pro-life, and black evangelicals became less so over the last decades of the twentieth century. Without a reliable cadre of vocally anti-abortion religious leaders and without everyday pro-life politicization in their holy spaces, black Protestants formed their own opinions about the issue. For those who opposed legal abortion, that belief did not seem to factor into their votes. One study from 1992 found that only 8 percent of black people considered a candidate's position on abortion salient when making their decision at the ballot box, as opposed to 26 percent of white people.[76]

As time went on, opposition to abortion grew more important to white evangelicals. The idea that life began at conception seeped into evangelical periodicals, radio programs, and magazines. Evangelical media moguls like James Dobson, Tim LaHaye, Jerry Falwell, and Pat Robertson all made opposition to abortion central to their publications and programs. Compiling and distributing biblical "proof" of abortion's immorality, these national leaders "pulled opposition to abortion into the very heart of what it meant to be an evangelical Christian," according to anthropologist Susan Friend Harding.[77] In the 1980s, pro-life politics entered evangelical lives through their televisions, mailboxes, and Christian bookstores.

In the 1980s and 1990s, white pastors got creative about how to convey the horror of abortion to their flock. For example, Keenan Roberts, an Assemblies of God pastor in Thornton, Colorado, came up with the idea of the Hell House in 1990. The Hell House was a pop-up, socially conservative Haunted House that welcomed guests in the run-up to Halloween. Visitors walked through a series of rooms with gruesome dramatizations of sins, culminating in a botched abortion. One visitor described the woman in the abortion scene as "a shrieking victim/patient" and the doctor as "a brutal, dirty sadist" who "cackled and threw 'fetus' pieces at the audience."[78] In the Hell House, sinners ended up in a fiery hell. According to its creator, the experience would lead visitors on a path straight to Jesus. Still, while conversion was the explicit goal—Roberts even promised a conversion rate of 25 percent—most audience members were already evangelicals or Pentecostals.[79] For them, the Hell House might have renewed their faith but it also reminded them that abortion would lead to eternal damnation. Roberts packaged and sold Hell House kits all across the country and hundreds of evangelical congregations began putting on Hell Houses every October.

In white evangelical communities, Hell Houses, *What Ever Happened to the Human Race?* showings, and numerous other anti-abortion actions led many to elevate the issue above all others. In the 1980s and 1990s, white evangelicals joined existing pro-life groups and formed their own new groups, rejuvenating and radicalizing the movement. By the 1990s, white evangelicals, who had been divided over abortion only twenty years before, opposed legal abortion on average more than American Catholics.[80] Through their opposition to abortion, white evangelicals would stand alongside Catholics and Mormons and claim the mantle of morality.

Beginning in the late 1970s, many sociologists and pollsters noted a correlation between the frequency of church attendance and pro-life belief.[81] These social observers concluded at turns that frequent attendees were more fervent, more dedicated to the denomination's theology, more committed to their religious identity, or more opposed to secular modernity. In explaining this phenomenon, most overlook how white anti-abortion activists turned the church into political space in the 1970s. Those who came to church more frequently experienced fetal politics as a central part of their faith experience. This was true for white Catholics, Mormons, evangelical Christians, and some mainstream Christians, though the shape of that religious and political syncretism was different in each faith. But by the late 1970s and early 1980s, many white Americans envisioned opposition to abortion as a central component of their religious devotions and identities.

ETHNIC MEXICANS AND THE PRO-LIFE MOVEMENT

There were important outliers to this general trend of religious politicization. If religious fervency and church attendance correlated to pro-life belief, why did devout, ethnic Mexican Catholics not join the pro-life movement? They should have been primed by their church hierarchy in ways similar to their white co-religionists, and yet, few joined the anti-abortion cause. Ultimately a different kind of moral politics took root in ethnic Mexican Catholic parishes, one that was often at odds with the imperatives of the church hierarchy and the anti-abortion movement.

Ethnic Mexican Catholics were, demographically speaking, ripe for pro-life politicization. White anti-abortion activists and social commenters regularly noted that Mexicans and Mexican Americans generally had "traditional" families and opposed abortion personally. In 1978, one white Catholic explained why ethnic Mexicans should be "right-wing": "Consider that we are talking about a people who are very conservative on social issues, strong family people, people for whom religion is not simply a private affair but an active force in community life, men who are *macho*."[82] Surveys generally backed up this observation, albeit with less reliance on racial stereotypes. A 1986 national survey found that 67.6

percent of the broader Latinx Catholic community believed abortion was always wrong, a rate significantly higher than the U.S. Catholic population as a whole. A Hispanic Pew poll in 2007 found a similar trend; 63 percent of Latinx Catholics believed abortion should be illegal.[83] This anti-abortion sentiment, however, never translated into significant political participation for the cause. The reason for this discrepancy lies, in part, in ethnic Mexicans' relationships to racial justice movements and to the Catholic hierarchy.

For many ethnic Mexicans, Vatican II altered local parishes for the better. The move to conduct mass in the "vernacular" meant that many parishes had to hold both English and Spanish services. Imbued by the spirit of Vatican II, American social justice movements, and Latin American liberation theology, many ethnic Mexicans called for more change in their local churches. They asked for respect of their religious culture, promotion of Spanish-speaking priests and ethnic Mexican bishops, and a reasonable division of resources between parishes dominated by Anglos and those dominated by people of color.[84] This increased empowerment within the church, along with other structural change, led to a "Latino religious resurgence" in the late twentieth century.[85]

This resurgence coincided with the Catholic hierarchy's renewed commitment to pro-life politics. Once anti-abortion activists motivated the Catholic Church to use their resources "in defense of life" in 1975, the hierarchy did so with abandon. Catholic parishes around the country began developing organizational infrastructure to oppose legal abortion. In the 1980s, the church hierarchy began to police and sometimes purge pro-choice Catholics from their institutions, demanding uniformity on the issue of abortion. Anti-abortion activism often subsumed the church's other ministries. To many observers, abortion seemed to become the "single issue" of the Catholic Church at the end of the twentieth century. One of the first signs of this political tunnel vision was the 1976 presidential election when the National Conference of Catholic Bishops supported Republican presidential candidate Gerald Ford. It did not seem to matter that the GOP platform ran counter to almost all of the conference's political positions. What mattered to the bishops was that Ford supported a constitutional amendment banning abortion.[86] In the long run, this singular focus on abortion reshaped the politics of the Catholic Church. It suppressed feminist Catholic campaigns for an acceptance of birth control and female priests and sidelined liberal campaigns against nuclear weapons and poverty. But it also pushed to the margins the reforms demanded by ethnic Mexican Catholics.

One parish in Denver shows how this institutional tension played out on the ground. Our Lady of Guadalupe was founded as a mission in 1936 to serve north Denver's growing ethnic Mexican population. Located in bottomland near the Platte River, the church met the needs of new migrants to the city who came from Mexico, New Mexico, and other parts of Colorado.[87] In the 1960s and 1970s, its parishioners dove into social justice politics, using the infrastructure of their church to aid a number of embattled movements. They focused on Chicano issues, especially the United Farm Workers' grape boycott. In the 1980s and 1990s, they continued advocating for field workers, while also working on issues related to the AIDS epidemic, gun violence, and U.S. intervention in Central America.[88] Early on, Our Lady of Guadalupe parishioners realized they were at odds with the leadership of the archdiocese. The church's priest, Jose Lara, remembered that in 1969 the parish became "like a center" for the United Farm Workers (UFW), who had come to town to stimulate support for the grape boycott. While Our Lady of Guadalupe enthusiastically offered aid, the UFW was not similarly welcomed by Archbishop James V. Casey. "There is no problem in California. Everything is fine," Casey explained.[89] The tensions between Denver's ethnic Mexican community and the archbishop only increased in the 1970s. Because of the parish's work with the Chicano movement, the archbishop openly distrusted the community, going so far as to allow the police to search the church for explosives in 1976. They believed that local Chicano activists were behind a string of bombings in the city.[90] According to a parishioner, one day the police "bust[ed] in," threw Father Lara to the ground and injured him, but found no bombs. Lara demanded the archbishop's resignation.[91] Though the archbishop reconciled with the parish, this did not make up for the long institutional neglect and hostility ethnic Mexican Catholics had experienced. Robert Trujillo told the *Denver Catholic Register* that in all his years of Catholic schooling, he "never once heard a priest take a stand against poverty and social injustices"; instead priests regularly explained that poverty and war were "penalties" for sins.[92] Father Lara realized in those years that "time after time, the church has not been leading in moral issues."[93] This was in a period when the Catholic Church in Denver and around the country was throwing its political weight behind what it considered the preeminent "moral issue" of the time.

Denver's Our Lady of Guadalupe parish did not join local efforts at abortion reform or the nascent pro-choice movement, but they did express a subtle, and illuminating, ambivalence about the church's role in the pro-life movement. In the 1970s, the archdiocese's paper, the *Denver Catholic Register,* regularly reported on abortion politics in the region and the nation; one reader called it "haranguing."[94] In this political climate, the parish never let their church be used for anti-abortion activities. Instead, parishioners and their priest chose to sideline the politics of sexual morality. Lara remembered that church members began to ask for forgiveness for breaking a picket line, rather than breaking natural law. To Lara, this was a victory. He said many other Catholics, "conservative people," confessed their "bad thoughts about sex . . . but [did] nothing for the downtrodden." At Our Lady of Guadalupe, he claimed, there had been a conversion "from that traditional morality to a practical morality of helping others."[95]

Perhaps Our Lady of Guadalupe's inaction on the issue of abortion can be explained the same way many explained ethnic Mexicans' dedication to liberal politics and the Democratic Party; they simply prioritized other issues. But the contours and history of Mexican Catholicism offer a more complex answer. Their brand of Catholicism was forged on the margins, at the edges of empires, often far from the heart of colonial religious institutions. Thus, ethnic Mexican Catholics developed a deeply embedded Catholic culture, but without a dedication to Catholic hierarchy or church doctrine.[96] This religious autonomy was only accentuated in the American West, where a dearth of clergy led to lay religious leadership and more democratized faith practices.[97] American colonial institutions and the Catholic Church tried to remake Mexican-American Catholicism in the late-nineteenth and twentieth centuries; specifically they tried to repress folk religious practices, restrict the use of the Spanish language, and generally remake it, according to historian Anthony Stevens-Arroyo, in the "likeness of European immigrant Catholicism on the East Coast."[98]

The practices surrounding the Virgin of Guadalupe, the Denver parish's namesake, illuminates the complex dynamics of Mexican Catholic devotion. As the story goes, Our Lady of Guadalupe, the Virgin Mary, appeared to Juan Diego, a Nahuatl-speaking man, near Mexico City in 1531, to encourage the conversion of Native peoples to Catholicism. For many ethnic Mexicans in the centuries after, Our Lady of Guadalupe was a sign of a special godly understanding of the New World and the sufferings and oppressions of the Mexican people.[99] In the twentieth century, many ethnic Mexican women took very different messages from the Virgin of Guadalupe than Anglo Catholic women took from the Virgin Mary; for ethnic Mexicans, she was not a symbol of virginity and selfless motherhood but a representation of God the mother.[100]

In 1976, Our Lady of Guadalupe parish in Denver enshrined this forgiving, matriarchal image in their church when Father Lara commissioned a Chicana artist, Carlota Espinoza, to paint a mural of the Virgin behind the altar. She modeled Our Lady of Guadalupe on a "North Denver Chicana," the angels on "neighborhood kids," and Juan Diego on "the janitor of the church."[101] In this mural, a relatable and familiar Lady of Guadalupe took the place at the head of the church that was usually reserved for an untouchable image of Jesus Christ. In fact, one observer felt that the whole church was infused with the "divine feminine"—a divinity that could be embodied by any female parishioner.[102] Forty years later a priest built a wall in front of the mural for this exact reason, explaining that the mural "detracted from the central focus" on Jesus, the divine masculine.[103] But in the 1970s, this mural reflected the religious community it served. As a *Denver Post* reporter put it, "The church was a symbol of the fight for equality and the mural was the emblem."[104] Just as fetus pins and fetus dolls became emblems of Catholic politics for white Catholics in the 1970s, the Virgin of Guadalupe with a Chicana face offered ethnic Mexicans an alternative moral vision.

White pro-life activists often did not recognize the differences between white and ethnic Mexican Catholicism. Mexican Americans' practice of Catholicism was a conundrum to them. In ethnic Mexicans' devotion to the Virgin of Guadalupe, they saw a dedication to female purity and motherhood. In ethnic Mexicans' commitment to Catholic ritual, they saw a traditionalism that seemed to predate Vatican II. Thus, white pro-lifers fell back on the assumption of so many Anglos before them: ethnic Mexicans were fundamentally anti-modern, unchanged by history. For white anti-abortion activists waging a battle against social change, this was admirable. However, they missed the ways that ethnic Mexicans' Lady of Guadalupe was different from the Virgin Mary; they missed the subtle revision of the concept of sin at the heart of many Chicano parishes; and they missed the ways that ethnic Mexicans encouraged social justice campaigns, campaigns from which the church's anti-abortion crusade often distracted. Anti-abortion activists followed a path blazed by centuries of white Catholics before them: they tried to shoehorn Mexican Catholicism into the mold of European Catholicism, and by doing so they missed an opportunity to forge an all-encompassing Catholic movement.[105]

Thus, the Catholic pro-life movement remained almost entirely white.[106] Emma Gomez and Libby Ruiz, discussed in chapter 1, were anomalies. This was not because all ethnic Mexicans supported legal abortion but because

Catholic institutions and the pro-life movement prioritized abortion over other issues that deeply affected people of color. One undocumented Mexican woman explained the tension in the church's politics: "They say the children in our womb are 'innocent life,' but the day they are born they call them 'illegals' and [tell them to] 'go home.'"[107] In the 1960s and 1970s, Latinx, especially ethnic Mexicans, demanded a place at their religion's institutional table. They were incrementally successful at getting the Catholic Church to acknowledge the needs of their communities and even, occasionally, the church's racism, but despite those gains the "Latino religious resurgence" often took a backseat to the pro-life movement.[108]

ECUMENICAL CHAPELS OF PROTEST

Despite the absence of religious people of color, most white pro-life activists remembered their movement as a vibrant religious coalition. From the vantage point of the early twenty-first century, Arizona anti-abortion activists Helen and Phil Seader contended that although Vatican II had argued for a reconciliation between faiths, this was not possible until different denominations found a common foe. "The churches couldn't do it on their own. Abortion did it. Abortion made the Ecumenical Council," Helen Seader claimed. "It was . . . abortion that brought us all together."[109] Activists sidestepped thorny religious differences and focused on common politics, all while building an ecumenical rhetoric and an ecumenical practice. Pro-lifers redefined an old term—Judeo-Christian values—creating a socially conservative umbrella under which very different faith traditions could stand. In protest spaces, especially outside of abortion clinics, they put ecumenical rhetoric into practice, creating a space where religion and politics merged. Unlike the movement's claim to be a racial coalition, its claim as a religious coalition was more than just words.

These ecumenical coalitions of religious conservatives were neither seamless nor conflict-free. In fact, they faced incredible challenges. From the 1940s through the 1960s, ecumenism had been mostly the preoccupation of mainstream Protestants, who believed common theological ground could lessen long-standing denominational conflict. In the same period, American intellectuals invoked the phrase "Judeo-Christian tradition" to distinguish the West and its divinely ordained ethics, nuclear families, and democracies from anti-Semitic Nazism and later atheistic communism.[110] As historian Neil J.

Young has shown, Catholics, evangelicals, and Mormons rejected attempts to find common theological ground in the immediate postwar period, with each group worried that such efforts would water down their claims to absolute religious truth.[111] These religious groups were less comfortable than mainstream Protestants with the monotheistic pluralism that permeated postwar American discourse.

Some of this reticence carried into the anti-abortion movement of the 1970s and 1980s. Right to Life groups tended to be dominated by Catholics, while groups like Operation Rescue tended to be dominated by evangelicals. In some large urban areas, crisis pregnancy centers—pro-life clinic-like alternatives to women's health clinics—were also split between those staffed largely by Catholics and those staffed by evangelicals. This segregation was not simply because people preferred their own, but because activists disagreed on whether proselytizing should be a central part of their work. Mary Menicucci, director of a Catholic-dominated crisis pregnancy center in Albuquerque, put her group's philosophy this way: "we pray to God about the girl, we don't preach" to her.[112] Evangelical activists often believed that the crisis of unplanned pregnancy was the perfect time to offer their religious testimony. Because of this disagreement, the Catholic and evangelical crisis pregnancy centers in places like Phoenix and Albuquerque often refused to work together. White conservative religious people faced real hurdles getting people from different faiths to participate in the same organizations and movements.

Ecumenical groups were not immune to such tensions. One major, divisive issue was what form religion should take in pro-life organizations. Many Catholics, especially those involved in Right to Life groups, were uncomfortable with open displays of religiosity. Ruth Dolan, a Colorado Right to Life activist and, in her words, the group's "token Protestant," recalled an argument in the early 1970s. At the time, she was on the board and in the process of drawing up new bylaws. One evening, she remembered, the board debated whether prayer should be required before and after meetings. Dolan was in favor, but the rest of the board was not. She remembered:

> And I gave a little speech that said well if we want to pass anything . . . we had to be on God's side and we better pray. . . . And they voted it down. . . . I was so mad I went into the bathroom and splashed cold water on my face because I don't think I can work with these people. . . . One man said, well I'm not against motherhood and apple pie but I'm afraid we'd offend an atheist. That's when I really blew my stack. [laughs] I don't care if you offend an atheist. I'm offended. God will be offended.

Dolan stayed in the group for the next three decades, taking solace that even though prayer was not in the bylaws, she "never went to a meeting where they didn't [pray]."[113] Regardless, the implication was clear: Catholics were less comfortable with mandating explicit religiosity in the organization's official documents. While the regularity of Christian prayer at meetings kept Dolan in the group, the debate shows how even a discussion of organizational bylaws could fracture a delicate religious coalition.

And yet, religious coalitions were absolutely necessary to the pro-life movement. They accentuated the claim that this was not a Catholic movement; they helped support the argument that theirs was a moral movement representing all Middle (white) Americans; and it helped build real political power that could sway elections. One strategy was simply to present an ecumenical face to the public. As activist John Jakubczyk remembered, in the late 1970s he and Carolyn Gerster represented the group at public debates because Gerster was a Protestant and he was a Catholic. Jakubcyzk argued that they put forward Protestants or atheists "as examples that the stereotypical, white, Catholic, over 30, over 50, over whatever, female . . . was not representative of the movement."[114] This was not limited to debates and speeches but infused almost all public pro-life presentations in the 1970s and 1980s.[115] This display of religious diversity was not superficial, like the movement's displays of racial diversity, though. In those years, the movement built real bridges between faiths, both in rhetoric and in practice.

The anti-abortion movement made religious coalitions, in part, through discursive bridge building, which would have been foreign to conservative religious groups just a few years before. In order to make a coalition without stepping on any theological toes, anti-abortion activists in the 1970s borrowed some of that earlier ecumenical rhetoric from mainstream Protestants. By then, the notion of a Judeo-Christian tradition had begun to fall out of favor, as some mainstream and liberal intellectuals argued it generalized and glorified what was a more complicated and oppressive American past.[116] At the moment when the term was receiving its strongest intellectual criticism, social conservatives embraced it. They argued that while Greeks and Romans had allowed abortion, monotheism had provided a radical break from that world. Anti-abortion activists contended that sexual modernity was a rejection of monotheistic morality and an insidious vehicle for reshaping a Judeo-Christian nation. For example, in 1978, Neal J. Maxwell, an important LDS Church leader, told an audience at Brigham Young University that they were facing the establishment of "irreligion as *the* state religion." He argued such a state-sanctioned irreligion rejected America's "rich Judeo-Christian herit-age" and disallowed political viewpoints rooted in faith, like "resistance to abortion."[117] For anti-abortion activists, "Judeo-Christian values" was an incredibly valuable tool; it was nationalistic and religious but also capacious: it could include not only Protestants but Catholics, Mormons, and Jews as well.[118]

Ecumenism was more than rhetoric, especially in small towns and cities where activists had to rely on a small cadre of religiously diverse people. This ecumenism was enacted in pro-life political work, perhaps most importantly in protests outside of abortion clinics. There, activists did more than put a religiously diverse face on the movement; they actually forged an alternative—and ecumenical—religious space. In clinic protests, activists turned anti-abortion ephemera into tools of religious devotion to produce a space where politics and religion merged almost seamlessly. From the outside, this reli-gious/political performance seemed like a representation of diverse but cohe-sive social conservative religions. To participants, the differences between denominations remained; and yet, even with the acknowledgement of such difference, activists mainly remembered these protest spaces as both holy and productively ecumenical.

Throughout the 1970s, activists worked to make protest spaces into reli-gious spaces through prayer. Regular observers and participants alike noted the centrality of prayer to pro-life protest. For Catholic activists, this often involved reciting the rosary, a set of prayers counted using a string of beads. Like the rosary itself, repetition was also key to this political devotion. One neighbor of an Albuquerque clinic noted that he was awakened in the morn-ing regularly "by the droning of the rosary being recited outside my win-dow."[119] In a 1976 Boulder protest, activists recited the rosary on "an infor-mal, indefinite basis" in order "to invoke 'god's Grace to change men's hearts' and to provide a 'shield of roses' to save the unborn."[120] The organizer of that protest extended the group's daily prayer into a nine-week novena, or period of persistent prayer focused on a specific petition, and noted that public prayer was a key way "to express their opposition to abortion."[121]

While prayers were targeted mostly at God and outside observers, they were important for activists themselves. A regular picketer outside Albuquerque clinics since the early 1980s, pro-life activist Phil Leahy recalled that "the prayer was so important for keeping us faithful because we would be out in front of . . . the abortion mills . . . and it was so sustaining."[122] For new activists, prayer was sometimes a gateway to other types of protest. Activist

Laura Bowman began praying outside Albuquerque clinics on Saturdays but she "had no interest in counseling [and] had no interest in getting in people's face." At that time, she "knew nothing about the pro-life movement." Through her experience outside clinics and her observation of "prayer warriors," however, she "slowly but surely" was drawn into "speaking to girls that were going into the abortion mills."[123] For Bowman at least, prayer was the first step toward more direct and confrontational types of activism.

While Protestants did not recite the rosary like Catholics, prayer was also important to them as a form of protest. Protestants often interjected more evangelical tempos into their public prayer. "Remember what you were like before you were born again," a Protestant activist in Tempe, Arizona, asked a crowd of two hundred protestors in the early 1980s. The crowd responded with a loud "Amen," while individual protesters "murmured 'Jesus'" and "swayed in prayer."[124] Such prayers were often paired with other practices of religious devotion, like the lighting of candles and singing of hymns.[125]

Both Catholics and Protestants hoped for conversion in these political/religious spaces. According to anti-abortion activists, an aura of godlessness hung in the air around the abortion clinic. Patricia, a regular picketer outside of a Tempe clinic, told a local reporter that "'You know, you are lonely without God. I can sense that about you.' She could sense that about everyone who went into the clinic, she said."[126] A place heavy with political and religious condemnation, the abortion clinic was a godless place that offered the possibility of redemption, according to activists. Phil Leahy recalled that protesters were heartened anytime they could convince women to, at least temporarily, delay an abortion. "First and foremost, we are there to save souls," he noted. He said that abortion providers, clinic staff, volunteers, and patients all had their eternal spirits on the line. "Where would they go when they die? . . . At least . . . our surface perception [is] that they would go to hell."[127] Colorado activist Tom Longua echoed Leahy's sentiments: "We know that by staying outside [the clinics] and putting this fear of God, fear of hell maybe, into some people's minds that some . . . have turned away. So have there been souls saved that otherwise would be going to hell? Yeah, no doubt. . . . That's success for eternity."[128] These activists did not specify a denominational avenue to eternal salvation. Refusing an abortion was enough, at that moment, to save a woman's soul. Women seeking abortions were facing damnation, according to activists, and only pro-lifers could save them.

For those passersby who did not immediately identify abortion clinics as sites of moral tragedy, creative activists helped them see the space with new

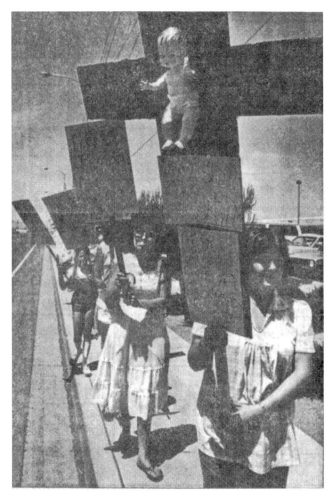

FIGURE 7. A protest outside a Tempe, Arizona, abortion clinic on Mother's Day, 1983. (Courtesy of *Easy Valley Tribune;* Planned Parenthood of Northern and Central Arizona Collection, Arizona Historical Society)

eyes. Most commonly, activists encircled clinics with signs citing scripture, commandments, or religious themes, paired with fetal imagery. At one 1983 protest in Arizona, for example, a pro-life activist walked around an abortion clinic with a large crucifix, but instead of Jesus being crucified, a baby doll, representing a fetus, took his place.[129] Fetuses were dying for America's sins. At another early-1980s protest in Arizona, a dozen crosses "in memory of 300 to 400 . . . children" lost that day occupied a nearby lot.

In the early 1980s, Arizonan John Jakubczyk was inspired to make this spatial redefinition feel permanent. At that time, few anti-abortion groups could sustain daily protests with their members alone. In Jakubczyk's plan, each group would take a day, so "anytime anyone's driving by, they see people praying and picketing and sidewalk counseling. And they'll think it's 24–7."[130] This idea—which Jakubczyk termed Project Jericho—spread nationwide when Joseph Scheidler, the head of the Pro-Life Action League, included it in his book *Closed: 99 Ways to Stop Abortion*. Through the perpetual presence of protestors, makeshift graveyards, political crucifixions, and other pro-life concoctions, activists recast medical spaces and surrounding areas.

Such beliefs and practices changed the protest space outside of abortion clinics into quasi-religious spaces. Phil Leahy recalled that the sidewalks and parking lots outside of abortion clinics where he worked always felt "chapelesque."[131] For him, abortion protest was a ministry whose home was the public space outside of Albuquerque's abortion clinics. These spaces, however, were different from other types of religious spaces, like churches, shrines, wards, temples, or even home altars. The public devotional spaces outside abortion clinics were always political. Even when activists demanded that anti-abortion politics be interjected into Sunday services at their churches, those spaces never became consistently political. Few devout Catholics could avoid pro-life politics in their parishes, but neither were they faced with those politics with every prayer, image, or sermon. The devotional space outside of abortion clinics was different. There, activists forged an ecumenical religious expression that was inseparable from the politics of abortion.

Many remembered this dynamic in the rescue movement of the 1980s and 1990s. Phil Leahy remembered that in these protests (and in jail later) activists explored each other's religious tenets and found common ground:

> There would [be] Protestants and evangelicals [there] and we would be saying the rosary and they would say, "What's this rosary all about?" and then we would have a chance to explain you know that we were Christ-centered like them . . . and so we had this exchange, you know. And then we would see their devotion to the Bible . . . and how they could quote scripture and had so many passages memorized, and so that was a real solidarity because we both sens[ed] the horrendous evil of abortion.[132]

This kind of ecumenical activity did not erase doctrinal difference or push activists to water down their denominational commitments, but it did make

"Judeo-Christian values" a reality for activists. It also created a foundation for an expansive "religious" morality that superseded deeply held antagonisms between faiths, at least in the area of abortion politics.

When activists made functional pathways to medical clinics into ecumenical religious space, they changed the geography of American cities. Fetal crucifixes, pop-up graveyards, and signs calling for God's wrath invited casual passersby to rethink previously generic city streets. Activists demanded that observers consider if these spaces were places where battles between good and evil were enacted. For the patients, volunteers, and employees of the clinics, the moralizing of the space had an even greater effect. Kayrene Pearson, a Congregationalist minister who was one of many clergy escorting patients through crowds of anti-abortion protesters into Boulder's clinics, remembered that "you have the feeling that guilt is placed on you" there. Even for clergy, she said, "It's a heavy, heavy environment to go into."[133] Common thoroughfares—the route to school, the path to work, the place one parked—were weighed down with promises of salvation and threats of eternal damnation.[134]

When activists infused mundane spaces with white ecumenical, conservative moralism, they also changed the boundaries of American religion. Pro-choice activists regularly demanded that religious ideals not be forged into public policy. Anti-abortion activists eventually responded to such arguments with a full-throated demand for religion in the public square. New Mexico anti-abortion activist Father Steven Imbarrato put it this way: "The ACLU [and others want to] get religion out of the public mindset. That is where we need to take this fight, down in Main Street USA and . . . on the sidewalks, right? . . . But we've got to step off the curb."[135] Religion was not supposed to be private or contained; it was supposed to be devotedly public and political. Religion, in this vision, denied relativism, and embraced an ecumenical but rigid moral code, where abortion was murder and an act against God. Through such rhetorical and political work, white conservatives named themselves as the defenders of religion and as those who would save the soul of America.

· · ·

Over the course of the 1970s, white pro-life activists made fetal politics personal to many religious Americans. Even for those who might have theoretically opposed abortion, they would not have experienced those politics in most of their religious spaces before the late 1960s and early 1970s. This was true even for those who witnessed social conservative activism in Catholic organizations in the 1960s. By the early 1980s, few white Catholics, Mormons, or evangelical Christians were able to avoid pro-life arguments and imagery in their daily lives.

Despite tensions within and between pro-life groups, evangelical, mainstream Protestant, Mormon, and Catholic activists were all linked in important ways. They all were pushing back against liberal co-religionists. Conservative Mormons faced other Mormons who claimed their religion was historically feminist. Conservative evangelicals overwhelmed moderates in their midst who thought an abortion should be a decision made by a woman, her husband, and her pastor. Conservative Catholics demanded that other Catholics recommit to "tradition" and "natural law," even as liberal white Catholics and Catholics of color pushed the church to abandon outdated ideas and to commit itself to a broader campaign for social justice. Faced with dissent and change within their own faith communities, many white religious people worked to place social conservatism in general, and anti-abortion politics in particular, at the heart of Christian religious practice.

As a result, the communities and regions filled with these populations felt transformed. Ted Haggard, pastor of the 11,000-member New Life Church, saw God all around him in the Mountain West; what he and others often really saw was the work of social conservatives. When talking of Colorado Springs, Haggard hailed its "spiritual depth," "health[y] churches," and a "better quality of life"—all the result of "local Christian opposition to the devil."[136] Certain regions, especially in the middle of the country, became imprinted with this combination of anti-abortion politics and conservative Christianity. These were places where people would hear pro-life sermons at church and sit next to like-minded congregants, where they might be able to protest outside an abortion clinic, and where elected officials would reflect "Judeo-Christian values." In such places, "moral" Americans remade Middle America.

By the early 1980s, white pro-life activists in the Mountain West and elsewhere had both politicized many of their religious spaces and sacralized their political spaces. Anti-abortion activists rejected the ideas that pro-life opinion was simply a religious minority's view or that anti-abortion politics violated the separation of church and state. Instead, they argued that opposition to abortion was at the heart of monotheism. They put these ideas into practice outside of abortion clinics across the country. They made their vision of religion's role in society a reality in the "public square" of protest. This pro-life Judeo-Christian ecumenism helped to ground white social conservatives' claim to moral authority in modern America. It augmented their claim to be modern-day "abolitionists." Over the course of the 1970s, activists built a place for conservative religion in mainstream American politics. In the 1970s and onward, they helped make abortion essential to how many thought about being a Christian in America. In the 1980s and 1990s, activists expanded their personal politics to focus on American women, children, and families.

PART TWO

———————

FOUR

Redefining Women's Rights

Reachout, a crisis pregnancy center in Tucson, was located in a small house in Sugar Hill, one of the city's few black neighborhoods.[1] Most women who came to Reachout had to walk or take the bus. They often waited their turn outside on the porch before entering the center where they were promised a free pregnancy test and counseling. But neither a glass of lemonade or a cool spot in the shade could cool those Tucson summers or ease the anxiety of an unplanned pregnancy. Reachout had begun in 1973 out of frustration. A small handful of friends, neighbors, and co-religionists had started a pro-life group called Conservation of Human Life in 1971, but they felt they had made little impact on the growing numbers of women accessing legal abortions.[2] Discouraged by their lack of success and inspired by Birthright, the crisis pregnancy center network begun in Canada in 1968, five women from Conservation of Human Life decided to form a clinic-like, pro-life alternative to Planned Parenthood. Once a pregnant woman entered Reachout, volunteers gave her a free pregnancy test. Then, while she waited for the results, anti-abortion activists used diagrams, photos, illustrations, videos, and stories about the process of fetal development to convey that life began at the moment of conception and that any interruption thereafter constituted killing. Activists employed these materials and promises of emotional support to convince women not to abort.

In centers like Reachout—called crisis pregnancy centers (CPCs)—anti-abortion women tried to stop abortion one woman at time. CPCs have been the "least publicized and the least understood" part of the movement, according to sociologist Ziad Munson, and yet they were also the part "to which the majority of all volunteer hours in the pro-life movement is devoted."[3] Activists flocked to this corner of the movement because so much rested on making fetal politics personal to American women. Activists dealt with small and inconsistent budgets and often weathered multiple moves in order to reach women before they had abortions. They used deceptive practices, often masquerading as abortion providers, in order draw these women to their doors. Many of their clients left CPCs traumatized or simply frustrated, while others imbibed the pro-life vision. Any concerns about deceptive practices were swept aside for the larger good of "saving babies."

In CPCs, white pro-life women positioned themselves as moral, not political, authorities. They presented themselves as mothers, friends, or medical professionals trying to show other women biological and gendered truths. Anti-abortion women conveyed that it was their experience as women that led them to their anti-abortion stance, not partisan politics. White women activists asserted their moral authority by claiming to have special access to universal truths, and they tried to use that moral authority to transform the women of color, poor women, and young women who were the majority of the clients at CPCs. Such work gave white, socially conservative women an important place in a movement that believed morality sprang from nature and common sense. CPC activism also had high stakes: it had the potential to save both fetuses and women.

This rhetoric of "saving both" masked a tension at the heart of CPC activism, one that feminists regularly identified: the needs of fetuses and the needs of women were sometimes at odds. In the first decade of their existence, CPCs prioritized stopping abortions. Activists attempted to solve just enough of a woman's immediate material and familial problems in order to get her to change her mind. In the 1980s, CPCs began to find these solutions wanting. CPC clients were not cooperating. Many CPC activists came to believe that they needed to delve further into women's lives through educational programs and therapy in order to reach them. Some activists left CPCs in this period because they believed that the centers had begun to focus too much on women at the expense of fetuses. Those who stuck with CPC activism believed that this deeper involvement would help "abortion-damaged" women and that those women, in turn, could become the faces of abortion's harm.

In the 1980s and 1990s, as CPC activists endeavored to quietly politicize women, radical activists grabbed the headlines with their national campaign of civil disobedience. Pro-life "rescues" drew activists from around the country to targeted cities, where they temporarily stopped women from accessing abortion. Journalists and scholars who have studied this movement often focus on this turn to radical activism, but trends at CPCs point to another, quieter transition in the last two decades of the century. There was an unspo-ken realization—in this part of the movement and others—that the threat to the fetus was not enough to galvanize the anti-abortion movement. Activists needed to make the fetus a core part of other identities, turning others into the victims of abortion as well. CPCs, in those years, tried to make resistance to abortion central to what it meant to be a woman.

If pro-life activists could convince American women that abortion was murder and that it damaged the woman as well as the fetus, then hypotheti-cally activists could stop abortion without changing the law. CPC volunteers put their hope in cultural politics, believing they could make women feel connected to fetuses. In order to do their work, CPC activists had to get more involved in women's messy and complicated lives. Over fifty years, some parts of their program changed, but one core piece did not. They believed that women's health was intimately linked to carrying a pregnancy to term. White women activists used modern rhetoric and technologies to convince their diverse audience of an old idea: that all women were the same, bound by their biological ability to give birth and their innate impulse to mother. Many CPC clients refused to change their minds about abortion or conform to these socially conservative visions, but many others did grasp ahold of these anti-abortion ideas and became activists themselves.

THE CHALLENGES OF "TOTAL TRUTH TELLING"

Crisis pregnancy centers were organizational havens for women in the anti-abortion movement. Often, the board of directors of a crisis pregnancy center was evenly divided between men and women, but the CPC founders, activ-ists, volunteers, and directors were almost always women. Women in the mainstream anti-abortion movement as well as those outside of it found their political home in these centers. There, white pro-life women could "mother" poor, young, black, and ethnic Mexican pregnant women and try to convince them, in turn, to become mothers. CPC activism was essential political work because lives hung in the balance, according to activists, and because such activism proved the universal applicability of their moral vision. Thus, early CPC volunteers persisted in their work despite serious organizational hur-dles and the potential moral hazards of deception. Small budgets, a lack of consistent space, or the problems of getting pregnant women in the door were not enough to stop CPC activists from the important work of "saving babies."

The first crisis pregnancy centers in the world were started in the late 1960s; activist Robert Pearson supposedly started the first in Hawaii in 1967 and Louise Summerhill founded Birthright in Toronto a year later.[4] The first CPCs in the Four Corners states took inspiration from these forerunners and were founded soon after. Denver's Birthright was the first CPC in the region, started in 1968 with the help of Frank Morriss, the *Denver Catholic Register* journalist profiled in chapter 1. According to Colorado activist Margaret Sebesta, Louise Summerhill agreed that Denver's was the first Birthright in the United States.[5] Tucson, Phoenix, Las Cruces, and Albuquerque all had Birthrights by 1972, and Salt Lake City soon followed in 1974.[6] Other early CPCs in the region, like Reachout, were modeled on Birthright.[7] In just ten years, between 400 and 600 Birthrights were founded around the country.[8] Other CPCs followed the model set up by Robert Pearson or cobbled together a program for themselves.

No matter the model, most early CPCs ran on a shoestring budget. Reachout had no private space for counseling and no offers of permanent housing for the first few months it existed. Reachout's activists met potentially pregnant women at a local restaurant, which afforded neither the privacy the women desired nor the legitimacy the activists needed.[9] But within the year, Reachout activists fell upon some good luck. Joan Doran, the wife of a prominent labor leader, offered the group a small home in Sugar Hill, a house they would use for little or no rent for almost two decades.[10] Others began in spare bedrooms or old ambulance garages.[11] For its first three years, Denver's Birthright consisted only of a small table and a red telephone in an activist's home.[12] Most CPCs relied upon cheap rent or donated spaces around their cities.

Activists often attributed their acquisition of donated spaces as random products of luck or circumstance, but there was deliberate logic to where those spaces were located. Reachout, like many CPCs, had a home in a neighborhood filled with women of color, a population white activists thought especially susceptible to abortion.[13] As in many other western towns, African Americans in Tucson were at the bottom of the racial ladder and were systematically denied equal education, employment, health care, and housing.[14] The Dorans donated their home to Reachout right when a new public housing project was lowering rental prices and drawing in new, poorer African Americans to the neighborhood.[15] The changes in Sugar Hill likely motivated the Dorans to donate their house to Reachout. Poor, urban women of color had long been associated with hypersexuality and what was termed "over-reproduction," and that association was only solidifying in the 1960s and 1970s. Many Americans believed "ghettos" were filled with women more prone to unwanted pregnancy and abortion, and thus in need of anti-abortion services. Thus, the donation of a house in Sugar Hill might have been spontaneous, but it was likely not random.

Reachout was more stable than most early CPCs. It was able to stay in that first location for almost twenty years.[16] Many other CPCs jumped around neighborhoods in their cities, following the goodwill of local pro-lifers. Birthright of Albuquerque was initially housed at the Newman Center, a student Catholic ministry, on the campus of the University of New Mexico. Then it moved into a spare room at a local Catholic hospital, where it stayed for over ten years. When the hospital could no longer allow them to stay rent-free, the CPC rented various homes from the same generous anti-abortion landlord.[17]

What early CPCs lacked in funds and spatial stability, they made up for in support from other activists. Most often, they worked in tandem with local Right to Life affiliates. When Denver's Birthright moved out of its founder's spare bedroom, it moved next to the office of Colorado Right to Life, because the group's new director wanted to support the CPC.[18] Right to Life newsletters advertised the centers, requested donations, and solicited volunteers.[19] CPC activists and Right to Life activists were often one and the same in these early years. Margaret Sebesta remembered that one of Denver Birthright's early problems was "how the same group" could run the CPC, "do the Right to Life organizing and take care of the family." Forget making bread and cookies "from scratch," she joked.[20] CPC women were not separate from mainstream pro-life activism, but rather an essential part of it.[21] Many activists worked to stop abortion through one-on-one counseling in crisis pregnancy centers, while also doing legislative or educational activism through Right to Life.

The symbiotic relationship between crisis pregnancy centers and Right to Life groups and local religious groups meant that CPCs were a remarkably consistent part of the American urban landscape in the late twentieth century. Despite moving from location to location, being staffed almost exclusively by a rotating cast of volunteers, and subsisting on small, intermittent donations, especially in the early years, most CPCs were incredibly resilient. All of the first CPCs in the Four Corners states still exist (as of 2017). Over the years, these forerunners were joined by many others. For example, in New Mexico, there were Birthrights in Albuquerque, Santa Fe, Gallup, Las Cruces, and Farmington by 1977.[22] In the 1980s and 1990s new CPCs—

founded by evangelical Christians—proliferated in the region and across the country. Many were a part of new umbrella organizations for CPCs, such as Carenet. These CPCs continued to sprout up in urban areas, but increasingly spread into suburban and rural areas too. By the end of the century, crisis pregnancy centers outnumbered abortion providers in the United States two to one—with roughly 4,000 CPCs and 2,000 abortion providers.[23] CPCs' persistence and numerical advantage meant that the centers reached an incredible number of American women every year.

Persistence and determination were not always enough to get women into crisis pregnancy centers; activists used deception to get women considering abortion to sit down with pro-life activists. Whether they were Birthrights, a local variant like Reachout, or an evangelical CPC like Carenet, all crisis pregnancy centers had the same essential components: they depended on vague advertisements, refused to refer women to abortion providers, and offered few, if any, medical services. These components remained the same from the early 1970s to the twenty-first century. Early on, one Reachout activist suggested that they make advertisements reading, "Is your pregnancy a problem? Call Reachout," and then put them around the University of Arizona and in the local newspaper. The ad would list a 24-hour hotline that women could call. "They didn't know where [we] were coming from," pro-life activist Helen Seader recalled. "Most of the girls called because they thought we were going to give them abortions." She added, "Everybody that called me wanted an abortion. Everybody."[24] In 1975, Reachout reported handling 20 to 30 calls a month while Birthright of Tucson reported getting 80 to 100 calls a month.[25] Once a woman called, CPC activists often convinced her to come to the center to get a free pregnancy test to confirm that she was, in fact, pregnant.

When women entered the CPC, activists offered them free pregnancy tests, but they also tried to offer a personal relationship with an anti-abortion activist. Laurie Futch, a Birthright activist in Phoenix, emphasized that the counseling in her CPC was always designed to feel like a kitchen table conversation between friends. "We just offered friendship to gals who were having a crisis," she said. "We always [tried] to have a homey place."[26] Futch and others asserted that they achieved this kitchen table feeling because they were not professionals. Activists were just homemakers, wives, mothers, daughters, or friends. When *National Right to Life News* profiled Birthright in 1976, the writer suggested that women came to CPCs precisely because the counselors were "just women": "Why should she be afraid to talk with Jane Doe Birthright? This is not someone she has to impress. This is not a brilliant professional. This is not a meaningful person . . . Just a housewife." A pro-life counselor was simply a woman who listened to another woman's problems and then, as *National Right to Life News* put it, "from the well of her womanhood experience she responds."[27] In CPCs, activists tried to play the role of mothers or friends to women seeking abortion.

Crisis pregnancy centers were largely woman-only spaces. This was not because anti-abortion men disregarded abortion-seeking women but because pro-lifers believed no man could speak from the well of his "womanhood experience." Men were left with peripheral and subsidiary roles, aiding in promotional and fundraising activities. White women had special roles in this corner of the anti-abortion movement; they had the experiential authority to speak to other women and the moral authority to intervene in intimate familial issues.

Even though crisis pregnancy center volunteers rejected the gendered alienation that came with being "professionals," they employed the authority of medicine to make their appeals. "Mother" was not the only social role these activists tried to occupy. Free pregnancy tests were the hook to get women in the door, and CPC counselors acted the part of health care providers when they took a woman's urine sample. This medical posture was easier for some activists than others. Emma Gomez, who was one of the few early ethnic Mexican pro-life activists and a founder of Albuquerque's Birthright, was a nurse.[28] Discussions of biology, bodies, and medicine would have come easily to her. However, most CPC volunteers had no medical training whatsoever. They simply acted the part of a medical provider.

CPC "counseling" was focused on fetal development, with counselors explaining what a fetus looked like, showing models or movies, and discussing heartbeats, fingers and toes, brainwaves, and fetal pain.[29] Later in the century, activists used movies and products developed by the movement to support their claims.[30] But in the late 1960s and 1970s, activists often used scientifically legitimate models and movies made by non-activists. In a crisis pregnancy center, these items took on new meaning.

Santa Fe's Birthright used a 1971 documentary made by Claude Edelmann called *The First Days of Life,* which chronicled fetal development from fertilization to birth using intrauterine photography.[31] Edelmann, a medical doctor, was a part of a largely pro-natalist, postwar scientific community that looked to the minute details of fetal development to solve an array of human problems. By the late 1940s, historian Sara Dubow argues, scientists and psychologists believed that fetuses not only had a "biological and physiological life," they also had "a biographical and psychological life."[32] These many fetal lives extended the responsibilities of the mother all the way back to conception and individualized the developing fetus. In the 1960s, new intrauterine medical technologies helped personify the fetus. Pioneering doctors breached the womb and, as sociologist Monica Casper has argued, brought "fetuses under modern medicine's gaze as a new category of patient."[33] Embedded in this fetus-focused medical culture, some doctors were ardently opposed to abortion, while others like Edelmann were not. He said he "never intended [his movie] as any kind of campaign for or against abortion." But Edelmann's work was clearly born from a medical world that fetishized prenatal life. His book included sentences like "there was a dramatic explosion of life" and "the human form is unfolding like a flower."[34] CPC counselors co-opted scientific work like this to make their pro-life pleas.

CPC counselors also made amorphous scientific claims. Counselors used language similar to that which filled the pamphlets they passed out, beginning sentences with phrases like "In the past few years, research by important medical doctors has proved. . . ." Such sentences ended with phrases like "life begins at conception" or "abortion could do permanent damage to your female organs."[35] Then, with fetal models and the endorsement of distant, faceless doctors, they made the argument that abortion was murder. In the 1980s and 1990s, CPCs became even more medical, sometimes in performance and sometimes in practice. Some CPCs simply had their activists wear lab coats.[36] Other CPCs began offering free STD (sexually transmitted disease) tests and ultrasounds to draw in women. One CPC director explained why: "If you can get a lady into an ultrasound room, then 90 percent will carry that baby to term."[37] In these spaces, activists would stand in for the doctors who—they believed—had failed these unfortunately pregnant women.

Central to all their assumed identities (doctors, friends, mothers) was activists' apolitical nature; their authority came from being outside partisan politics. All CPCs contended they were apolitical. Some merely suggested their pro-life stance was not a political one. But others, like the simply named Crisis Pregnancy Center in Phoenix, said they were actually not against abortion or even interested in the battle over abortion; they were just offering alternatives to it.[38] These arguments were so successful that often journalists suggested that Birthrights were nonpartisan, separate from the abortion wars.[39] Those claims clearly disguised how every crisis pregnancy center was explicitly part of the anti-abortion movement, from funding, to volunteers, to materials and ideology. But the claims also show how white socially conservative women thought about truth and politics. In this particular logic, activists suggested that politics constituted an opinion, a judgment or spin, whereas white social conservatives were providing facts or "universal truths." As one CPC activist put it, "We are anti-manipulation here. It is . . . non-judgmental, total truth telling. . . . [A woman's] dignity is sacred to us. So we are not going to diminish her dignity by trying to put our agenda on her."[40] Another pro-life author argued that there was "no preaching, no moralizing" at crisis pregnancy centers.[41] Crisis pregnancy center activists set this groundwork in order to make claims about the ahistorical, apolitical "truth" of fetal life. Activists were truth tellers, while other women ignored the truths their bodies and souls told them. Arizona activist John Jakubcyzk explained, "Women deep down know that it's a baby. They know. Even the pro-choice women know. They just find justifications, rationales, whatever and they do it."[42] In CPCs, it was white pro-life women's job to reconnect "lost" women to this biological truth.

Not all were convinced by these apolitical "truth tellers." Many did not change their minds about abortion. Some days, Helen Seader recalled, "I wasn't sharp enough to save babies . . . there were days when they decided no . . . they were going to have the abortion and that tore you up. You went home and said, where were you good Lord? What could I have said? What could I have done?"[43] In fact, by Reachout's own accounting, in 1985, almost 35 percent of clients left the clinic undecided or still wanting an abortion. Over 55 percent came specifically for the free pregnancy test and never intended to have an abortion. That year, fewer than 10 percent of clients who came for pregnancy tests told Reachout volunteers they had changed their minds about abortion.[44]

While many women left CPCs simply unconvinced, many others left traumatized. One such case made it into the Arizona's court system in 1986. That year, pro-life activists found a lost woman in the parking lot of a Tempe medical complex that housed both an abortion clinic (Family Planning Institute) and a crisis pregnancy center (Aid to Women Center). According to the woman, people in lab coats asked if she was looking for the abortion provider. She said yes and the activists took her to the CPC; there, they locked her in a room with a "vivid" video depicting a third-trimester abortion. Aid to Women activists argued that the woman had not been locked in the room, but rather that the door had jammed. The judge thought differently. The court found the CPC director guilty of false imprisonment, ruling that it did not matter whether the door jammed; the victim was

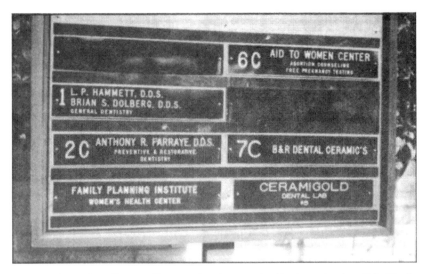

"restrained by deceit." "I want[ed] to make sure what happened to me doesn't happen to other women," explained the plaintiff. "It was a terrible experience."[45] Unfortunately, such things did happen to other women.

The Aid to Women Center was not the only CPC to face legal trouble because of its deceptive practices. Beginning in the 1980s, local courts in a handful of states demanded that CPCs clarify their purpose and distinguish their differences from nearby abortion providers.[46] Women traumatized by crisis pregnancy centers also got hearings in the U.S. House in 1986 and 1991, when Rep. Ron Wyden of Oregon led House subcommittee hearings on the practices of "bogus abortion clinics."[47] In the 1991 hearing, witnesses argued that their experiences at CPCs had been laced with manipulation. One woman testified that CPC activists, impersonating abortion providers, asked how her parents would feel "when they found out that [she] had murdered their first grandchild." Another disclosed that she was forced to watch a graphic film that claimed abortions caused "women to bleed to death [or] never have children again." The executive director of the National Coalition of Abortion Providers testified that it was a common CPC tactic to give women inaccurate information about the gestational age of the fetus, all in an attempt to delay their decisions until it was too late for a legal abortion.[48]

Fifteen years later, not much had changed. A congressional report in 2006 showed that 87 percent of CPCs offered misleading information about the health effects of abortion.[49] In the 1980s, Reachout's director responded to the national "negative publicity" by saying, "Our detractors would have the public believe that showing a girl 'those awful pictures' is terrible while the actual abortion itself is totally acceptable."[50]

From the 1970s onward, in the Four Corners states and around the country, white anti-abortion women in CPCs sought out women in order to tell their reproductive truths. Sometimes they played the part of sympathetic mothers, other times, authoritative doctors. If they needed to leave out certain facts—that they usually had no special medical equipment, that they would not refer women to get contraception or an abortion, and that they had no legal responsibility to be medically accurate—they would. Because ultimately, CPC activists believed this would protect fetal life and that doing so would benefit all women. If they could convince American women, they believed abortion would end. From the 1970s onward, though, CPC activists wrestled with what it meant, in practice, to "save both" woman and fetus.

SAVING BOTH

Making fetal life personal to a pregnant woman might have seemed, initially, like an easy task to anti-abortion activists. While almost any woman could find herself at a CPC, the centers usually dealt with women who did not have independent access to health care, either because they were too young or too poor. White CPC activists thought that remaking poor women, young women, and women of color who came to them would not be too difficult, but in practice the "kitchen table" conversations were often not sufficient. CPC activists regularly had to get involved in women's lives. Early activists waded in only ankle-deep. They offered minor material or familial support in order to get a woman to change her mind about abortion. The women who came to CPCs refused to conform to pro-life imaginings and displayed much deeper problems than activists could address. When clients resisted, some CPC activists began to wonder if these women were the poor women and women of color in need of a savior, or "bad" women corrupting society.

CPC activists often offered some kind of familial support partly because many of their clients were very young. Activists envisioned these women as especially likely to get pregnant, vulnerable to coercion, and in need of pro-life "mothering." In popular culture from the 1970s onward, the pregnant teenager became one of the most potent images of the sexual revolution's errors: excessive, adolescent sexual activity unhindered by forethought, contraception, personal responsibility, or the bonds of marriage.[51] Thus many early CPC efforts focused on them. Helen Seader remembered her earliest activism as a protest against Planned Parenthood "taking our girls" to California for legal abortions. Her group began notifying parents through church bulletins that if their daughter was pregnant, she could end up "with a doctor or with an agency that might refer their girl for an abortion."[52] Once Reachout officially formed, its founders ran advertising campaigns in high school and university newspapers, and placed notices in university bathrooms, dorms, and school clinics.[53] CPC activists, in their own minds, kept pregnant teenagers from making bad situations worse. Activists had to convince a young woman that being a single mother or giving her child up for adoption were better options than having an abortion.

The anti-abortion movement's legislative arm promoted state laws that would require a minor to notify her parents before having an abortion, or force the abortion-seeking adolescent to get parental consent.[54] In almost all the thirty-seven states that eventually passed parental notification or parental consent laws, a minor could go to a judge and get a waiver in order to get an abortion without her parents' knowledge. In many states, these waivers were extremely hard (even traumatic) to get. Nevertheless, anti-abortion activists saw this waiver system as representing the continued erosion of parental rights at the hand of a perverse, liberal state.[55]

At the same time, CPC activists worked on familial levels to address pregnant teens. If the state was not going to support parents' control over their dependents, then crisis pregnancy centers could counter the power of Planned Parenthood by briefly standing in as a girl's parent and trying to stop her abortion. Once CPC activists convinced a girl not to terminate her pregnancy, *then* they encouraged her to talk to her parents and gain their support for her pregnancy and future child. In Tucson, Helen Seader often went with teenagers to break the news. "There was no good [way] to tell [a] mother that [her] thirteen-year-old was pregnant," she recalled.[56]

CPC activists only selectively used the language of "parental rights." They knew that many parents supported their child's choice to have an abortion or that parents might suggest abortion as the best option for a pregnant teen. Crisis pregnancy centers created that "kitchen table" atmosphere not just as an emotional tactic, but because they saw some parents as part of the problem. According to activists, parents, along with boyfriends, were the ones allowing or even pressuring young women to ignore their maternal inclinations.[57] CPC activists, then, tried to stand in the parents' stead to protect teenagers from the state, and stand in the state's stead to protect teenagers from parents.

The other group CPC activists envisioned as their primary clients was poor women. They set up shop in poor neighborhoods and advertised on public buses, at bus stops, and in free newspapers.[58] They always emphasized their "free" services in order to draw these women to their centers. In CPC activists' minds, poor pregnant women just needed a little material aid so they could be freed from financial constraints. For abortion opponents, poverty was a minor hurtle that could easily be overcome, because people "always get by." Maternity clothes, a bassinet, or some diapers might be enough to convince the fiscally desperate to try to "get by." "All our volunteers wanted to help the poor girls," Helen Seader recalled; "They're so poor. They're so needy."[59] "Poor girls" tugged on the heartstrings of pro-life activists, while also fitting into their image of the woman victimized by society.

The romantic "poor girl" was not always the one that CPC activists encountered, however. Many anti-abortion activists were more comfortable with needy women when they remained at a distance. Donating bassinets and diapers was easy charity. Getting up close and personal with women in hard times was more difficult. Many CPC supporters refused to put women up in their homes or even in CPC offices when they needed a place to stay. Helen Seader recalled that activists would often respond, "Will they steal my money if I keep them in my house?" Helen's husband Phil added, "[Many activists] wanted an FBI examination."[60] The Seaders, who were willing to bring women into their home, differentiated themselves from those who would not. Many activists wrestled with whether the women they ministered to were the down-on-their-luck kind or the thieving kind. Pro-life rhetoric demanded that abortion-seeking women were the former but "bad" poor people also had a place in the anti-abortion worldview. Were these women society's victims or potential criminals? Pro-life culture pulled activists in different directions on America's poor.

That nagging concern that CPC clients were the "undeserving poor" was also born from the fact that centers often served poor women of color. In these western cities, poverty and racial discrimination worked in tandem, so that crisis pregnancy centers served a disproportionate number of women of color. Reachout, located in a black neighborhood, probably saw a lot of

African American women. Activists at other CPCs in the Southwest noted that most of the people they saw were Latina.[61] Mary LeQuiu of Carenet in Albuquerque added that at her CPC, they saw a lot of "immigrants from . . . Mexico or South America, either documented or undocumented. We deal with a lot of undocumented."[62] Many anti-abortion activists imagined women of color as naturally inclined to motherhood. This centuries-old stereotype had been used to connect women of color to "nature" rather than "civilization," and served to erase their reproductive labor. For anti-abortion activists who pointed to the corrosive quality of modern society, this imagined "natural" inclination was a benefit.

The "natural mother" stereotype warred with another in the minds of 1970s conservatives, producing some uneasiness about proximity to the poor. In 1976, presidential nominee Ronald Reagan told the story of a black Chicago woman who had taken advantage of federal programs, illegally obtaining thousands of dollars. His famous invocation of the "welfare queen" was a part of a broader white concern that people of color gamed the system and lived off of those who worked.[63] This concern arose during Colorado's 1965 birth control debates, for example. While CPC activists rarely promoted the punitive solutions that other conservatives did, some did agree that women of color had a cultural flaw. "I certainly see . . . the deterioration of the culture, as far as mores and what is acceptable, and complete ignorance of how important marriage is for themselves and for society," Laurie Futch noted about her Latina clients.[64] This "deteriorating culture" might have motivated someone like Futch to adjust her counseling programs. For other CPC activists, like the ones the Seaders encountered, that racial stereotype might have led them to worry they were bringing thieves, not earth mothers, into their home. Their resistance also suggests that CPC activists wrestled with broader questions: was material aid enough to reform these women? And were CPC activists truly stopping abortions?

These questions plagued activists and led them to have doubts about their centers' practices. Since their inception, most CPCs had featured a donations closet where items were gathered to help support women who decided to carry their pregnancies to term. Gradually these services expanded, and CPCs offered clothing, diapers, and furniture to poor mothers. By the mid-1980s, over half of Reachout's clients came for the donations closet, not because they needed a pregnancy test or were thinking about abortion.[65] In 1989, 47 percent were returning clients. It is unlikely that these women were repeatedly considering abortion; most were likely there for the donations.[66]

In many CPCs, managing donations for women who were not even consider-ing abortion became the majority of the center's work.

Activists began to wonder if pregnant women were abusing their services. A few, they believed, took more than their fair share. Mary LeQuiu in Albuquerque recalled, "I mean, everything in the closets is donated, 100 percent donated and you'd have one client come in and wipe the place out."[67] Another CPC activist remembered thinking of clients: "She makes me so mad, she takes only new things!" and "She just uses us to get free stuff."[68] Activists—who themselves relied upon deception—fretted that some preg-nant women were abusing their trust. And in a certain sense they were: women in need were taking control of the charity, denying activists the opportunity to link their donations to pro-life messaging. Most of the women who used the donations closets did not change their minds about abortion. Most were just seeking help in an uncharitable world. Thus, CPC activists were right to question if providing material support was effectively challenging legalized abortion.

By the end of the 1970s or early 1980s, many CPC activists sought new ways to "save both" woman and fetus. Many acknowledged that their famil-ial and material solutions to women's problems were insufficient. They were distributing free pregnancy tests, cribs, and layettes, but were they stopping abortions? Were poor women, young women, and women of color embracing white social conservatives' ideas about when life began and about woman-hood? Many said that not enough women who visited CPCs were being swayed, so activists changed their tactics. They borrowed from psychology and second-wave feminism in order to make fetal politics more personal to American women.

ABORTION AS TRAUMA

In the last two decades of the century, one of the most profound changes in the anti-abortion movement was an increased emphasis on the pregnant woman as the other victim of abortion. By the 1980s, abortion-seeking women were no longer just victims of coercion or poverty, they were victims of abortion itself. If they received an abortion, they risked being psychologi-cally traumatized for a lifetime, according to anti-abortion activists. As a result of this changing rhetoric and activists' concerns about the centers' inef-fectual practices, CPCs re-envisioned many of their programs. Activists

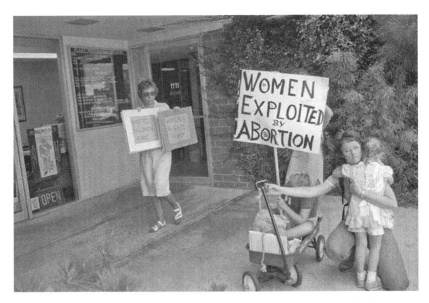

FIGURE 9. Anti-abortion activist Debbie Thyfault (right) focused on the harm abortion caused women in a protest outside an abortion clinic in Torrance, California. Dr. Lynn Negus (left), a professor of medicine at University of Southern California, responded with a pro-choice counter-protest, 1985. (Courtesy of AP Images)

retained their focus on fetal imagery, biological arguments, and promises of emotional and material support, but they also added extensive education and counseling programs to their repertoire. In these new programs, CPC activists attempted to change women's psyches to address how liberal society had affected them. This new combination of programs, activists hoped, would allow them to truly "save both."

These new programs at CPCs were developed in accordance with a new political and psychological diagnosis put forth by the pro-life community: post-abortion syndrome. By the late 1970s, American audiences were knowledgeable about the mental repercussions of trauma, as the media detailed the experiences of Vietnam veterans with post-traumatic stress disorder (PTSD). Anti-abortion activists claimed that the mental repercussions from abortion were similar, including high rates of depression, attempted suicide, substance abuse, and violence.[69] In 1981, Vincent Rue, a psychotherapist, coined the term post-abortion syndrome during a congressional hearing on "Abortion and Family Relations" and pro-life psychologists David Reardon and Anne Speckhard took up the torch of the abortion-damaged woman. Both Reardon and Speckhard helped develop the diagnosis, arguing that because of "post-abortion stress," women re-experienced the trauma of their abortion through flashbacks, hallucinations, and nightmares.[70] Radical activist Norman Weslin explained it in more graphic terms: he said women with this syndrome woke "in the middle of the night, screaming, with dragons clutching at her stomach, and seeing phantom babies."[71] In this diagnosis, anti-abortion activists imagined a new kind of victimhood for women who had abortions, one where their unknowing perpetration of a moral crime led to long-term psychological damage.

This diagnosis was strikingly at odds with American medical and psychiatric thought in the second half of the twentieth century. Beginning in the 1950s, some psychiatrists began to argue that carrying an unwanted fetus to term, not abortion, could have massive repercussions on a woman's mental health.[72] By the 1980s, most psychiatrists and their professional association, the American Psychiatric Association (APA), agreed that abortion did not cause psychological trauma. To be included as a post-traumatic stress disorder, the stressor would have to be an experience "that would be markedly distressing to almost anyone."[73] In 1989, Nancy Adler of the APA told *Time* magazine "that despite the millions of women who have undergone the procedure since the landmark ruling *Roe v. Wade* . . . there has been no accompanying rise in mental illness." The APA followed up with thorough studies in the next few years that found that severe negative reactions to abortions were rare and "best understood in the framework of coping with normal life stress." "Distress is greater before abortion," the APA proclaimed. The American Medical Association joined the chorus in 1992 when it published a literature review on the pro-life diagnosis that began, "this is an article about a medical syndrome that does not exist."[74]

With the creation of post-abortion syndrome, anti-abortion activists made abortion into a critical psychological event in the life of American women, not just a medical reality for the life of fetuses. Thus, crisis pregnancy centers had to expand their mission. CPCs began to work on educational and therapeutic levels to educate American women about the social systems that led to abortion and the trauma it caused. Lisa Sutton of Tempe's Crisis Pregnancy Center explained, "The pregnancy obviously isn't the whole problem. We don't want to put a Band-aid on and send her out with a bullet hole. We want to dig the bullet out."[75]

One way that CPC activists sought to "dig the bullet out" and transform women's psyches was by changing their donation system. Rather than allowing women to assess their own needs and take whatever they deemed necessary, many CPCs in the 1980s began insisting women earn donated items. Dinah Monahan of Show Low, Arizona, often gets credit for developing the program. She was the daughter of Virginia Evers, the creator of the Precious Feet pin. In the early 1980s, Monahan and her parents ran a crisis pregnancy center in rural eastern Arizona. Before the creation of Monahan's program, her center provided the typical CPC fare: pregnancy testing, counseling, and donations. Additionally, they offered childbirth and parenting classes, and "education in the biblical concept of the 'sanctity of life.'"[76] But there was no link between their classes and their charity. In those early years, Monahan, like so many CPC activists, felt like "we were simply accommodating our clients, not transforming them."[77]

From this experience, Monahan created a program, "Earn While You Learn," where women earned points or "mommy dollars" by attending classes. The subjects of these classes ranged from prenatal and newborn care, to abstinence, "the developing pre-born," and "sexual integrity."[78] The dollars, in turn, could be used to purchase donated items in a "baby boutique."[79] She implemented this program in her crisis pregnancy centers, including the only center in the country on an Indian reservation, and eventually marketed it to CPCs across the nation. Over the years, her educational program turned into a forty-five lesson course in nine modules, in both English and Spanish, with homework corresponding with each lesson.[80] Albuquerque activist Laura Bowman said that the program taught women "how to be better women and better mothers and better wives."[81] Both Catholic and evangelical CPCs embraced Monahan's program or something similar. Through such programs, activists could change women's worldviews, not just their minds about abortion.

With these programs, many CPC activists felt like they had finally found a solution to their problem of irresponsible women. One activist noted that the women "felt better about themselves because they earned it. So it wasn't the entitlement kind of thing. They were also much more respectful. So it engaged them in positive behavior."[82] This program reasserted activists' power over material aid—getting "entitled" women to "earn" their charity. It righted the momentarily inverted power relations between activist and client—making sure clients, often women of color, did not take advantage of their white benefactors. Most importantly, it inaugurated a massive re-education campaign for poor and young women. CPC activists could help make these women into "good wives and mothers." Through such programs, CPCs could save women before they were "traumatized" by abortion.

Beyond these new education programs, CPCs also revamped their counseling programs—and here they borrowed feminist tools. One activist recalled that in the 1980s, "people began to realize that they needed to address the pain that women felt who had chosen abortion."[83] So pro-life groups created programs to deal with the trauma they believed women experienced through abortion. CPCs in the Four Corners states organized post-abortion groups and taught local religious leaders how to do post-abortion counseling with members of their congregations. (By the mid-2000s, the Catholic Church ran some kind of post-abortion counseling in at least 165 of its dioceses.)[84] CPC activists also participated in groups like Women Exploited (WE) and Women Exploited by Abortion (WEBA) and retreats like Rachel's Vineyard, a scripturally based post-abortion program where women were taken "step-by-step . . . through all of the deepest possible wounds" abortion had caused for them.[85] Though WEBA was started by an Iowan in the early 1980s, it quickly spread across the country. Arizona alone had five chapters by 1985.[86]

These programs, ministries, and retreats were a kind of pro-life consciousness raising. Second-wave feminists had created consciousness raising as a process by which a woman's personal experiences were translated into political engagement against sexism. Post-abortion counselors used a similar technique to different ends.[87] They probed into the personal trauma, depression, guilt, and melancholy in a woman's life and gave it a social explanation. They gave those feelings an origin point: abortion. Unlike consciousness raising, women in post-abortion counseling were not allowed to direct the sessions but instead were led to inevitable conclusions. "We didn't get into . . . [what] their mother did to them . . . or if they were bipolar," one counselor explained. "We really stayed focused on the abortion issue."[88] Here, unlike in other realms of their activism, anti-abortion activists did make the personal political, rather than the other way around. They took women's actual experiences and gave them political meaning.

The premise underlying post-abortion counseling was that women who had abortions were in denial. These women could be healed only by confronting this denial, retrieving traumatic events, and working through their grief.[89] In the first half of the 1980s, post-abortion counseling in an Arizona CPC used a religious manual that called on a woman to confess her abortion to God as a moral crime, calling abortion a manifestation of Satan's hatred for children. Once a woman asked for forgiveness for her sin, the manual suggested that her psychological and mental problems could be alleviated. In one story, one of the co-authors, minister Bill Banks, recalled that a woman from a "southwestern state" with an incurable bone infection came to him for healing. Once he guessed that she had had an abortion and convinced her to confess her sin to God, Banks maintained, "not too surprisingly, she was able to walk without any pain at all, and she left the room CARRYING HER CRUTCHES!"[90] The authors connected abortion with physical and psychological problems, but the language of sin, forgiveness, and scripture dominated their counseling techniques.

By the late 1980s, CPCs in the region began to move away from counseling with openly religious appeals and began instead to use psychologically focused techniques advocated by the group Post Abortion Counseling and Education (PACE).[91] PACE was a ministry of the Christian Action Council, a pro-life lobbying group founded in 1975 by pediatrician and future surgeon general C. Everett Koop and theologians Francis Schaeffer and Harold O. J. Brown.[92] In 1980, the Christian Action Council became Carenet and their PACE program followed a much more therapeutic model than previous manuals. Many CPC counselors may have counseled extemporaneously, adapting programs as they went along, interjecting their own beliefs and their own experience with trauma or abortion, but most probably followed PACE manuals closely, believing they were doing delicate work with delicate psyches.[93]

The first step in PACE's post-abortion counseling was to identify the syndrome in the woman. Each priest, group leader, or crisis pregnancy center counselor had to figure out whether an individual fit the diagnostic criteria. The criteria were, in a word, broad. If a woman experienced the break-up of a romance, was preoccupied with children, or was angry at men—and she had an abortion—she was probably suffering from the syndrome. If a woman was pursuing academic or professional success, was adamantly pro-choice, or was questioning God—and she had an abortion—she was potentially traumatized.[94] In other words, one woman's liberation was another's diagnosis. If a woman had any unresolved feelings about her abortion, ranging from mild guilt to a sense of shame to regular re-experiencing of the procedure, she probably had post-abortion syndrome. Together, these criteria included almost any woman who had had an abortion (which would come to include roughly a third of American women). These guidelines turned very common female experiences in the 1980s into symptoms, signs of a psyche gone awry.

Post-abortion counselors were often dealing with women who had already identified themselves as hurting, depressed, or feeling guilty, but pro-life activists also claimed that post-abortion syndrome could manifest itself in complete repression of any negative feelings. Because so many women denied their trauma, it was important that activists engage in public education so that healthy, happy women could consider if they were deluding themselves and were, in fact, deeply unhappy and traumatized. Beyond CPCs, anti-abortion activists in the 1980s and 1990s talked about this syndrome almost anywhere they did educational activism: schools, churches, public forums, protests, and legislatures. In these years, they used media like radio and television to promote their political diagnosis. In the framework of post-abortion syndrome, pro-life activists implicitly asked, could the increasing rate of divorce, the phenomena of middle-class single motherhood, and the popularity of feminism itself be products of mental illness?

In order to overcome a woman's proclivity for denial and repression, PACE counseling demanded that a woman re-experience her abortion. The woman had to detail the physical and emotional experience of that day, the sensations of pregnancy and abortion, the pulse of fetal life and its death, and the interactions with those involved in the abortion. Through the power of suggestion, counselors helped these women find answers to questions that they may have had at the time or that they asked now. Does a fetus experience pain or distress? The manuals responded, "The woman becomes acutely aware of her perceptions of the fetus as an unborn child with the capacity to feel, perceive, and signal its distress," and she re-experiences "a sensation of death." Were health care providers insensitive? Many were insulting, insensitive, and abusive, manuals asserted, but ultimately the biggest problem was that providers caused the woman and her fetus pain.[95] Once explored, the counselor could then "organize" these facts. This "reorganization" would necessarily make the connection between a woman's current anxieties, insecurities, or sadness and her abortion.

Breaking through a woman's repression and denial was accomplished more easily in a group setting, according to manuals, because one woman's awakening could cause a collective emotional landslide. Manuals called this "tailgating": where "one woman's therapeutic experience provides the vehicle for the experience of others." One manual offered an example. In one group session, a woman who was ambivalent about conceiving again was given a doll and asked to "externalize her feelings about her aborted child." Even without the words "aborted child," this doll probably connected abortion to a sense of lost maternal purpose, since many women throughout the twentieth century had learned their social roles as mothers in part through playing with dolls. Once the counselor asked the woman to connect her aborted fetus to her "aborted child" through the body of the doll, she expressed deep feelings of remorse and sorrow. Then other women mirrored this transformation, "mov[ing] from an intellectual exploration of their abortions to a much deeper awareness of the depth of denial and repression of their feelings."[96] Manuals warned that although this new awareness was possible through individual counseling, it was harder without the emotional responses of a group.[97]

To make peace with her "transgression," counselors suggested that the woman engage in role-playing to repair her damaged relationships. First and foremost, she was asked to repair her relationships with God and with her aborted fetus. Then, and less important, she might role-play reconciliation with her parents, her partner, or her health care provider. To reconcile with the divine, the woman was asked to play both parts: God and herself. While the counselor was never supposed to explicitly speak for God in such role-play, the counselor did tell the woman what God wanted to hear. The manuals offered this template: "Heidi, can you tell God exactly who it is that you killed?" "Heidi, can you ask God to forgive you for killing Brittany?" Eventually, this would lead to the woman's confession: "Please God forgive me for killing my baby" or "Please God forgive me for letting them kill Abigail." In this process, the counselor was supposed to reshape the woman's view of God (if it was askew). If a woman saw God as a judgmental father, manuals instructed counselors to tell her that God is forgiving. If a woman mistook divine love for open-ended acceptance, manuals told counselors to remind her that God has a strict law, which had been broken, and that he demands atonement. Along the way, "a Christian counselor can offer ... peace by introducing the woman to her Savior, Jesus Christ."[98] Activists tried to avoid the expectations of psychiatry by renaming the practice. As one Colorado post-abortion counselor explained, "we didn't call it therapy.... We called it education."[99]

This "education" loosely adapted the framework of PTSD counseling but reversed its core principles.[100] Post-abortion counseling made women see themselves as fully culpable perpetrators rather than helping them manage destructive, self-blaming cycles. Post-abortion counseling's resolutions were in the realization that abortion was murder and a crime that had to be forgiven by the fetus and by God, rather than a long-term improvement in daily life. Because post-abortion counselors were Christian pro-life activists, they took for granted that an acceptance of abortion as a moral crime and an acceptance of Jesus Christ in women's lives would lead to emotional well-being.[101] Such counseling became a core part of CPC activism from the 1980s onward.

Not all CPC activists were happy with this new focus on women's psyches. Some activists gradually pulled away from the centers during this period. Helen Seader, who would go on to be a part of the rescue movement, recalled the reasons for her departure from Reachout: "It was just that when they got away from the initial thing about saving the babies, that I thought, I was tired."[102] Many of those who stayed believed that they had finally figured out a program that would "save both." In fact, women activists continued to flock to CPCs throughout the 1980s and 1990s. The departure of Seader and others like her shows, however, that a problem remained at the heart of CPC activism: could activists balance the needs of both women and fetuses? In this new era, was the movement's first priority to prevent women from experiencing psychological trauma or was it to keep them from terminating their pregnancies?

In the 1980s and 1990s, this tension was expressed most clearly in the debate over whether to use graphic photos and videos of abortions. In those years, radical pro-lifers were remaking their protests, increasingly using bullhorns, pickets, "sidewalk counseling," and large, gory photos both to convince women not to abort and to create a media spectacle.[103] As the nation watched increasingly radical activists humiliate, harass, and traumatize women seeking abortions, activists within CPCs debated these tactics. Birthright in Canada split from many U.S. Birthright groups over the issues of how to counsel, whether to show videos, and whether even to use the word "abortion." Other crisis pregnancy centers refused to use pictures of aborted fetuses, turning increasingly to educational material that highlighted "living" fetuses. Still other CPCs popped up whose primary goal was to get women into intimate settings with gory photos or videos.[104] Many of the longest lasting CPCs, however, sidelined graphic photos in the 1980s, envisioning themselves as part of a truly "pro-woman," nonjudgmental women's rights movement.[105] One Arizona activist responded to CPC critics in 1985 with the declaration that her center did not "persecute abortion-exploited women."[106] Even as those who left crisis pregnancy activism questioned whether the centers were still "saving babies," a new breed of activist joined the ranks of CPC volunteers: the "post-abortive" woman.

"POST-ABORTIVE" ACTIVISTS

In 1985, WEBA member Pam Laub told her abortion story to the Health Committee of the Arizona House. She said that twelve years earlier, when she had the procedure, doctors did not tell her that she would experience a lot of pain and "almost [bleed] to death." In other forums, Laub added that the doctor had sexually assaulted her during the procedure. The violation of her body (in the assault and the abortion) was paired with the violation of her psyche. She said a lack of information and a "denial of post-abortion trauma" were "trademarks of the abortion industry." She explained the purpose of her activism: "People like me are living proof that abortion causes far more problems than it solves."[107] Laub was not alone; she was one of many white women politicized by post-abortion counseling in the 1980s and 1990s. Though CPC activists hoped their new educational and therapeutic programs would prove the universality of their political and gendered ideals, it actually proved how racially specific their vision was.

While post-abortion groups in the Four Corners states did not keep racial statistics (or any statistics at all) on its members, the most vocal members of these groups, those who testified to state legislatures and spoke at rallies, and have made it into the historical record, were all white.[108] In the late 1980s, David Reardon, an early proponent of post-abortion syndrome, did a national survey of 252 WEBA members across 42 states. With this study, Reardon aimed to prove that women who had abortions regretted their decisions and suffered psychological trauma after the procedure. Of course, many critics pointed out that the women's membership in WEBA presupposed their experience of trauma. But the survey also exposed the demographics of WEBA membership (or at least the demographics of the supposedly representative survey). Almost 87 percent were white.[109] Such stark numbers reveal that the audience that was receptive to "post-abortion syndrome" was a racialized one.[110]

If many WEBA members were like Helen, a participant in Phoenix's WEBA group, their politicization shows that social conservatism and post-abortion syndrome offered a salve for some white women's deteriorating economic and social circumstances. Helen had been a "small-town . . . soft-spoken, blond . . . cheerleader" when she came to study at the University of Arizona. There she had fallen in with the "wrong sort of crowd" and quickly became pregnant. Her two subsequent abortions were paired with a decline in her social status. She married young, quit school, and ended up in a "podunk freeway town." She had avoided birth control because "nice girls don't do 'it'" but then did not receive the life nice (white) girls were promised. She eventually became a mother of three but was plagued by regret about her abortions. Eventually, Helen was "brought . . . back to the Lord" and began volunteering at a crisis pregnancy center.[111] For white women like Helen, abortion—and the sexual modernity that made abortion an option—seemed like good explanations for the hard road they had walked in their lives.

At public events, in legislative hearings, and in crisis pregnancy centers, "post-abortive" activists like Helen argued that abortion was murder. They all told a similar story: their abortion provider had failed to discuss fetal development, he or she had ignored the profound physical and emotional damage of abortion, and patients suffered as a result. They argued that they had never received "genuine help" until they found post-abortion grieving retreats and groups.[112]

Such activism was not a by-product of post-abortion counseling, but rather one of its central goals. Tucson WEBA's president claimed that one primary objective of the program was to help each woman "look beyond the scope of her individual abortion experience and to be able to reach out and help other women."[113] Thus, many of these women got involved in pro-life activism, especially at CPCs. As one woman who had gone to Rachel's Vineyard recalled, "that experience freed me so much that I wanted to go out and really help women . . . who are thinking about abortion and that brought me to a pregnancy center."[114] Another WEBA participant, after realizing her abortion had been a mistake, regularly prayed, "God, please bring me a woman considering an abortion."[115] In 1984, Arizona WEBA president Karen Sullivan reminded *Arizona Right to Life Newsletter* readers that this activism was not confined to CPCs: "Members [of WEBA] want to influence legislators and the general public with first-hand testimony."[116] A woman's abortion placed her on the same level as those who were considering abortion and her trauma was proof that abortion was a physical and moral abomination.

For many women, this kind of advocacy came with repercussions. Looking back on the 1980s, anti-abortion activist John Jakubcyzk believed that the movement was not prepared to deal with these women who joined the cause. "One of the sad things in the early days is that a lot of women who had suffered from abortions got involved but they hadn't healed yet. And they burned out. And it was tragic."[117] Many were unable to handle getting involved in other women's lives and in their reproductive decisions, when they had not yet recovered from their own.

Very few women of color offered to be the faces of "post-abortion syndrome." Through multiracial spaces like the Catholic Church and CPCs, large numbers of women of color in the 1980s and 1990s heard the pro-life pitch about the emotional damage of abortion. Undoubtedly some of these women were receptive to the message and yet, few joined even this corner of the anti-abortion movement. For many, legalized abortion did not seem like a complete explanation for their economic and social need, their pregnancies, or their options. Members of communities politicized even in minor ways by racial justice movements would have been less convinced by a movement that largely ignored the problems of racism and classism. CPCs ministered to poor women of color, but then attempted to politicize them only as women for whom abortion was the source of all their problems. Thus, pro-life activism within CPCs and within post-abortion groups remained as white as the rest of the movement.

By the twenty-first century, crisis pregnancy centers had made fetal life incredibly personal to many women. For some of the CPC clients who had "kitchen table" conversations over fetal models and pregnancy tests, abortion became an immoral choice. For some of the women who came to CPCs in order to get "free" clothes and furniture, required classes changed how they thought about being a "good wife and mother" and made abortion central to that new ideal. For some of the women who did post-abortion therapy, their lives were re-narrated around the single traumatic act of abortion. For all of these converts, anti-abortion activists changed what it meant to be a woman. They made the supposedly intrinsic knowledge of fetal life central to the female experience. Once that link was made, CPC activists had the potential to not only stop abortions but make more activists.

Those white women who became "post-abortive" activists had a measurable effect on their communities, their state, and their nation. Pam Laub, who testified to the Arizona House in 1985, helped get an anti-abortion bill passed. She spoke of her trauma to a legislature already primed to pass anti-abortion bills. That year, a prominent pro-choice Republican had just lost his seat and a reporter noted that "it was his pro-choice stance on abortion that got him ousted." The same year, a handful of virulent anti-abortion representatives joined the Arizona legislature—including Trent Franks. The pro-life movement had helped elect a willing audience for Laub's appeals.[118]

To that receptive audience, Laub spoke in favor of an "informed consent" bill which would make it mandatory for doctors to detail the risks of abortion and suggest alternatives like adoption. It also required that women be told of the "method of disposing of the fetus."[119] Anti-abortion activists in the legislature and those outside of it made the argument that the bill would protect women.[120] Such women-centered pro-life narratives helped pass that bill in Arizona and many others like it across the country in the next three decades. As historian Karissa Haugeberg has shown, this rhetoric eventually helped crisis pregnancy centers get an incredible number of state and federal dollars in the twenty-first century. Through a single government program, CPCs received over $24 million between 2001 and 2005.[121] CPC activists convinced many Americans—and often the U.S. government—that it was they, not abortion providers or feminists, who truly protected women.

. . .

This work affected all parts of the United States but had a more profound impact on the American West, especially as CPCs moved into rural areas. By the early 1990s, abortion was "virtually unobtainable" outside the region's urban areas. The number of abortion providers in rural areas had dropped 51 percent in the previous decade. That left rural westerners, especially those in remote areas, with incredibly long drives to get reproductive health care. The drive was often only the first hurdle. This was still true twenty years later. As of 2014, 78 percent of Colorado counties, 80 percent of Arizona counties, 91 percent of New Mexico counties, and 97 percent of Utah counties had no abortion provider.[122] The huge majority of those counties, however, had a crisis pregnancy center. In rural areas, CPC activists could become friend, mother, doctor, and political mentor to those who had no other option.

From the early 1970s onward, CPCs sought to stop abortions, but by the 1980s this part of the pro-life movement became much more ambitious. Activists educated women in conservative religious morals and anti-abortion logic, in addition to prenatal and newborn care. With the help of pro-life psychologists, they positioned women as victims of abortion, psychologically damaged by committing socially sanctioned murder. With this theory in hand, activists attempted to "raise the consciousnesses" of women so that they could become the faces of abortion's damage. They worked to make abortion personal to the people who made the decisions about abortion. As crisis pregnancy centers proliferated in cities, rural areas, and college towns across the country, activists worked in parallel ways on another group supposedly "victimized" by abortion: American children.

FIVE

———

Politicizing the Young

On a January day in 1988, two hundred Utahns packed Salt Lake City's Capitol Rotunda to mourn the fifteenth anniversary of *Roe v. Wade*. They started the annual Right to Life rally with pro-life songs from a children's choir. Once the children were done singing and had begun fidgeting in their seats, the keynote speaker addressed the audience. "Isn't it wonderful that their parents didn't abort them so we can hear them sing today?" asked activist Penny Lea of Pensacola, Florida. Next, she foretold a terrible future for the children present and for America's youth as a whole. "Abortion is the root of a modern American malaise and has helped create a nation of sad, frightened youths, many of whom turn to suicide," she said. With these children's lives now bookended by narrowly averted "murder" and looming suicide, Lea plunged them into history. "The children of today are troubled because they feel as though they are survivors of a holocaust that dwarfs the Nazi campaign that exterminated the Jews in World War II," Lea claimed. "These children we see here today are survivors. . . . They have never known a nation that hasn't killed children." With the burden of survivor's guilt on their shoulders, how could America's children be anything but depressed? Lea concluded her remarks with a call to arms: "Unless abortion is stopped, . . . we will end up aborting this nation."[1] In this fiery speech, Lea portrayed children as psychologically damaged, perpetually at risk, lucky to be alive, and harbingers of America's end. As "survivors of the abortion Holocaust," children and young adults were the casualties of feminist sins and government policy gone awry. However, young people were more than symbols in the anti-abortion movement of the 1980s and 1990s. Adult activists increasingly sought out children and teenagers to be an audience for their pro-life appeals, remade youth spaces into pro-life spaces, and worked to create a new cadre of activists. Adult activists hoped these "survivors" would be the future of their movement and the future of a better, more socially conservative, society.

While many Americans had deep anxieties—even panic—about children's safety at the end of the century, no movement better capitalized on the concerns about innocent, victimized children than the anti-abortion movement.[2] Because of their focus on victimized fetuses (called "children" by activists), actual children were a part of pro-life protest from the very beginning. In the late 1960s and 1970s, children were presented in anti-abortion narratives as inherently depoliticized. They stood in for everything good, simple, and innocent in a world depraved. Ultimately in many pro-life morality tales, children embodied both an imagined pre-adult innocence and an imagined pre-1967 national innocence. It was this imagined past that pro-life activists asked their followers to recreate: one in which Americans were committed to nuclear, patriarchal families and religion; "truth" was uncontested; and abortions were illegal. Unfortunately, activists argued, pro-choice culture had already begun corrupting these innocents. In order to counteract this corruption, anti-abortion activists had to wage a counter battle, politicizing children in order to make them innocent again.

The place of children in the anti-abortion movement changed in the 1980s and 1990s. In these years, adult activists gradually entered youth spaces—like schools and homes—and remade them into pro-life spaces. Most of this organizing was focused on teenagers, but in many cases it incorporated younger children as well. Activists from around the country traded tools and tactics in this work, meaning that Mormon children saw the same pro-life films as Catholic children in Sunday schools, and white children, ethnic Mexican children, and black children all held the same mass-produced fetus dolls in their hands. Movement tracts often implied a white audience, made up of both white endangered children and white saviors of people of color. Using the political slippage between fetus and child, activists asked all children to represent fetuses, commit to pro-life politics, and take that commitment to their classrooms, their legislatures, and their city streets.

By the 1980s and 1990s, white young people were increasingly responding to adult activists' political invitations. Just twenty years before, Americans had watched young people on the left—most especially civil rights activists—transform American life and politics. Many assumed, as a result, that youth were predisposed to liberalism. While conservative youth certainly existed in the late 1960s and early 1970s, they "didn't rock the boat enough to leave a traceable wake," according to historian Gael Graham. By the end of the century, anti-abortion activism, the broader conservative movement, and flourishing religious cultures would change that trend.[3] In the anti-abortion movement, white young people found a political issue that blended conservative morality with more modern sensibilities. In this movement, they could express their beliefs that secular society had undermined the relationship between men and women, the nuclear family, and Americans' religious faith. They could show that white people were victims of a national genocide and those victims were reflected in their own faces. They could convey these conservative principles all while being a part of American consumer culture and—perhaps most importantly during the rights revolution—a modern "civil rights movement." By the end of the century, adult activists had successfully built a base of young activists who would claim to be a "pro-life generation."

SCHOOL

One of the most important sites of anti-abortion activism was the nation's public schools. After World War II, Americans expected schools to provide more than a curriculum in reading, writing, and arithmetic and lessons in civic values. Part of schools' new social function was to provide a public forum where students could learn and form opinions about politics. Historian William Reese sums it up this way: "In one breath the public demand[ed] higher academic standards and basics, and attention to just about every divisive issue."[4] Beginning in the late 1960s, anti-abortion activists played both sides of this equation: condemning what they saw as secular humanism in public schools (which supposedly sidelined the educational "basics") and at the same time bringing politics into classrooms as a key piece of their own educational activism. As with CPCs, public schools offered white socially conservative activists an opportunity to pitch to a broad multiracial audience and prove the universality of their politics. They suggested that liberals and feminists—those white elites and "bad" people of color—had put children at risk of death from legal abortion and also of becoming perpetrators of abortion. Young people could avert these destinies for themselves and forestall them for others by joining the pro-life "civil rights movement."

The topic of abortion entered public schools even before the *Roe v. Wade* decision. Beginning in the late 1960s, as public conversation about the ethics of abortion escalated, some junior high, high school, and college teachers asked their students to learn about the issue and form an opinion. Students regularly wrote to pro-life and pro-choice groups, state legislators, and governors for information on abortion ethics and law to include in school projects.[5] Once *Roe* was decided, discussions of abortion expanded out from social science classrooms to health and biology courses, as teachers began to include this now legal alternative in their sex education classes. Most of these teachers were likely not activists for either side but instead wanted their students to learn about a contemporary moral, political, and health issue.[6]

Because of these pedagogical openings in public junior high and high schools, beginning in the late 1960s, pro-choice and pro-life activists came to those schools to offer their viewpoints. While the decentralization of public schools and relative autonomy of teachers make it difficult to trace such everyday activism, what is clear is that anti-abortion activists made school education an essential part of their movement. Colorado activist Margaret Sebesta remembered that going to public high schools was one of the first things her group did after it formed. She recalled that they "got the bum's rush over at East High School" in Denver because someone in the office "didn't want us to go to the classrooms" but they "just persisted." Finally they got to the classroom and "gave our first talk. . . . We did a lot of that."[7] In subsequent years, the educational committees of many pro-life groups focused in large part on such school presentations. In 1972, one pro-choice clergyman in Colorado noted, "Right now the fight is in the schools where groups on both sides go to speak."[8]

Anti-abortion activists sometimes came to classrooms and schools by invitation.[9] When invitations were not forthcoming, insistence also got activists into schools. Nancy Ellefson, an anti-overpopulation activist, recalled that in the early 1970s, when she spoke to students about overpopulation, the local Right to Life group would come to the school and demand equal time. Because Ellefson's talk did not deal with abortion, she felt that students were getting only one side of the issue. At that point, Planned Parenthood would not help, she recalled, so "I took a self-taught, crash course in the abortion issue . . . and I started doing talks on abortion." Soon after, Ellefson and one of her friends on the local Planned Parenthood board joined forces and formed New Mexico Right to Choose.[10] Thus, at least in New Mexico, school classrooms were some of the first local sites where the public experienced pro-life and pro-choice activism, some of the first public forums where pro-life and pro-choice became a political dichotomy.

It is possible that in those early years, public schools had fewer rules about the presentations activists gave. After all, many teachers and school administrators were probably unfamiliar with the emerging language and performance of the abortion debate. Because of this, anti-abortion presentations in the region's public schools could have been more graphic, more religious, and more uncompromising in these early years. According to Nancy Ellefson, in the early 1970s pro-life speeches consisted of a "gory little slideshow," probably based at least in part on the pictures from John and Barbara Willke's *Handbook on Abortion*.[11] They might also have been similar to the presentation put together in the early 1970s by two women who were directors of a California pro-life group, United Parents Under God.

The United Parents Under God presentation was made for junior high and high school students and was supposed to be distributed across the country. It drew heavily on the Willkes' *Handbook*. Pictures of aborted fetuses and their imagined lost life stories (with "feet [that] will never kick a football ... run on a playground ... or play hopscotch") were the centerpiece of the presentation. Next to pictures of aborted fetuses were pictures of two prematurely born infants of color (the only people of color in the presentation) who were supposedly in danger of abortion. With murder hovering in the air, activists asked their teen audience, "Is someone you love next?"

According to the presentation, young people were physically and intellectually vulnerable to pro-choice views because they inhabited "atheistic" classrooms "where evil can no longer be called 'evil.'" "You are quite literally 'trapped' in a completely 'pagan' situation in our secular society and schools and we must reach you anyway we can," they were told. According to pro-lifers, liberal white elites had been brainwashing children and young people through the media, public schools, and many other institutions. "[W]omen's liberal abortion speakers," political scientists ("who typically work for the STATE" and for whom the "ends justify the means"), and new "secular-science textbooks" were all trying to frighten teenagers "into killing [their] OWN OFFSPRING," activists said. They claimed that pro-choice people, like Hitler, promoted a super race and would eventually call for the elimination of the elderly, the sick, and their political opponents. Pro-life women—"ordinary women ... who LOVE you" according to the California presentation—protected children while feminist "witches ... distort[ed] God's purposes of sexuality."[12]

This anti-abortion educational program was made for a white audience. Almost all the pictures in the presentations were of white people. The students in school assemblies, the pro-choice political scientists, the "true" scientists, the thoughtful mothers sitting around a table discussing the issue, and young new pro-life activists were all pictured as white. In the United Parents Under God presentation, the abortion debate was visually represented as an argument between white Americans. The only exceptions to this were the two infants of color, one supposedly born at 20 weeks' and one at 21 weeks' gestation. The authors of the presentation used these pictures to contest the limit of fetal viability (defined as the gestational age when a fetus has a 50 percent possibility of long-term survival outside the womb). *Roe v. Wade* had made viability an essential issue in abortion law, setting it at 28 weeks' but possibly at 24 weeks' gestation.[13] The only people of color in this presentation were those on the cusp of "humanness" and presumed to be at risk of abortion (though the two pictured infants, no matter at what gestational age they were born, were the results of wanted pregnancies.) Activists made the point that these two premature infants of color were the people that pro-lifers recognized as fully human and pro-choice people considered less than fully human. Thus, the authors made people of color the objects of salvation by white (Christian, pro-life) activists.[14]

However, white children were also threatened by black people in this presentation. The authors explicitly compared abortion to mandated school busing, thus hailing their white audience using the politics of racial conservatism. This pro-life material contended that busing for the purposes of racial integration, like pro-choice sex education, undermined (white) parents' natural rights. They recounted a story of a Michigan judge who removed a girl from her parents' home because they refused to allow her to be bused to a "high-crime area."[15] Now black people were no longer victims to be saved but threats to white children and a broader social order. Using the racial code of the busing debate, these authors posed the state and public schools as confounding nature. "Nature," here, was racial segregation and forced reproduction, though activists left this unsaid. In this manual, as in other parts of the movement, activists positioned themselves as a moral middle, threatened from white elites and black rabble-rousers, on a campaign to save people of color, the nation, and themselves.

Certain aspects of the United Parents Under God's manual were common in pro-life presentations in the Four Corners states, while other aspects were sidelined. It is likely that school presentations there maintained an emphasis on visuals, biological discussions, subtle or overt condemnations of abortion providers and feminists, and comparisons that likened legalized abortion to slavery and the Holocaust. The strong Christian tone of the United Parents

Under God manual was probably less common or quickly dropped in presentations to public schools. Colorado activist Meme Eckstein recalled of her presentations in schools: "In the Catholic school, we could talk about God" but in public schools they confined themselves to explaining what is "abortion and post abortion."[16] New Mexico Right to Life activist Dauneen Dolce agreed: "We [were] certainly not going to go into a school and talk religion, I can tell you that."[17] Other pro-life groups, outside of Right to Life, would have been more comfortable with religious language but would have had less access to public schools.

At private religious schools, white anti-abortion activists and teachers had much more latitude. For example, in 1985, an eighth-grade history teacher at Redeemer Christian School, an evangelical school in Mesa, Arizona, connected eighteenth-century religious revivals in England to the modern abortion controversy. Teacher Wayne Neiman told students that during the revivals, "individual spiritual awakening spread through the culture," and that the students could be agents of change. To "protest the greatest injustice in twentieth-century America," the class took a field trip to a crisis pregnancy center in Tempe, watched *The Silent Scream* (a film supposedly depicting a fetus screaming during an abortion), and picketed a local abortion provider with handmade signs.[18] Pro-life educators at private schools could include mandated pro-life activism as a part of the lesson.

While anti-abortion activists in public schools could not show the explicit *Silent Scream*, they had other pro-life films at their disposal. In the early 1980s, anti-abortion activists began to combine the slide shows that had served them so well with new tools: movies made expressly by the pro-life movement to appeal to younger and less politically savvy audiences. One shown often in the early to mid-1980s was a 28-minute film called *Matter of Choice*. The movie begins with a newspaper editor assigning a vaguely pro-choice journalist a story on the ethics of abortion. The journalist meets first a disreputable-looking abortion provider (a white elite) and then a former provider, now pro-life activist, who rebuts everything the first interviewee said. Then, the journalist (and the audience) watches a first trimester abortion. Eventually, the journalist realizes that abortion is murder when, while driving, she almost runs over a child. The film moves from a sense of ambiguity on the issue of abortion to the "facts," leading to the journalist's (and hopefully her audience's) inevitable conclusion. "As you watch her investigate, you learn all the basic facts about abortion," one promotional tract for the movie claimed.[19] Through the eyes of this "impartial" journalist, the movie walks viewers through "both sides" but concludes with the clear "truth" of prenatal life.[20]

In public schools, anti-abortion activists often showed this film to health classes.[21] In that setting, depending on how the teacher framed the lesson, *Matter of Choice* might have come across more as objective truth than political opinion. The film's setup already gestured to impartiality, with the journalist confronting ostensibly unbiased evidence. In the context of a health, biology, or sexual education class, this journalistic "objectivity" was combined with the scientific authority that imbued classroom space. Here the truth claims implied in the school setting worked to activists' advantage, helping making the fetus into a baby, and abortion into murder.

This type of education did not make newspaper headlines the way protests did, but it did reach an incredible number of young people every year. In the early 1980s, Arizona Right to Life began to note in their newsletter the classes and schools at which their southern division gave talks. In one nine-month period in Tucson, the group's educational division went to sixty classes in health, government, child development, marriage and family, social studies, and biology at eight different public high schools.[22] In one school year, in a single school district, pro-life activists probably spoke to between 1,300 and 1,800 students. This was not unique to Arizona. New Mexico Right to Choose noted that they were going to "over a hundred classrooms a year" and each was likely matched with an anti-abortion presentation.[23] Anecdotally, many pro-life activists throughout the region remember school presentations as a common, everyday part of their activism.[24]

Anti-abortion activists got a variety of responses from students. Of course, pro-life groups were much more likely to record the encouraging ones. In one Tucson Right to Life newsletter in 1988, a writer noted that the group often solicited reactions from students on their presentations. "The replies . . . are overwhelmingly positive in nature and reflect a very real desire on the part of the students to have this information available to them," the writer reassured membership. A few students wrote to thank Right to Life speakers for their help in bringing pro-life perspectives to schools. What "a wonderful job and a great presentation you gave," one Tucson student said. "I'm just glad that there is someone like you to stand up for the children that cannot for themselves."[25] In 1980, two Tucson students pushed a bill prohibiting public funding for abortion through the state's model congress. At least in this case, adult activists had not only attracted children to the pro-life cause but also created anti-abortion leaders.[26]

One activist in the 1980s had a more nuanced recollection of her school visits. Joan Poulin, educational director of Arizona Right to Life, reported that in public schools the "'me first' ethic is always disheartening." Still, she continued, "my faith in human nature is renewed when I see so many of our young people honestly wrestling with the complexities of the issues."[27] "Me first" was a euphemism, in pro-life rhetoric and elsewhere, for a generational selfishness supposedly endemic to those born in the late twentieth century. Activists believed that this ethic was the central motivator for young people's support of abortion rights, since abortion was the ultimate expression of errant individualism. Thus, Poulin may have been alluding to encounters with students who defended their right to access legal abortion. Her use of "me first" suggests that she may have encountered reticent, or even dismissive, teenagers more often than future activists. In this less optimistic narration of school activism, Poulin took heart not in conversions to the cause, but in serious consideration of the issue.

New Mexico pro-choice activist Nancy Ellefson argued that overt pro-life and pro-choice political presentations in schools, at least in her state, all but ended in the late 1980s: "What we noticed was the number of requests for speeches in the schools had dropped off." They asked the teachers why. "And they said, if we have you in, we have to have Right to Life in. We hate their presentations so much. To keep them out, we have to keep you out." By 1988, New Mexico Right to Choose noted that requests for school presentations had dropped from over a hundred a year to "a handful." Instead, the group made booklets listing abortion providers and reproductive resources that teachers could hand out at their own discretion, and thus teachers could avoid giving anti-abortion activists a public podium.[28] Their words suggest that, at least in New Mexico, the place of overt activism in public schools changed in the late 1980s. This was also the case elsewhere. In 1989 in Phoenix, Arizona, one school administrator said "'Right to Life' [could] not by invited into their classes at this time"; "they were skipping the topic of abortion "until a committee decide[d] what is to be included in the curriculum."[29]

Even if anti-abortion activists got fewer invitations for presentations, some public school teachers continued to use pro-life material in their classrooms in the 1980s and 1990s. In 1993, in Colorado Springs, dozens of parents protested when a teacher showed their seventh-grade children a video clip of an abortion with an anti-abortion voiceover in a sex education class. As one local reporter put it, the parental protest started a community-wide debate over "academic freedom, providing balance on controversial issues, and the role of religion in public schools." Some parents also criticized the sex education teacher, Linda Coates, for telling Bible stories in class, arguing that the Bible condemned homosexuality, and not showing the abortion film to parents in advance (as dictated by school policy). Coates had her supporters, however. One hundred and fifty parents lined up to defend the teacher and the anti-abortion film. Some argued that the anti-film parents were imposing their views on the pro-life "majority" and that the film did provide balance "since the news media is excessively pro-abortion."[30] These conservative parents imagined school less as an objective mediator on important public debates and more as a local conservative counterpoint to society's overt liberalism. But the school district disagreed. The district moved the teacher out of the science department into social studies, and the school rededicated itself to parental previewing of all sex education material.

Perhaps, in the mid-1980s and 1990s, public schools and many public school teachers became less comfortable with activist presentations on the subject of abortion. Perhaps teachers and administrators became less willing to navigate the quagmire of objectivity, balance, and parental rights when it came to outside activists. Perhaps strongly pro-life teachers had to take it upon themselves to integrate anti-abortion materials quietly into their lessons. It is likely that all these things were true. What is certain is that in the 1980s and 1990s, anti-abortion activists shifted their focus from straightforward anti-abortion political presentations in public schools to abstinence education.

Beginning in the 1980s, after decades of contentious local debates, those opposed to comprehensive sex education gained access to federal dollars. In Ronald Reagan's first term as president, conservative U.S. senators helped pass the Adolescent Family Life Act (AFLA). The bill allocated funds to programs that worked to prevent adolescent pregnancy by promoting "chastity" and "morality," rather than contraception. Sociologist Janice Irvine notes that the law was "rigidly anti-abortion," because it "imposed speech restrictions on grantees about abortion" and "mandated parental consent" for teen's participation "*unless* the parents supported abortion." To qualify for funding, groups had to involve religious groups. And to meet the expectations of the law, those groups would have to be pro-life.[31] Thus, anti-abortion groups—made up of white conservative moralists—became essential participants in many of the nation's new sex education programs.

White religious and conservative groups all over the country used AFLA funds to develop pro-life, abstinence-only sex education curriculums, often just retooling old pro-life presentations. In the late 1980s, with the support of the local Right to Life group, 1,800 Tucsonans signed a petition asking the school district to adopt the Sex Respect curriculum, a national abstinence-based curriculum. Sex Respect had been developed in 1983 by the Committee on the Status of Women, a conservative pro-life group in Illinois using AFLA funds.[32] Like many abstinence education programs, Sex Respect emphasized innate male and female gender attributes and responsibilities and exaggerated the fallibility of birth control, while condemning or disregarding homosexuality and abortion.[33] In Tucson, residents were invited to a one-day workshop at a local crisis pregnancy center, and, by Right to Life's accounting, many left encouraged "by the possibilities suggested by this new approach to education about human sexuality."[34] Though Tucson's school district did not adopt Sex Respect, the program was embraced by many school districts and touched thousands of public school students across the United States; by 1992, 1,800 schools had adopted the curriculum.[35]

A variety of other abstinence programs were promoted on a much smaller scale. In 1997, Arizona Right to Life teamed up with Passion and Principles, an abstinence-only education program created by and primarily taught by one white woman, Karie Weston. Weston, by her own accounting, had lost her virginity at fifteen ("an incredible gift I could never get back"), gotten pregnant, and had an abortion. Years later she diagnosed herself as suffering from post-abortion syndrome. She wrote, "the truth was revealed to me through a series of video tapes" and "twenty-one years later I realized I, too, was a victim." From this pain, she put together an abstinence-only curriculum to teach "young people today ... the truth, the hard truth!" She concluded: "It is now my life's work to fight against the lies told on behalf of abortion and the truth about abstinence and adoption."[36]

Passion and Principles focused primarily on what Weston called the "4 As": abortion, adoption, abstinence, and all of your life (as a single parent). Like other abstinence-only education programs, Weston's talk focused on risks, calling premarital sex "deadly," a brief moment in time that could have "devastating effects."[37] She combined this with a discussion of her own story and skits that, as Arizona Right to Life put it, "visually impact young people with the truth." These skits included "'The Gift Wrapped Box,' signifying the treasure of a sexually pure lifestyle; 'The Broken Heart,' showing the painful reality of ripping one's heart apart through premarital sex; and 'Tumbling Dice,' proving once and for all that 'safe sex' is a lie."[38] At one Phoenix high school, Passion and Principles set up a wedding booth where students came

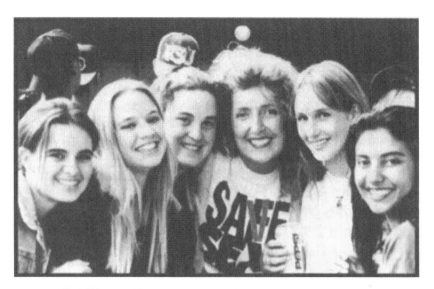

FIGURE 10. Karie Weston with teenagers she met through her abstinence education program, Passion and Principles, 1997. (Courtesy of Arizona Right to Life; University of Arizona Library Special Collections)

"to experience what was worth the wait."[39] Together these demonstrations used visual metaphors to convey the emotional and physical risk inherent in premarital sex, and the morality, honesty, and wholesomeness inherent in a heterosexual marriage. Patriarchal nostalgia was a part of every aspect of Weston's presentation.

At the crux of Weston's presentation was the protection of the fetus. Abortion was her first "A," and the other three were either better or worse solutions for or ways to avoid unplanned pregnancy. Abortion was the problem her program was trying to solve. In many of her presentations to public and private schools, Weston gave out Precious Feet, the pin of feet the size of a 10-to-12-week-old fetus created by Arizona businesswoman Virginia Evers, as well as Young Ones, plastic fetal dolls that were models of an 11-to-12-week-old fetus.[40] In the 1980s, a pro-life Wisconsin couple, Dave and Bonnie Obernberger, had created the Young One doll. The Obernbergers had come up with the idea of a doll because their pamphlets were not having the desired effects.[41] The Young One cost 30 cents each in quantities fewer than 2,000, and only 22 cents in quantities over 10,000.[42] Embodying the "unborn," the fetus doll was both precious and cheap. While the Obernbergers marketed Young Ones to all corners of the pro-life movement, the dolls were probably most often used in situations like Karie Weston's: to educate children and young adults. Anti-abortion educators could avoid using potentially controversial pictures and give their students a fetus to take home with them.[43] In educational settings, the dolls served as a bridge from girls' presumably innocent childhood to an adolescence filled with possibilities for sex and pregnancy. But the doll also had an important duality for activists: it was both a potential baby and potential murder victim. While the dolls were more sterile than gory pro-life photographs, the manikins demanded that young people think about murder and innocence. The juxtaposition of the clean, white plastic body and a presentation on the "violence" of abortion was the crux of that pro-life lesson.

Made of cream-colored plastic, the fetus doll was white and had the beginnings of a penis. By connecting a 12-week-old fetus to the ultimate universal subject, the doll argued for its humanity through the re-creation of existing racial and sexed social stratification. Through its whiteness, the doll gained additional social privilege, while reminding its child owners that white people too were victims of discrimination. Through its maleness, the doll gained social privilege, denying feminist assertions that women's lives were primarily at stake in arguments over reproductive rights. Finally, through its constructed biology (its belly button without an umbilical cord), the doll gained social privilege through its connection to a born baby, demanding the same rights accorded birthed humans.

One pro-life author noted that the Young One was a "powerful message," because "unlike most handouts, carelessly tossed aside, he simply could not be discarded—or disregarded."[44] However, activists were not totally right about this. In 2010, two Roswell, New Mexico, high schools banned the distribution of fetus dolls because of "doll-related disruptions." Students dismembered the dolls, putting the heads on pencil tops and sticking the pencils to the ceilings. Students also used them to plug toilets, lit them on fire, and turned them inside out to resemble penises.[45] These students—at least—did more than discard the dolls; they inverted the pro-life message the dolls embodied.

But how was the Young One received by ethnic Mexican and black children, often the majority in southwestern schools? Perhaps they internalized the racial and political messaging of the doll, becoming part of the long history of children of color asked to treasure white bodies.[46] Or perhaps this was a moment of alienation for students of color, especially those politicized by racial justice movements. While there is little evidence of students of color's reactions, the movement's eventual production of fetus dolls of color suggests there was some pushback. In the late-twentieth century, major toy companies—with pressure from racial justice movements and politically influenced small businesses—began to produce "ethnically correct" dolls to encourage children of color to identify with their dolls and to help them associate people of color with beauty.[47] Much more was at stake for anti-abortion activists. For them, life was at stake. By the early twenty-first century, pro-life activists followed the toy industry's turn to multiculturalism, and began producing fetus dolls in multiple shades to use with children and adults.[48] This shift in colored plastic, however, did not change the racial politics of the movement. Fetus dolls of color fit in a movement that regularly co-opted racial justice movements and portrayed people of color simultaneously as victims to be saved and potential threats. When Weston brought these fetus dolls to schools, she inserted pro-life political culture—and its attendant racial politics—into the heart of adolescent life.

Weston's program also demonstrates the close relationship between many abstinence-only programs of the 1980s and 1990s and crisis pregnancy centers. Weston's activism was a product of CPC activism, especially their promotion of the idea of post-abortion syndrome. Once self-diagnosed as a victim, Weston directed her activist energy not at women considering abortion, but at young people. She used the ideas and educational tools of CPCs as the foundation for Passions and Principles. In addition to this ideological connection, Weston also developed a reciprocal relationship between her program and local CPCs. After one school presentation, she stopped at a crisis pregnancy center on a whim and convinced a young woman not to have an abortion. The next day she brought this young woman to another school to "share her decision" with an audience of high school students.[49] Thus, the CPCs, at least in this instance, provided Passion and Principles with a real woman who rejected abortion. Through this relationship, Weston helped to politicize two constituencies: one pregnant woman became an anti-abortion activist (at least for a day) and high school students learned about abortion from two pro-life women who had faced the decision themselves.

Weston was not alone in embodying such connections. In fact, many CPCs took up abstinence education directly. In Albuquerque in the mid-1980s, for example, the local Carenet, part of a larger chain of crisis pregnancy centers, developed its own abstinence education program. According to Mary LeQuiu, a Carenet activist whose children went through the course, the program included a variety of lessons from "risk avoidance [of] things like drinking, drugs, sexual behavior" to "abortion techniques" and "fetal development." In their abortion unit, the abstinence educators, according to

LeQuiu, noted "a cloud of ignorance about abortion in general, particularly abortion risks."[50] Lessons on fetal development and the risks of abortion were, of course, CPC activists' forte. At least part of this abstinence curriculum was probably taken wholesale from pro-life political materials and the school presentations given earlier in the decade. LeQuiu contended that at one point in the 1990s, the Albuquerque Carenet abstinence program was reaching 10,000 New Mexican high school students each year.[51] By 2005, CPCs around the country had received $130 million in federal money for abstinence education.[52]

With abstinence-only education, white pro-life activists found a federally sanctioned and subsidized home in the nation's public schools. In the 1990s, abstinence education obtained support across the political spectrum, partly because white conservatives had been so successful at maligning comprehensive sex education and partly because most Americans approved of its focus on abstinence. But most Americans also wanted sex education that included discussions of HIV/AIDS, STDs, contraception, condoms, and sexual orientation. Even in Arizona, a 1985 poll showed that 93 percent of respondents supported teaching comprehensive sex education to high schoolers and 73 percent to elementary school children. National polls taken throughout the 1980s and 1990s showed similar numbers.[53] But as Janice Irvine notes, by the late 1990s, "many students heard only about abstinence." A 1999 study of all U.S. school districts showed that only 9 percent of children lived in districts that required comprehensive sex education. All other students lived in districts with a mish-mash of other policies or no policy at all.[54]

But in terms of abstinence education, place mattered. It was students in certain parts of the South and West who were mostly likely to hear only the abstinence-only message. In 1999, the Guttmacher Institute found that 55 percent of school districts in the South and 40 percent of the districts in the Mountain West taught that contraception was ineffective and abstinence was the only safe way to avoid pregnancy and disease (compared to 20 percent in the Northeast). In these regions, many children heard only about the value of waiting, likely from a local anti-abortion activist.[55]

No longer political partisans visiting for a day, paired with pro-choice speakers, white pro-life activists in the Four Corners states and around the country now came to schools as abstinence educators. And with the change of title, they gained the legitimacy they needed to tell "the truth" to children and young adults. No longer did activists need to combat the "pagans" or "secular humanists" teaching children. Now, they were the teachers.

While the very public space of federally funded schools was always a primary concern of anti-abortion activists, they looked as well to politicize private space—or as activists put it, to instill "values" in their children. Some of the most important organizing of children took place in the most "private" of spaces: the home. For adults who had committed their free time to a political movement, it was only natural to incorporate those politics into their home life. These pro-life lessons came in both quotidian and extraordinary forms. In their homes and in their communities of like-minded white people, activists made opposition to abortion into more than a political cause. It became a lifestyle for many children of conservative parents.

Early on, anti-abortion parents probably talked to their children about abortion using literature made for adults. But in the 1980s, parents had new tools for those everyday talks. One example of this material is a 1986 pamphlet targeting young children, entitled "You Are Special." Throughout the pamphlet, the author asked children to connect with the fetus they once were. In a section titled "Tiny You," the pamphlet explained, "You began as a single cell when a sperm from your dad and an egg from your mom joined together. At that moment, everything that was you was already there." The author linked children's lives to abortion: "Sometimes parents get confused and scared when they find out they're going to have a baby. . . . They don't know their baby is alive. They choose abortion. Abortion means that they force their baby to die when it is still growing and living in its mother's womb. At abortion clinics babies die before they have a chance to be born."[56] Compelling the child to envision his or her own potential death, this pamphlet pushed the young reader to identify with all aborted fetuses.

Beyond pamphlets, Christian publishers and pro-life distributers began marketing a number of books parents could read to their children about sex and, implicitly or explicitly, abortion.[57] Virginia Evers's Heritage House sold many of these books to pro-life consumers. Books targeted at younger children included *Why Boys and Girls Are Different, Where Do Babies Come From?, Before I Was Born,* and *How Did God Make Me?* Offerings for parents of older children included *How You Are Changing, Sex and the New You,* and *Love, Sex and God.* All formatted to help parents answer children's questions about sex, these books offered age-appropriate biology lessons along with conservative lessons on gender and sexuality. Promotional material for *How Did God Make Me?* said the book would allow "your son or daughter [to] discover exactly what life is like in the womb." *Before I Was Born* told children "why God made boys' and girls' bodies different" and explained "God's plan for loving marriages and families." According to Heritage House, these educational materials helped parents move beyond the "sweaty palms and lump-in-the-throat approach."[58]

All these books, published in the 1980s and 1990s, included some points in common. First, children's bodies and personalities came from God. Biology lessons proved first and foremost the existence of God's hand in creation. Second, these books emphasized children's acceptance of themselves. For example, *Where Do Babies Come From?* encouraged children "to accept sexuality naturally, as another gift from God."[59] This was not sexual liberation for kids, however. Pro-life parents were not suggesting that God made all sex acts and sexualities, and therefore all were acceptable. They argued just the opposite. They maintained that God made boys' and girls' bodies different, created puberty, and sanctioned heterosexual marriage for a purpose. This was the "natural" sexuality children should accept. These books linked sexed bodies to fixed gender roles to heterosexual marriage and reproduction in a logical continuum, each authenticating the other. Here biology and God worked in tandem to prove that sex difference, gender difference, heterosexuality, and uninterrupted reproduction were natural and divinely ordained.[60] If children and young adults loved or lusted outside this logic loop, they might risk not "walk[ing] with God for a lifetime."[61]

While white pro-lifers and social conservatives advocated teaching all young people about sex and reproduction in the home, boys and girls often got very different lessons. For example, the movement made specific talking-points cards, one set for girls and another for boys. The cards aimed at girls said that while boys just wanted sex, girls wanted "a lasting relationship." Girls did not really have a physical yearning for sex, but rather an emotional one. Encouraging virginity, either primary or "secondary" (when a person recommitted to sexual chastity after having sex), the card asked girls to find their self-respect and commit to remaining "chaste" before marriage. Boys got a very different message. They were the hormone-driven, sexually frustrated yang to the girls' emotionally driven yin. Because boys were biologically driven without any innate understanding of emotional connection, the boys' card had to explain "intimacy in a relationship." Boys were also asked to remain abstinent until marriage—not pure, not virginal, not chaste, just abstinent. A pro-life bumper sticker echoed this message: "Real Men Don't Need 'Safe Sex'[:] They Choose Abstinence."[62]

These gendered lessons extended beyond the printed word to toys. In addition to the cheap, plastic Young Ones, some children had access to other types of fetus dolls. In the 1990s, Heritage House developed what it called Touch of Life Babies, which were heavier models of fetuses with real-feeling skin, and marketed these models as great for kids.[63] Heritage House envisioned this toy primarily for girls. The advertisement for the doll featured a picture of a ten- or twelve-year-old girl cradling her Touch of Life baby. Opposite the picture were testimonials. One happy (adult) owner named her Touch of Life babies, had a baby shower, wrapped them in swaddling blankets, and put them each in their own cribs. Perhaps parents and activists asked young girls to treat their fetuses similarly. Activists who gave out less expensive fetus dolls (like the Young Ones) in group settings often recounted offering them first to girls, then being very pleased when boys wanted them as well.[64] Activists likely believed that girls had the responsibility and natural inclination toward parenthood that could be elicited through the use of the doll. That boys sometimes wanted to "parent" a fetus was a happy, if unexpected, outcome. By replacing a baby doll with a similar-sized fetus doll, pro-life activists made the claim that babies and fetuses were the same. And a girl, as the primary consumer of these dolls, was both prospective mother and a once-endangered, now-grown-up fetus.

Of course, some of the most common educational moments came during quiet times and conversations between parents and children. One activist noted that all his children, no matter their age, said the same prayer before bed: "And Lord, shut down the abortion clinics!"[65] While most of these private prayers and conversations are not recoverable, at least one offers insight into some of the gendered lessons parents imparted to their children. Activist Dauneen Dolce recalled important conversations she had with her four sons as they were growing up. Dolce reminded them that while they did not have to carry a fetus, they had the same responsibility to it. She told one son, "If you came home and you got a girlfriend pregnant, I don't want you to say she's pregnant, you're going to say we're pregnant." She emphasized, however, that while he had the same moral responsibility as the young woman, he did not have the same rights. "I told him she can kill your baby without you saying anything." Dolce concluded that giving full legal rights to the woman to terminate her pregnancy "change[d the relationship between] men and women."[66] For Dolce, the heterosexual unit was bound by reproductive responsibility, legal and moral. Legalized abortion had freed women and men from that responsibility, causing a ripple effect through the many "natural" roles of women and men. Worried that her sons would imbibe this "new" culture of masculine irresponsibility, Dolce lectured them on the value of moral accountability. But she also told her sons that they were helpless; any errant girlfriend had the legal right to take that moral responsibility away from them and force upon them the emasculating choice of abortion.

In many pro-life families, anti-abortion ephemera slipped into children's everyday lives, sometimes in unforeseen ways. June Maskell, the daughter of a Colorado activist, remembered an anti-abortion tape was always on rotation in her family car. She recalled, "There was this one really weird, creepy song where there was a little kid's voice that was being aborted: 'Mom don't take me away. I could be someone special.' It was supposed to be a voice from the womb." Additionally, Maskell remembered that she sometimes found fetuses in unexpected places. "In my dad's glove compartment, he had thin mints and those little fetuses," she remembered.[67] Some pro-life goods were purposefully placed while others simply overflowed into the nooks and crannies of children's lives. In both cases, parents could not always control how their children interacted with fetuses. What one child might find inspirational, another might consider "weird" and "creepy."

Younger children might not even have understood pro-life lessons. In 1973, an *Arizona Republic* reporter quizzed an eight-year-old boy who was helping picket a Phoenix abortion clinic. He was the son of Carolyn Gerster, the former president of Arizona Right to Life and then vice president of National Right to Life. When asked if he knew what an abortion was, he replied that he did: "Abortion is when you kill babies about ten weeks after birth." But then he "tucked his chin and whispered [that] he wasn't sure why he was marching."[68] The confusion on the boy's part on whether abortion occurred before or after birth shows, in part, how successful activists were at blurring the boundary between fetus and newborn child for so many young people. It also demonstrates that children were not always a reliable audience for pro-life appeals.

Anti-abortion politics thus became a part of everyday life for many children, but some of the most powerful organizing took place around the most out-of-the-ordinary events in a child's life. John Jakubczyk, a longtime pro-life activist in Arizona, remembered one of the saddest moments for his family: his wife's miscarriage nineteen weeks into her pregnancy. To grieve the loss, Jakubczyk crafted a small coffin and held a private wake for the family. He said, "All the little kids got to see their brother. And then we had a little memorial service, right around the corner here at St. Francis, at the cemetery.

And then later, about a month later, we had a mass. We had about three [to] four hundred people at the mass." Many of those who attended, Jakubczyk explained, were women who had had a miscarriage or an abortion that they regretted. Though Jakubczyk had been a pro-life activist for many years, he said this miscarriage made abortion more personal to him: "Whether the loss is accidental or, you know, on purpose or through coercion or whatever, there is a loss there."[69] Such ceremonies were not unusual for families dealing with grief from a miscarriage, but Jakubczyk did something much less common. He linked the miscarriage of a wanted pregnancy to the willful termination of an unwanted pregnancy. Through familial grieving, perhaps abortion was now personal to his children as well. This event was not unique to the Jakubczyk family; former Pennsylvania senator and presidential candidate Rick Santorum did something very similar when his wife miscarried in 1996. They too brought the body back to the house for their kids to see, as he said, that it was not a "fetus" but a "baby."[70]

In the 1980s and 1990s, home lessons in "values" were no longer limited to the dinner hour or the weekends. With an explosion of homeschooling, many now had all week for such lessons. While schools became sites of escalating battles over prayer, sex education, racial integration, evolution, and citizenship, many conservatives chose to leave the battlefield entirely—and took their children with them. In fact, social conservatives, especially the evangelical ones, left public schools in droves in the 1980s and 1990s. Between the early 1970s and the early 2000s, the numbers of children being homeschooled mushroomed from 15,000 to somewhere between 1 and 3 million.[71] These white conservative children were removed from multiracial public schools and enmeshed further in the religious and political worlds of their parents.

Though a conservative homeschool movement did not begin until the 1980s, conservatives' exit from public schools was foreshadowed decades before. Historians have documented the intensity with which white people around the country, especially in the urban South and North, protested mandatory city busing programs—programs intended to desegregate urban schools and level the educational playing field.[72] Similar, if less famous, protests happened in the Four Corners states as well.[73] Starting in the mid-1960s, Denver implemented a two-way busing plan, where white children were bused into schools dominated by children of color and children of color were bused into schools dominated by white children. White resistance to the program included legal strategies such as the 1969 election of an anti-busing school board, but it also included violent resistance such as the 1970 bombing of two-thirds of the school system's buses. When these efforts failed to end mandatory busing in Denver, many white city residents did what others did around the country. They moved to the suburbs.[74] But some decided that rather than move, they would homeschool their children. Former Colorado state senator and homeschooling parent Kevin Lundberg remembered that the busing system was the reason he and his wife decided to homeschool their children: "I couldn't countenance the idea of sending a kindergartener across town. . . . It wasn't a matter of prejudice of any sort. Well yes there was a prejudice and the prejudice was I wanted my son to have the best education possible."[75] This logic was common in anti-busing arguments. The "best education" available was often in white neighborhoods, and thus children in those neighborhoods had a right to it. Opponents did not acknowledge that segregation, economic disparities, and social injustice had created both school excellence in white neighborhoods and school deterioration in the neighborhoods of people of color. Children, in busing opponents' minds, especially white children, were bearing the burden of federal experiments in social engineering. Or, as one Denver commenter put it, children "have become pawns in what can only be called a monstrous game of musical schools."[76]

For many conservatives, public schools had changed profoundly in the 1960s. White elites and people of color were socially engineering schools in racial, sexual, and gendered ways, according to them. In 1962 and 1963, the Supreme Court ruled that official school prayer, school-sponsored religious activities, and classroom Bible readings were unconstitutional. As the decade continued, some parents became further enraged that their children were receiving sex education—pro-life activist Carolyn Gerster called it "indoctrination."[77] These critiques only intensified as the century wore on. Groups like Concerned Women for America and Christian Coalition regularly warned their members that public schools were places where the federal government could steal the hearts, minds, and even the bodies of their children. Public schools gave children condoms, whisked them away for abortions, and taught them about "diversity," homosexuality, and "unbridled sex," conservatives argued.[78] Even as some parents complained to their children's teachers, pushed pro-life school board candidates, and advocated abstinence education, others chose to avoid public schools altogether.

Statistical data on homeschoolers suggests that they were overwhelming white, middle class, and religious. A 1995 sociological study found that 98 percent of surveyed homeschooling families were white, most often with young, married parents and a male breadwinner. The survey also showed that these families made slightly more money than the average American family and were highly religious—91 percent claimed that religious commitment was "very important" to them.[79] In the 1990s, the Home School Legal Defense Association, an advocacy group, sponsored a study concluding the overwhelming majority of parents who homeschooled their children were evangelical Christians.[80] Another survey said that most families home-schooled in order to provide "religious or moral instruction."[81] One New Mexican father explained their choice to homeschool this way: "We're trying to keep our kids from perverted sexual and moral views. . . . The schools can't teach morality. They teach safe sex."[82] Here the phrase "perverted sexual and moral views" most certainly referred to acceptance of teenage and premarital sex, birth control and abortion, and homosexuality. "Moral instruction" at home was the solution for an increasing number of Americans.

With full parental control of curriculum and reduced outside influences, homeschooling allowed for children's politicization. This runs counter to one of the major social critiques of homeschooling, which was that homeschooled children would not participate in civic or community activities. Critics complained that if children retreated from the democratic space of public school, they retreated from American democracy as well. Those who have studied homeschooling, however, have found the opposite: homeschoolers participated extensively in civic and political activities. For example, a 1996 National Household Education Survey showed that children schooled at home or at private schools were 9.3 percent more likely to be politically active than their public school counterparts. They were also 13 percent more likely to donate to political causes, 10 percent more likely to attend a public rally, and 26 percent more likely to volunteer for organizations. Two sociologists studying homeschooled children concluded that these students participated so much because they formed strong social networks and because they created *"shared moral cultures* that facilitate social solidarity and trust."[83]

Shared "moral" cultures, strong religious affiliation, and opposition to "liberal" or "secular" schools meant that homeschooling parents and home-schooled children were much more likely to participate in conservative and pro-life campaigns than in other types of political activities. Denver home-schooling parent Kevin Lundberg argued that the homeschool setting led to politicization: "They weren't taught to be a political activist but they were naturally within that setting. . . . Parents who get involved in teaching their kids directly learn an awful lot about a lot of things and become committed to those things. . . . They're in the rough and tumble world of ideas with their kids. And being essentially Christian in nature the homeschool movement is by necessity not just pro-life but active pro-life." He contended that parents did not homeschool their children in order to make activists, but rather it happened organically. And while the anti-abortion and homeschool movements were different, "they were the same people doing the same things," he remembered. "So you know if you want to find a place where there are pro-life people, go to a homeschool anything and you'll find them there."[84] June Maskell echoed Lundberg's assessment; Maskell went to public school but most of the other children of pro-life activists, she said, were homeschooled.[85] Some activists credited homeschooling with not just young people's participation, but their passion. Reveling in all the young activists at a 1993 rally, radical activist Norman Weslin focused on homeschooled children's enthusiasm, writing that they expressed their commitment to the "pre-born . . . in such a beautiful 'lived-experience' way!!"[86] Homeschooled children took the "rough and tumble world" of socially conservative ideas and put them into practice in the anti-abortion movement.

This movement to mobilize youth did not operate in a vacuum. In fact, especially for evangelicals, it was a piece of a broader project to bring conservative Christianity into the everyday lives of children. Utilizing the tools of popular culture, adult evangelicals helped create a vibrant conservative youth culture, believing it was more important to change hearts rather than votes. In this youth culture, abortion played a central role. Of all religious beliefs, it was the issue of abortion that "crystallized" evangelical youths' difference from their secular peers, according to historian Eileen Luhr. Anti-abortion belief became a litmus test for this community; for example, Christian rock bands had to express pro-life sentiments to play at evangelical concerts. Many in turn played explicitly anti-abortion songs, talked about abortion in fan magazine interviews, and encouraged young people to offer their own pro-life testimony.[87] Thus the pro-life movement and the evangelical community had a symbiotic relationship at the end of the century. The anti-abortion movement gave evangelicals a defining moral issue while evangelical popular culture offered a hip vehicle for the movement's ideology that reached an even broader youth audience.

In the 1980s and 1990s, with the help of consumer culture, white conservative parents had made anti-abortion politics into a lifestyle for their children. This lifestyle was a counterpoint to what activists saw as liberalizing influences in public schools and the media. Norman Weslin diagnosed the problem this way: "The news media seeks to seduce our youngsters into their

Culture of Death."[88] When social institutions no longer maintained the "common sense" of white privilege and patriarchy, socially conservative activists had to do more than sign a petition or picket a clinic. A pro-life educator offered the movement's solution: "I feel I have a personal mission to teach youth that life is a precious gift. I believe education is a major key to closing the doors of abortion clinics."[89] With anti-abortion books, films, stickers, T-shirts, and toys in hand, parents could increasingly integrate their politics into the everyday lives of their children. With the help of socially conservative consumer goods, parents helped create alternative political cultures for their children to inhabit.

THE STREETS

"So many of the women going in for abortion are teenage girls, and so few of us are objecting," fifteen-year-old Camille Remmert told the crowd at the 1991 Colorado Rally for Life. Remmert had come to this realization while picketing her local abortion clinic. She told the teens in the audience that they needed to get involved by joining her on a picket line, volunteering for a pro-life teen group, and writing their legislators. "We are the future of this country and they would be foolish not to listen to us," she said.[90] Remmert was, in fact, part of a growing number of white teens and children publicly protesting abortion and picketing clinics on a regular basis. Outside clinics, some carried anti-abortion signs with slogans like "Abortion Kills Children," hoping their identities as a young people would accentuate this pro-life claim. Others, like Remmert, specifically named themselves as near victims of abortion, carrying signs like "I'm Glad I Wasn't Aborted" and "Survivors of the Abortion Holocaust."[91] Such activism shows how successful anti-abortion adults were at politicizing and mobilizing youth at the end of the century. Moreover, the overwhelming whiteness of these new activists shows how racialized the pro-life message was, even as anti-abortion activists made their political pitch in multiracial spaces like public schools.

While adult pro-life activists had dreamed of this type of activism since the late 1960s, anti-abortion groups put more effort into organizing young people in the last two decades of the century. One Colorado feminist, working undercover at the 1985 National Right to Life Convention, noted that the group was concentrating largely on the "youth and the grassroots." At the convention, this observer noted "a lot of young people in their 20s and 30s, and even quite a few teenagers." The convention's program included work-shops on the pro-life youth movement. In one workshop, a "school teacher" instructed parents on how "to teach the pro-life message in the home, start-ing with toddlers." The pro-choice spectator also saw a host of anti-abortion books and films targeted at teenagers, which she said were "too numerous to list."[92]

Many of those materials were coming from pro-life businesses, which were increasingly marketing to children. In 1981, Heritage House, the Arizona pro-life retailer, had very limited materials designed for children and young adults.[93] By the late 1990s, Heritage House's products for children had grown exponentially. The retailer sold gold-foiled Precious Feet stickers; abstinence stickers; child-centered balloons, including ones that read "I'm a Child Not a Choice"; and at least six different child- and teen-focused T-shirts, including one with a seal protesting to save "baby humans" (an answer to environmen-talists who sought to save seals). This was all in addition to children's books, abstinence education material, bumper stickers, and Touch of Life dolls.[94] Thus, adult activists asked children to be prolific consumers of pro-life arguments and material.

In most advertisements for pro-life material, the children pictured were white. They graced the cover of the catalogs, films, and books; advertised the T-shirts; and cradled the Touch of Life fetus dolls. Representations of chil-dren of color were rare, but a handful showed up on the pages of the catalog. Children of color showed up on the covers of a book on single parenthood (entitled *Do I Have a Daddy?*), a pamphlet on adoption, and a book on teen pregnancy. By re-associating people of color with single parenthood and other forms of "errant" heterosexuality, white pro-life activists entrenched stereotypes about women of color under the guise of racial representation. Children of color also appeared as members of diverse groups of children on covers of books targeted to children and teens. With these covers, pro-life cultural purveyors imagined a more multiracial young audience for their materials than many activists had in the past.[95] Though activists' multicul-turalism in this venue, along with many others, did not change understand-ings of racism and racial difference, the (white) creator was at least portrayed as anti-racist. As with earlier pro-life forms of racial liberalism, overt racial conservatism lurked close by.

In the same 1999 catalog, Heritage House advertised *Death of Truth,* Dennis McCallum's book responding to multiculturalism, in which he criti-cized the focus on power and inequality in American society, "the 'political correctness' movement," "extreme" cultural tolerance, and the decentering of "Truth" (articulated as Christian, Western cultural values).[96] At the end of the century, even in its child-centered corners, the movement maintained its exclusionary relationship to people of color, even as it articulated its own version of multiculturalism. It attempted to represent people of color more often and continued to co-opt the language and symbols of civil rights movements, while overtly criticizing discussions of racial inequality and difference.

This exclusionary relationship did not mean that no anti-abortion parents of color conveyed political messages to their children. In 2006, a twenty-three-year-old ethnic Mexican woman from near Albuquerque reflected on her own abortion and how she explained it to her pro-life mother: "My Mom used to protest [outside of abortion clinics]. (Laughs). So, we aren't supposed to [have abortions]. That is why I told her there was something wrong with the baby. She would disown me if she found out what was going on."[97] The movement's racial messaging discouraged but did not preclude the activism of this young woman's mother. Her story also shows that the broad targeting of children and young adults by the pro-life movement did not ensure that they would become and remain pro-life. Of course, this young woman was not alone in her quiet dissent from her parent's politics. With one in three American women getting abortions on their lifetimes, it is certain that many daughters of anti-abortion parents went on to get abortions themselves.

Children of activists rebelled in other ways as well. June Maskell, for example, rejected her father's pro-life politics in both small and profound ways. She had protested outside of Planned Parenthood with her father up until the age of nine, but as a teenager she slowly began moving away from her father's politics. In high school, her father told her she could have a car as long as she put an anti-abortion bumper sticker on it. She recalled, "I taped it to my window and I would take it down every day" before she got to school. Later in life, she broke from her father's politics in bigger ways. She ran for city council and later for the Colorado House and Senate as a pro-choice candidate endorsed by National Abortion Rights Action League (NARAL) and Planned Parenthood. For some pro-life parents, this would have been a bridge too far. In fact, Maskell recalled that some of her father's friends suggested he disown her. Maskell and her father instead struck a delicate balance; she protected his time to go protest at clinics and he watched her children while she passed pro-choice bills and won "awards from Planned Parenthood." Despite their political disagreements, Maskell credited her father with her life in politics. "He was an activist. . . . He wants to save the world and make it better and I do too. And I got that all from him."[98] In this family, political rebellion and inspiration were two sides of the same coin.

Even as some children of the movement strayed, large numbers of children and young adults in the 1980s and 1990s did follow their parents' lead and join the fight against legalized abortion. The group that exposed the success of these organizing efforts to the general public was Operation Rescue. As radical groups gained more attention in the late 1980s and 1990s, young pro-life activists too gained a spot in the national limelight. In these years, radical groups engaged in publicity stunts, attacks on abortion providers, and civil disobedience. Every abortion clinic in the United States experienced some kind of structural attack, or, as anti-abortion activists termed it, "brick and mortar" violence.[99] There was also a dramatic upsurge in personal violence against abortion providers, including eight murders.[100] The most famous radical pro-life group of its time, Operation Rescue pioneered the "rescue," in which thousands of pro-life activists would descend on an American city, creating human blockades in order to stop women from accessing abortion clinics. In cities like Atlanta (Georgia), Buffalo (New York), and Wichita (Kansas), Operation Rescue converged for months, tying up the city's police department and the local jails, and making it incredibly difficult for anyone to get near an abortion clinic.[101] The soldiers in this newly militant pro-life movement included not just seasoned adult activists, but many children and young adults.

In 1991, during Operation Rescue's blockades of abortion provider George Tiller's clinic in Wichita, children took center stage—and young children, at that. During those months of protest, stories of child radicals stood out from the rest. One day, in order to stop women from entering the clinic, one fifteen-year-old girl and five of her seven siblings, "one as young as ten," ran in front of an approaching car and sat down. Their mother quickly joined them.[102] Another day, the *New York Times* reported that one "little girl" protesting at Tiller's clinic was removed but not arrested by police. An adult activist comforted her: "It's all right. . . . There will be another time to get arrested."[103] National Public Radio recounted that one mother proudly confirmed that her children had been arrested many times. Other children reportedly "stood nearby in the shade of an oak tree singing children's hymns." Operation Rescue defended the presence of children, declaring, "Those children who were in front of the cars are not any older or younger than the girls who go in there to get abortions without their parents'

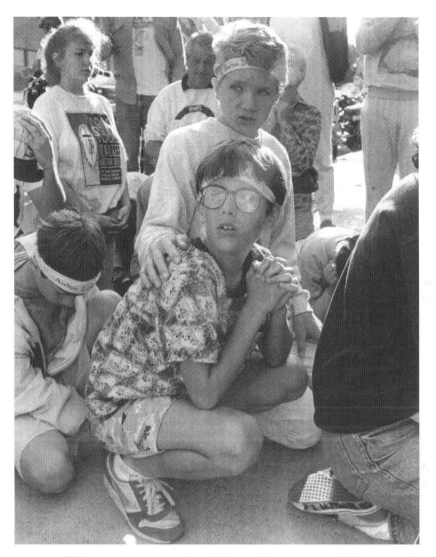

FIGURE 11. Children praying and protesting with the radical rescue group Missionaries to the Preborn outside a Milwaukee abortion clinic, Metropolitan Medical Services, 1992. (Courtesy of Susan Ruggles/SLR Images; Wisconsin Historical Society)

permission." Eventually, one Operation Rescue activist was sentenced to a year in prison for "ordering children to block cars trying to get into Dr. George Tiller's clinic."[104] While all parts of this movement had politicized and organized young people, Operation Rescue drew public attention to the success of those efforts.[105]

Unaware of how central child organizing was to the movement as a whole, many singled out Operation Rescue as particularly misguided in its inclusion of children and young adults. A 1993 *Rolling Stone* magazine article exemplified critics' use of the presence of children at protests to demonstrate the perversity of the radical movement. The author set the scene for a protest on a hot day in Melbourne, Florida:

> Women with the blood of the lamb in their eyes trampled all over neighbors' lawns, shoving plastic fetuses into the hands of small children and beshrewing them to burn in hell. And 10 feet from the room where women lay groggy after their abortions, born-again teens stood on aluminum ladders and cried out in angry, plangent wails: "Mommy, Mommy, why did you kill me? Why did you let them pull my head off with pliers?"

Once Randall Terry, the leader of Operation Rescue, arrived, the energy of the crowd intensified. "Catching sight of their hero, young girls in T-shirts that read I SURVIVED THE AMERICAN HOLOCAUST shrieked and breathlessly clutched their hearts, as if the fifth Beatle had arrived," the author recounted. When Terry began his fire and brimstone speech, parents pushed their children to block access to the clinic, break the law, and get arrested:

> The older kids went solemnly, already adroit, at the age of 9 and 10, at the business of political arrest. Other children as young as 6, however, sobbed and bit their hands in horror, begging their mothers not to make them go. With a knee in their back, though, and the fires of hell in their ears, on came the smallest of Florida's evangels, tottering, arms out, like tipsy zombies, groaning for their sweet friend Jesus to save them.

In this recounting, the author focused on the children to demonstrate the movement's radicalism, or as he put it, a movement "as cultic and ceaseless as any jihad launched by Tehran."[106] The young people in the story came across as either fanatical, brainwashed, hysterical, or coerced. Though unhinged and violent adults swirled around this story too, it was the children who truly embodied the excesses and dangers of the rescue movement. With such exoticizing characterizations, many Americans came to see this expression of the pro-life cause as less like the civil rights movement it claimed to be and more like a religious cult, indoctrinating the young with radicalism and violence.

Operation Rescue garnered criticism not just for the children in their ranks, but also for those they sought out. In the Four Corners states, Operation

Rescue and other radical groups came most often, though not exclusively, to Colorado. Warren Hern, a proud and outspoken doctor who provided third-trimester abortions in Boulder, as well as Denver abortion providers, drew this radical group to the Front Range. National Operation Rescue activists were aided by a fervent Colorado-based Operation Rescue affiliate. Between the late 1980s and late 1990s, Operation Rescue had a significant presence in the state, protesting at clinics and outside local high schools. In 1997, its members came to Denver high schools armed with blown-up photos of bloody, dismembered fetuses. The group said that, at schools, they used "the goriest abortion posters [they] can find."[107] The executive director of Operation Rescue Colorado at the time said the group targeted high schools because "that's where the battle 'for hearts and minds of kids' begins."[108]

Many criticized Operation Rescue's presence at local high schools. Colorado NARAL argued that "it is irresponsible to target teenagers, who lack the maturity and skills to handle Operation Rescue's trademark aggressive demonstrations."[109] Many were especially angry that middle school students and their younger siblings saw the group's graphic material. Parents couldn't have been reassured when there were reports of young teens crying while others were "ripping and tearing" the group's posters.[110] Locally and nationally, many Americans echoed these concerns. Some criticized the presence of children at protests, suggesting that they might be damaged because they were too young to understand the consequences of their actions, the complexity of the issue, and this level of social conflict between parents, friends, and the police.[111] Others argued that Operation Rescue's tactic of protesting outside abortion providers' homes and the schools of doctors' children was just plain wrong.[112] All such tactics seemed to violate the division between the adult and public world of abortion politics and the private, protected world of a child's home and school.

It was in these years that the pro-life movement's focus on children and young people ran most afoul of public sentiment. Activists had long capitalized on cultural anxiety about childhood and innocence. But in the late 1980s and 1990s, the movement that was supposedly "saving children" now looked like it was endangering them. A movement that had hoped to recreate what it saw as a pre-*Roe* national innocence—a whitewashed and patriarchal past—now looked like it was exploiting American youth and spreading the distress of the abortion wars into the private, protected worlds of childhood. In consequence, many Americans reasserted a hard division

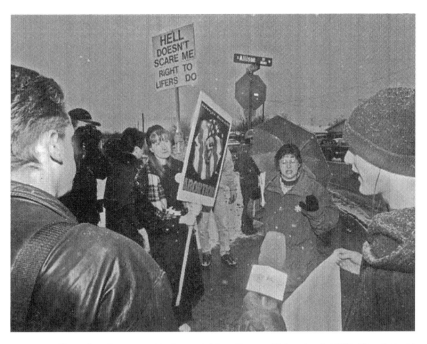

between public and private, putting children firmly in the private sector and abortion debates firmly in the public sector.

What observers missed was that many young people willfully joined this movement and found meaning in it. Pro-life adults brought their ideology into youth spaces and encouraged the young to participate, but their activism is not enough to explain the fervency of white pro-life youth. Like their parents, many young white people felt adrift in modern American society, felt like that society had lost its moral compass. Lauren Sandler, a journalist who enmeshed herself in evangelical youth pro-life culture, said that most teens thought of themselves as "soldiers in a holy war, a culture war, a civil war for souls on American soil." She continued, "They enlist for belonging. They enlist for love. . . . Many, though, are just kids who need a community organized around an ethic that provides their lives with purpose."[113] In the antiabortion movement, and in their broader religious cultures, white conservative youth found an explanation for their alienation, one that linked conservative religion, gender, and race. The movement also offered a modern vehicle—a civil rights movement—for their white conservative politics. The abortion issue helped articulate young people's difference and offered an opportunity for them to missionize to their peers and change the world.

By the end of the century, children and young adults were not confined to the movement's radical corners. Some probably joined because they saw a pro-life activist give a presentation at their school or church. Others were surely motivated by abstinence education programs or homeschool curriculums. Still others probably took to heart their parents' life lessons about sex, abortion, and responsibility. A fetus doll, a friend's T-shirt, or a passing glance at a gory photo outside their school might have convinced them. Children had long been named the hope of a pro-life future and the innocent victims of feminism and secular humanism. Many took this political inspiration and incorporated it into their core identities as young people. In fact, surveys at the end of the century showed that support for abortion rights had been decreasing among American youth since the early 1990s, from 67 percent in the early 1990s to 54 percent in the early 2000s, according to one.[114] Thus, they came to the rescue movement not as anomalous individual kids kneed in the back by radical parents, but as an overt constituency of the movement and an enthusiastic cadre of activists.

Of course, adult pro-lifers had other explanations for this swell of youth activism. As one activist put it, "They've had friends that have had abortions. They've seen the pain."[115] Or, as another activist theorized, children were more likely to be pro-life because they saw their mothers mourn previous abortions: "One little boy said every spring my mama cries and cries and cries and it's because I don't have a little brother or sister."[116] For anti-abortion activists, young people joined the cause because they had seen the trauma of abortion. Whether children were envisioned as invited activists or simply traumatized observers, adult activists increasingly took heart in the young people among them.

. . .

In the last decades of the twentieth century, anti-abortion activists regularly talked about the haven of childhood but they saw that haven as embattled and already deeply corrupted. And thus, right from the beginning of their movement, anti-abortion activists worked to politicize children. Activists campaigned to reeducate American youth, those most susceptible, they thought, to the political messaging of pro-choice activists and the "liberal" media. Anti-abortion activists remade youth spaces—from school to home—

into pro-life spaces, politicizing children so that they could help move the United States back to an imagined pre-1967 innocence. This work affected places like the Mountain West more than others, as willing school boards gave pro-life activists and "abstinence educators" more access to their children. The movement's mass-marketed political tools meant that Mormon, evangelical, and Catholic children and white, ethnic Mexican, and black children saw the same photos, heard the same pleas to chastity, and held the same fetus dolls in their hands, even if members of these groups did not always receive those political appeals in the same way. It was white young people who took these pleas and put them into action. Often in this work, activists successfully blurred the boundary between fetus and child, implicating real children in legalized abortion. They made children into abortion "survivors" and tried to give them a personal relationship to legal abortion. In the late 1980s and 1990s, the American public witnessed one of the outcomes of this public and private political work in the spectacle of pro-life "rescues."

Though the practice of rescue cast a cultural shadow over the larger pro-life movement, the attention child activists garnered did not change the tactics of the movement as a whole. Children remained the hope for a pro-life future, a new corps of activists, those at risk of corruption, and living symbols of those aborted. A 1998 issue of the Arizona Right to Life newsletter demonstrated just how important the images and the activism of children and young adults had become. While the issue contained stories about legislation, euthanasia, and elections, its pictures were all of children. An image of a baby graced the cover under the headline "The Real Face of the Pro-Life Movement." In the middle of the newsletter, a young girl with a dog advertised pro-life calendars and a young family with three teenagers and a baby promoted abstinence education. In an article about the Right to Life booth at the state fair, four little children held fetal models and asked, in the caption, "Were we really this little when we were in our mommy's tummy?" At the bottom of the page, another picture featured a pregnant mom showing her young son what his soon-to-be brother looked like in-utero. The article told of a four-year-old girl fascinated by a Precious Feet pin, willing to spend her single dollar to have it. But the last photo of the issue displayed the real hope of the movement: two teenage girls smiled for the camera while doing data entry for the group.[117] In this newsletter, children were the faces of the movement, the marketing tools, the objects of education, and eventually— hopefully—the activists.

SIX

Making Family Values

In a 2010 interview, two anti-abortion activists remembered fondly a story of an abortion averted. Some of the details were a little hazy, but Helen and Phil Seader agreed on much of the story from thirty years before: Helen was working one day at a crisis pregnancy center in Tucson when a young, "bright" woman contacted her. The man who impregnated her, a "bright" man who worked for the newspaper, wanted her to have an abortion. The two came to the center, and Helen brought in a pro-life doctor to talk to the couple. After describing the process of fetal development, the doctor looked at the young man and said, "so you're a bully." The man sat on the couch stunned and quiet. Finally he said, "You're right. You're describing to me a human being." Because of this meeting, the woman did not have the abortion. Helen concluded, "And they got married and . . . they had two more babies and everything. They had a good life." Their work in stopping this abortion had set the couple on a path toward marriage, other children, and perhaps even happiness: a "good family" and a "good life."

But there was a caveat to this tale of familial bliss. Phil Seader added that the young woman "did [leave her husband] for a while" for a "mountain man." Helen, a consummate storyteller, took up the amended account. After the couple married, they had problems. One day the woman showed up at the Seaders' door and dropped off her child, saying "You made me have her." The woman had already been living with the "mountain man" and, according to Helen, "her life was falling apart." The young woman, her new partner, and some others had set up camp at the bottom of the Tucson Mountains. Supposedly, the woman was feeding her child wine and doing drugs while living there. After about four months of taking care of the child, Phil and Helen Seader invited the woman and her estranged husband over for dinner.

"They got [back] together and were doing fine. They had other children," the Seaders concluded. The story's lesson remained the same, in other words. Even with the addition of child abandonment, homelessness, and adultery, these activists resolved once more that the couple "got a good life."[1]

In this story of the "bright" couple and the mountain man, the Seaders illuminated the politics of family within the pro-life movement. The Seaders believed that they saved the woman from emotional and physical damage and redirected her initial partner's bullying tendencies, his authoritarian masculinity. Carrying the pregnancy to term helped reorder gender relations that were out of whack. It was not significant that the "bright" couple's family was unconventional, to say the least. In another context, this was exactly the type of family social conservatives would have blamed for the deterioration of society. But for the Seaders, other pro-life activists, and many family values conservatives, abortion changed the story and changed the family. A woman or couple who avoided abortion could become an exemplar of family values. In the "family values" coalitions of the 1980s and 1990s, anti-abortion activists helped make "life" one of the defining characteristics of the "traditional family."

Anti-abortion activists did not immediately turn to "family" as the rationale for their cause. In the 1960s and early 1970s, supporters of legal abortion talked more about families than did those who opposed it. Abortion reformers and later abortion rights activists often argued that the birth of an "unwanted child" made for dysfunctional and abusive families.[2] Unwantedness was the cause of juvenile delinquency and adult crime. Forced reproduction was ruining many American families, according to abortion reformers. To rebut such arguments, anti-abortion activists used the language of individual and human rights. Activists connected an "unwanted" fetus to other "unwanted" people. Anti-abortion activists claimed that abortion, like all other social hierarchies, prioritized certain human lives over others and thus fundamentally disrespected human life. It became a core tenet of pro-life ideology that only people who opposed abortion truly cared about "the unwanted."[3] Rather than relate abortion to the American family, as abortion reformers did, early anti-abortion activists focused on the fetus as an isolated and autonomous individual threatened by a hardened society.

Ten years later, social conservatives changed course and put "the family" at the center of their campaigns. In the 1980s and 1990s, "family values" became political shorthand for a very specific constellation of issues: opposition to the Equal Rights Amendment, homosexuality, comprehensive sex education, pornography, feminism, secular public schools, and abortion. Their politics, conservative activists claimed, derived from a commitment to the "traditional family." This familial unit was self-sufficient, loving, and hierarchical, with a working father, a stay-at-home mother, and sheltered children. All members had defined roles that fit them psychologically and biologically. In the socially conservative worldview, the traditional family promoted heterosexuality, marriage, individualism, patriotism, independence, innocence, and Christianity in all its members, and abstinence in the young and single. As other historians have argued, this family was not a historical constant, but rather a historical composite put together by conservative activists for a contemporary audience.[4] None have acknowledged, however, anti-abortion activists' unique contribution to the political creation of the "traditional family."

White anti-abortion activists put the "unborn" at the heart of the family's structure and its reason for being. The late-twentieth-century "traditional family" was really a fetus-focused family. As religious studies scholar Seth Dowland has argued, social conservatives, especially evangelical Christians, defended the "traditional family" from the government, most often using the language of liberty.[5] However because those conservatives made fetuses central to "traditional families," they also used the language of rights. Pro-life activists changed the "liberty" of choice into irresponsibility, and the "rights of the unborn" into a family values mantra. The fetus brought an amorphous, if powerful, dedication to "personal responsibility," "life," and even "justice" to the core of the traditional family. It made heterosexual reproduction the family's defining act and its divine, natural validation. In the aftermath of *Roe v. Wade,* it also helped create the family's adversaries: feminism, secularism, the media, and the federal government.

Like so many other creations of the pro-life movement, this fetus-focused family was a product of white nostalgia. Social conservatives usually envisioned the "timeless" traditional family as having its heyday in the 1950s, often in segregated lily-white suburbs. This family came under threat in the 1960s as young people embraced civil rights, feminism, and New Left politics. People of color were never a part of the family's nostalgic image and only appeared as part of a cabal of corrupters. On the ground in the 1980s and 1990s, anti-abortion activists pitched the whitewashed fetus-focused family as one all people regardless of race could and should aspire to. In practice, activists tried to get both white women and women of color to fit into its rigid mold. As in other parts of this movement, these efforts at racial inclusion were paired with concerted attempts to silence the voices of poor people and people of color who had alternative definitions of family. In fact, in the New Right's broader politics it was women of color who would remain the faces of corrupted and corrupting modern families.

As they had with women and children, white anti-abortion activists worked to insert the protection of fetuses into the heart of the family—and by extension the family values movement. Activists made the pitch in intimate spaces and more formal political spaces that the health of the American family depended upon ending legal abortion, and in so doing, they often drowned out the voices of many. These cultural politics in turn got a national stage through conservative media juggernauts, like the nonprofit Focus on the Family. This organization, led by southerner-turned-westerner James Dobson, helped market the socially conservative vision of "family values" to people across the country.[6] Other "family values" issues would come and go—concerns over pornography, funding for the arts, the Equal Rights Amendment, and gay teachers, to name a few. All had their heyday in the last decades of the twentieth century. Opposition to abortion, however, remained one of the few constant commitments of the "traditional family" from its political inception until well into the twenty-first century.

UNWED PARENTS ANONYMOUS

In the last two decades of the twentieth century, the movement's singular focus on abortion motivated activists to alter their vision of the family. If stopping abortions was the primary goal, many activists could not be picky about what kind of (heterosexual) family a child should be born into. In crisis pregnancy centers, for example, anti-abortion activists had to make peace with single motherhood and some other nontraditional familial situations. This did not mean anti-abortion activists abandoned the fantasy of a heterosexual, patriarchal family bound by legal marriage. They idealized marriage but could not mandate it. This also did not mean single mothers were always on sturdy political ground in socially conservative circles. Many activists still railed against one-parent households and tried to get children out of them. But in the age of legal abortion, these were secondary goals. If fetuses were part of the family—the unit's raison être—stopping an abortion by definition preserved a family, however the household manifested. And sometimes that had to be enough.

Anti-abortion activists had to reconsider the woman-headed household because of the *Roe v. Wade* decision. The court had defined abortion, in the first two trimesters, as an issue of an individual's right to privacy. As a result, a woman—not her husband, parents, or doctor—had the singular right to decide whether to carry her pregnancy to term. Throughout the last decades of the twentieth century, pro-life activists tried to curtail this singular right, explicitly by pushing spousal and parental consent laws and implicitly by limiting federal and state funding for abortions. Despite these efforts, the court continued to protect, in some form, a woman's right to terminate a pregnancy. Because of *Roe,* anti-abortion activists were hamstrung. Thus, the family relationship that was most important to this movement would always be that between pregnant woman and fetus, or, as activists named them, a mother and her child.

Unwed Parents Anonymous (UPA), a group begun by Arizona pro-life activist Margot Sheahan, illuminates how conservatives both imagined the fetus-focused traditional family and allowed that family to encompass non-nuclear, often alternative households. In 1979, Sheahan founded the organization that she described as a "self help group for unwed mothers, unwed fathers, maternal and paternal grandparents, and anyone who is affected by the birth, or impending birth, of an out-of-wedlock pregnancy."[7] A white Catholic who had moved for health reasons from Canada to Arizona when she was twenty, Sheahan was deeply embedded in the pro-life movement by the mid-1970s. In fact, she became the president of Arizona Right to Life in 1976. Sheahan recalled that she joined the movement for two reasons. In 1960, she had a miscarriage and experienced a tremendous sense of personal loss, already connecting to the fetus as her child. Then, in the mid-1960s, Sheahan and her husband took in pregnant teens who later gave their children up for adoption.[8] Not only did Sheahan acknowledge the plight of unfortunately pregnant young women, she advocated pro-life compassion toward unwed mothers. As Arizona Right to Life president, Sheahan contended that her dual commitment to the rights of the fetus and the rights of the mother "to be nurtured and loved throughout her pregnancy" defined her political tenure.[9]

It took a personal familial crisis, however, for Sheahan to channel her compassion into a self-help group. "Suddenly our own family was called to experience the problem of unwed parents—through one of our children," she wrote later.[10] In the late 1970s, her teenage daughter, Angela, became pregnant. Sheahan explained Angela's pregnancy as a product of her historical moment;

she was a teenager when "contraception, abortion, premarital sex and free love were hailed as 'liberation.'" Sheahan and her husband could not believe that their "beautiful, perky, popular little girl" had become another statistic. Sheahan's white, middle-class daughter had been corrupted by the era. At the time, Sheahan herself was in a twelve-step program of some kind, which inspired her to follow the format of Alcoholics Anonymous in order to aid unwed parents.[11]

In the group she founded in 1979 and ran until her death in 2005, Unwed Parents Anonymous, Sheahan helped develop a conservative, white notion of family for a modern sexual age. The group provided a space for single parenthood within pro-life and socially conservative circles. Sheahan noted that the group never pushed unwed parents to marry. "The group does not believe a marriage should patch up a situation, but should be based on mutual love and a life commitment," she told one reporter.[12] UPA also focused on the complicated problems of unwed pregnancy: teenage naïveté, young men's "playboy" sensibilities, dysfunctional relationships, dating difficulties, overwhelming guilt and anger, and economic and social pressures. While accepting the many paths to single parenthood, UPA narrated it as an inferior family structure built out of personal and social dysfunction. "It is disturbing to witness the large number of women who choose to raise their child in a fatherless home," Sheahan wrote.[13] Single parenthood was a condition to be borne, not a legitimate personal choice. Yet even while single parenthood was a step out of the "natural order," it also was an opportunity for personal development— an opportunity, that is, to remake oneself and one's child into a family.

At the heart of UPA's message was chastity. UPA argued that the root of the problem of unwed pregnancy was premarital sex.[14] Contraception and abortion had promised "consequence-free encounters," to use Sheahan's words. Contraception was like a drug; a casual user could quickly become an addict.[15] For Sheahan, single parenthood was a product of social liberalism and late-twentieth-century society more broadly, rather than biological inferiority or mental illness (the causes offered earlier in the century). Sheahan portrayed premarital sexual relationships as chaotic, irresponsible, absent of intimacy and love. Marital sex, on the other hand, was "the ultimate communication of true love," a communication filled with responsibility that went "beyond sexual exploitation."[16] The only solution to the personal and social problem of unplanned pregnancy, then, was chastity. UPA defined chastity as more than sexual abstinence. To be truly chaste one also had to be modest, decent, refined, "simple in style," clean, attractive, and "totally honest and assertive in all relationships."[17] Such descriptors had long been used to define appropriate womanhood, and also to differentiate white women from women of color, and poor women from middle- and upper-class women. Here Sheahan repackaged these older but powerful notions and presented them as a universal goal for all women.

Promoting chastity was as much a solution to legalized abortion as a response to unwed pregnancy. In her book on UPA, Sheahan regularly mentioned that many participants had had prior abortions. "It is the great unspoken pain that hangs over our meetings; though seldom mentioned, it is always there," she wrote.[18] Sheahan provided "representative" stories of UPA participants, which all portrayed abortion in the same way: as a convenient way to avoid responsibility, followed by the realization of fetal personhood, profound regret, and emotional damage. Abortion flouted nature because, Sheahan contended, "every pregnant girl, deep down, wants her baby."[19] The group never offered abortion as a solution for pregnant women, because it was a "cop-out" and carried "tremendous negative moral implications."[20] In the words of one reporter, Sheahan kept the group going by "her sheer force of will and her untiring dedication to the life of the unborn."[21] She would not have disagreed. In almost all Sheahan's writings and interviews, she argued that UPA was a part of her broader pro-life project.

Abortion was both the "damage" that brought people to single parenthood and the political force that unified members. One former participant noted that "there are girls here, at UPA, from scores of different circumstances with one common bond—choosing 'life' for our children even though they are born out-of-wedlock."[22] Sometimes a member's opposition to abortion only developed once she or he came to UPA. Sheahan contended that in 1985 six hundred women had sought advice about whether to carry their pregnancies to term; she said only one went on to have an abortion.[23]

Margot Sheahan and Unwed Parents Anonymous reveal the evolving politics of family within the pro-life movement. Individuals learned commitment and responsibility in nuclear families. They had sex within the confines of marriage, where children—sexuality's "beauty, . . . meaning, . . . burden, and . . . wealth"—could be central. The family was thus "the singular bastion of hope in a world that is play acting other forms of getting along."[24] Though activists glorified this particular familial model, they did not insist upon it. Ultimately the women who came to UPA were redeemed through avoiding abortion and subsequently choosing chastity, not adoption or marriage— the ways white women were redeemed from unwed pregnancy earlier in the century.[25] Sheahan reminded her pro-life audience that "most unwed mothers hope to marry someday," but she also chronicled success among unwed mothers who never got married. In fact, in Sheahan's book on the group, *The Whole Parent,* very few of the composite stories or firsthand testimonials end in marriage. All include some form of increased self-respect, personal responsibility, and reverence for life. For Sheahan, women outside the "natural order" could create good families as long as they avoided abortion and remained chaste. What this means is that in the 1980s and 1990s, the fetus became the emblem not only of the tragedy of a disordered world but also of the redemption of that world through the family.

While UPA existed, a young woman who chose to raise her own child was praised just as much as if she put the baby up for adoption. That changed in the twenty-first century, especially in evangelical circles. Around 2007, evangelical theologians, organizations, and churches began pushing domestic and international adoption as a way for Christians to demonstrate their devotion to the "unwanted." They made adoption into a ministry. This was born in part from pro-life activism; one theologian argued that adopted children "had escaped the abortionist's knife . . . to find at your knee the grace of the carpenter's son." Moreover, in the 1980s and 1990s, a small number of CPCs across the country had rushed women into putting their children up for adoption, then orchestrated placement of those children with evangelical families. The adoption craze in evangelical communities in 2000s and 2010s meant that more evangelical CPCs sidelined their tacit acceptance of single motherhood and adopted more coercive adoption practices. CPCs' adoption enthusiasm however did not translate into higher numbers of women choosing adoption.[26] Because most women did not see "God's calling" in adoption, the anti-abortion movement could never fully displace single motherhood as the most palatable alternative to abortion. For those who prioritized stopping abortions above all, one-parent households had to remain "good families."

Individual people of color who avoided abortion could also be a part of "good families." In fact, Sheahan offered her socially conservative familial model as a way to remake errant families of color. In *The Whole Parent,* Sheahan included a composite story from "Barbara and Paul," who testified to how UPA had reshaped their "Mexican families." Those families had been too "macho" but became comfortable with displays of affection with the help of UPA.[27] The one story Sheahan chose to include in the book about people of color showed how the fetus-focused family could remake the excessive masculinity long associated with ethnic Mexican men. Pro-lifers in other parts of the movement believed the fetus-focused family could also remake women of color. For example, in the 2010s, one crisis pregnancy center in Albuquerque had a wall filled with pictures of women of color and their children, whom the CPC had supposedly saved from abortion.[28] These women and their children, to CPC volunteers and other pro-lifers, were now good families.

Individually, women of color could head the "right" kind of family. However, when the pro-life movement and the New Right telescoped out to talk about single parenthood at the symbolic level, women of color became the faces of family dysfunction. Through the figure of the "welfare queen," white conservatives condemned black women and their children and used those families to undermine public support for a variety of policies supporting the poor. As historian Rickie Solinger has explained, "The politics of reviling and punishing poor mothers for being unemployed, while at the same time making it more difficult for them to receive the education and training necessary to secure family-sustaining jobs, was a hallmark of the Reagan years."[29] The politics of the "traditional family" expose how the corrupting people of color—those who helped undermine society's morals—and the "right kind" of people of color—those white pro-lifers could save—were the same people. They simply existed on different registers of the movement's symbolic politics.

The inclusion of women-headed households and the inclusion of "good" women of color (at least on the individual level) was a product of necessity for the pro-life movement. UPA allowed for the participation of all those touched by unwed pregnancy, including men, women, and grandparents. But fathers, Sheahan recalled, rarely showed up.[30] She added too that "Some fathers . . . take little interest in their children and go to great lengths to avoid paying child support," and she lamented a generation of "fatherless boys" who disregarded "male authority."[31] In the rhetoric of the broader anti-abortion movement, men appeared only peripherally in search of a parental responsibility denied to them by women and the state. For example, Arizona Right to Life used Father's Day in 1980 to protest outside an abortion clinic because "fathers have no rights over unborn children."[32] While activists bemoaned the absence of men's rights in abortion decisions, the Supreme Court firmly settled the issue in the 1976 *Planned Parenthood of Central Missouri v. Danforth* decision and the 1992 *Planned Parenthood of Southeastern Pennsylvania v. Casey* decision. In the 1976 case, the court ruled that states could not require a husband's consent to an abortion. Sixteen years later the court ruled that a Pennsylvania law requiring the spouse to be notified before an abortion placed an "undue burden" on women accessing the procedure.[33] These decisions did not stop anti-abortion groups from pushing spousal consent and notification bills on the state level, but they did mean that activists gave such laws less attention.[34] UPA and other parts of the movement were deeply concerned about the effect abortion had on men's rights and masculinity but, out of legal necessity, these concerns remained on the movement's margins.

White pro-life activists helped conjure the "traditional family" in the late 1970s and 1980s by adding the fetus as one of its primary members and by making pro-life arguments central to its politics. The fetus-focused family entered Americans' lives in formal political spaces and more intimate spaces, like self-help groups. For the more than 2,000 Arizonans that joined Unwed Parents Anonymous over its thirty years of existence, Margot Sheahan hoped to help transform a personal crisis into a possibility for personal growth, but she also helped transform conceptions of family, from the nuclear family with a breadwinner at its heart to the "traditional" family with the fetus at its heart. Such politics would become a central part of the "pro-family" coalition. When the family values movement began to coalesce, pro-life activists brought to the party their newly fashioned old-fashioned family.

NEW MEXICO CONFERENCE ON FAMILIES

One important flashpoint for competing notions of family was the 1980 White House Conference on Families, a set of national and state-based conferences where President Jimmy Carter envisioned Americans could discuss how to strengthen families. His plan, which included many local and state conferences followed by three national conferences, would not come to fruition until the end of his presidency. Carter had envisioned the conferences as creating a middle ground between liberals and the nascent social conservative movement, but that was not to be. At all levels, the Conference on Families highlighted deeply entrenched social divisions rather than facilitating political reconciliations. The state conferences, especially, offered places for white social conservatives to flex their political muscles, all while molding and imposing their definition of family. This was nowhere more true than in New Mexico.

In New Mexico, white social conservatives did more than dominate the discussion and debate feminists; they imposed their definition of family on a variety of people with a variety of different concerns. Pro-life activists led the charge, rallying their troops to make sure New Mexicans went to the national conference in Los Angeles representing the "traditional family." Here, the fetus-focused, conservative, idealized family trumped all other concerns, including the demise of ethnic cultures, economic decline, juvenile crime, alcoholism, and women's oppression. Appropriating the language of genocide and anti-racism, white pro-lifers used their socially conservative multiculturalism to drown out people of color, poor people, religious liberals, and feminists.

Headed by Democratic governor Bruce King's wife, Alice King, the Council for the New Mexico Conference on Families organized the state's conferences. Each of the seven districts in the state was responsible for holding city, county, and district hearings. Twelve state delegates then went to the national conference in Los Angeles.[35] The council hoped that the state conference would stimulate unity and activism within New Mexico, acknowledging problems for a wide variety of families and offering solutions. At least one New Mexican argued that the conference and its attendant hearings were an "extraordinary effort at 'government of the people, by the people, for the people.'"[36] And in certain parts of the state, democracy looked triumphant. Many of the local and district conferences, held in March 1980, occurred without major disruption, especially in the sparsely populated central and southern parts of the state, where attendees were fairly evenly divided between Anglos and ethnic Mexicans. In these meetings, no particular political view dominated the list of issues, and participants offered a mix of familial concerns and an array of political solutions.[37]

Meetings held in other parts of the state, especially the northern parts, however, were divided and contentious. In district 1, which included two counties in the northwestern part of the state, there was a clear division between the speakers at the local meetings. Encompassing San Juan and McKinley counties, this region included Diné (Navajo), Zuni, Anglo, and ethnic Mexican people, people whose lives had been shaped by uranium mining and the Cold War extractive economy.[38] In the immediate postwar period, many saw the uranium industry as an economic boon in an area otherwise plagued by poverty (especially among Native peoples). Towns had grown exponentially as the Cold War brought migrants to the state's extractive hinterlands. But by the 1970s, it was clear that the uranium industry had taken its toll. Medical experts soon found that Diné uranium miners were contracting lung cancer at incredible rates, and in 1979, a uranium mill in the

Navajo Nation spilled over one thousand tons of radioactive waste, making it the largest such spill in U.S. history.[39]

By 1980, this region was economically thriving only for a select few. For most residents, it promised poverty, isolation, pollution, and exploitation. Some of these economic, environmental, and social divisions could be seen in the district Conference on Families. The meeting was bilingual, with roughly half speaking in English and the other half in Navajo. At least one attendee, the vice president of a chapter of the Navajo Nation, noted that he had never seen a meeting where "there were Indians and non-Indians in attendance."[40] If the meeting proved anything, however, it was how different the interests of the Native American people in the region were from those of local Anglos.

Participants discussed education, health, social services, and government. Of the first ten speakers, all of whom focused on education, seven spoke in English and three in Navajo. All of the English speakers addressed the same general theme: public schools were corrupting children and thus the family. As an arm of government control, schools were no longer Christian or patriotic, but rather were indoctrinating children in evolution, sex education, and "values modification," the speakers contended. An English speaker representing "a group of Christian women" argued that schools should be free of both secularism and gay teachers, and ultimately that "more freedom should be return[ed] to the individual."[41] Almost all English speakers blamed public schools (and the government) for moral decline and deteriorating families.

The testimony of the Navajo speakers articulated a different vision, despite the Diné's vexed history with formal schooling. In the first half of the century, a minority of Navajo children had attended industrial boarding schools for Indians, institutions designed to sever children from their parents, language, and culture and prepare them for primarily unskilled, low-paying wage labor. Many Navajo parents had resisted this system, avoiding schools altogether or else sending their children to mission or day schools nearby.[42] In the postwar period, increasing numbers of Navajo children went through formal education and many saw hope for advancement and maintenance of their identities in community-controlled schools.[43] At the district 1 conference meeting, one Navajo speaker, a self-identified recovering alcoholic who had been "saved by Christianity," testified on the value of education. He had been forced to work for his family herding sheep and was not able to go to school, but he noted that he "yearned for knowledge . . . transmitted by formal education." Another Navajo speaker said he hoped that tribal leaders, government agencies, health officials, and families could work together. United, they could "guide [their] children to be responsible citizens" and "gain pride" in themselves.⁴⁴ Though Diné people had a much more complicated relationship with schooling than local Anglos did, they refused to join the English-speaking conservatives in demonizing teachers and public schools.

The meeting's discussion on health focused on abortion, due to the English speakers in the room. Those attendees advocated making divorces harder to get, defunding Planned Parenthood, and requiring parental consent for contraception, but spent a majority of their time discussing the "evil and wick[ed] practice" of abortion. One English speaker discussed at length the role of abortion in the deterioration of the family. The federal government, he said, killed some children and indoctrinated others. He suggested that this was undermining the family's right to reproduce, both physically and ideologically. He argued, "Abortion is the invasion of the family['s] basic right—life and the right to live . . . in peace."⁴⁵ This speaker made "life" the central right of the family and thus abortion into the primary problem. Navajo speakers disagreed. Almost all of them used their time to talk about the need for programs to promote clean water, electricity, holistic health practices, education, and health services for disabled people. The Diné, like other Native people, had borne the brunt of racist, destructive, and misguided federal programs. But without economic privilege and the political illusion that society was organized as a meritocracy, the Navajo speakers had a more clear-eyed view of federal programs than the English speakers, seeing both their benefits and detriments. Rather than promote the fiction that the federal government could be completely removed from their daily lives, the attending Diné used the conference proceedings to try to influence the shape that future government intervention might take.

In another part of northern New Mexico, a conservative group also attended county and district meetings with more controversial results. In district 2, which included Taos, Santa Fe, Los Alamos, Rio Arriba, Mora, Colfax, and San Miguel counties, anti-abortion activists controlled many of the preliminary hearings.⁴⁶ This was especially true in Los Alamos, a county dominated by the Los Alamos National Laboratory and the highly educated, mostly white migrants who came to work for it. The roughly ninety attendees at the Los Alamos meeting advanced a socially conservative agenda, identifying as their top three concerns abortion, government usurpation of parental rights, and expanding definitions of family. Abortion was their number one issue by far; it received double the votes the number two issue got.[47] District rules required that Los Alamos residents bring these topics to the district meeting, where all the counties together would decide their most important concerns and elect their representative to the state meeting.

Many prepared for a political standoff at the district meeting. Before it began, one state Conference on Families council member warned, "I realize that the intentions of the pro-life people are good, but they may not realize they are shutting out other voices." A staunch pro-life state representative and one of very few prominent anti-abortion *hispanos,* Silas García responded, "Programs which promote abortion and promiscuity among our young people hurt the family. . . . Other issues will come up and may be expressed, and they are important. . . . But the root of the problem is in morality."[48] For good reason, many came to the meeting worried that the results would not fully reflect the diversity of New Mexico's families.

By all accounts, pro-lifers dominated the district meeting for Taos, Santa Fe, Los Alamos, and Rio Arriba counties.[49] One conservative recounted how "the speakers were ten-to-one against abortion."[50] Los Alamos and Santa Fe counties were slotted for the afternoon, and their representatives "gave numerous and repetitive presentations opposing sex education, ERA and abortion."[51] A district 2 council member complained about the "premeditated effort to dominate the Los Alamos, Santa Fe time allocation by a group of people hoping to prove the main concerns of the northern district were anti-abortion, anti-sex education and anti-Equal Rights Amendment at the district conference."[52] Many others complained that this group was "rude and pushy," and had not been present for the testimonies from the other counties.[53]

Eventually, through their sheer numbers, the Santa Fe and Los Alamos representatives dominated written and oral testimony as well as the voting for the topics that went to the state conference. Between written and oral testimony, 230 spoke against legalized abortion. The next highest number of testimonies on a particular issue was 83.[54] This group elected Mary Bond, a Los Alamos anti-abortion activist, to represent the entire district.[55] Bond received 83 votes, and her nearest competitor earned only 32.[56] Though many had arrived at the meeting concerned with a wide range of issues, social conservatives overwhelmed other attendees and voted that abortion was the primary threat to the American family.

Some protested the results of the meeting, especially those from Rio Arriba, a county that borders Colorado and includes a diverse array of residents, from the impoverished, largely *hispano* town of Española in the south to the Jicarilla Apache Nation in the north. Rio Arriba, though economically poor, had a rich and complicated history. American conquest of the region had impoverished Rio Arriba's indigenous and *nuevomexicano* population and, in the mid-twentieth century, the Los Alamos National Laboratory exacerbated the county's poverty, drawing many *nuevomexicano* residents into low-wage jobs long distances from their homes.[57] By the 1980s, Rio Arriba county was one of the poorest in the state.[58] Over 27 percent of its families were living in poverty in 1980, more than double the national poverty rate at the time.[59] Thus at the time of the conference, Rio Arriba residents had a long history of dispossession (often by their Anglo neighbors) and a long list of present concerns, concerns that went unanswered at their district meeting.

Ten participants from the county (which included both *nuevomexicanos* and Anglos) wrote a Santa Fe newspaper that their interests had been silenced at the meeting. In the testimony from Rio Arriba and Taos counties, residents had spoken on issues of "early childhood services, problems of the aged, health care in isolated areas, the effects of uranium mining, disruption of the family, needs of the handicapped, [and] problems of child abuse and child neglect." Representatives from Los Alamos and Santa Fe counties had completely ignored such issues. This political division, the ten argued, had class and racial connotations. They also contended Mary Bond could not "represent honestly the concerns of Taos and Rio Arriba counties with its Chicano and Indian majority." Their plea concluded with a rhetorical question: "Is it not absurd to send a member of one of the wealthiest counties in New Mexico (Los Alamos) to represent one of the poorest counties in the nation?"[60] For these people, the pro-life cause represented a campaign by the privileged that silenced voices for racial and economic justice.

Nevertheless, the group from Los Alamos and Santa Fe had broken no rules. Conservatives reminded the protestors and the larger New Mexican audience of just that fact. Mary Bond herself noted that conference procedures had been set long before. District committees had reached out to a variety of organizations and had publicized the local and district meetings. Every county had been allotted the same amount of time to testify, and representatives all had the same opportunity to vote. Bond and others from Los Alamos contended that people only complained "when they saw they were losing the ballgame."[61] Ultimately, conservatives had played by the rules, even if they had undercut the conference's broader purpose. The rules favored the voices of the economically privileged, those who could take the time to

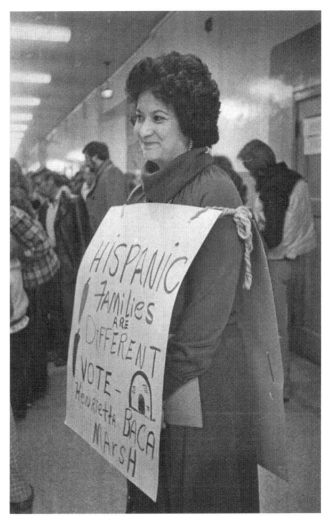

FIGURE 13. Henrietta Baca Marsh participating in the Conference on Families in Colorado. Her sign made a claim similar to one made by many New Mexico participants: that people of color had special familial concerns, 1980. (Courtesy of Getty Images; *Denver Post*)

attend meetings until the very end. Because economic privilege frequently fell along racial lines in this region, and despite the conference committee's best intentions, it was less likely that ethnic Mexican and Native people would have their interests represented. In district 2, white conservatives showed that majoritarian rules could be used to push a narrow political program rather than represent the complexity of New Mexico's families.

These meetings foreshadowed the dynamics of the state conference in Albuquerque. There, many attendees observed that a contingent of participants wearing red roses—a sign of the anti-abortion movement—took over almost every session.[62] Attendees in Albuquerque were supposed to determine what issues were most important to the broad categories of interest the rest of the state had voted on. In many workshops, one journalist recounted, "the effect of the voting . . . was to entirely change the intent of the topic, thanks to the red roses."[63] For example, in district meetings under the topic "Family Crisis/Violence," many had expressed concern over child abuse, spousal abuse, alcoholism, drug abuse, and incest. In the state conference workshop on this topic, however, attendees disregarded these issues and instead voted to express concern over government interference with child discipline and rising rates of divorce. A minority report disagreed, saying "violence is the threat to the integrity of the family, not services to aid the victims."[64] The workshops on the topics "Families and Major Institutions" and "Families and Government" came to be forums on the criminalization of abortion, prohibition of state funding for abortion, and parental consent for contraception and abortion. One journalist noted as well that issues discussed at district meetings—including "widespread unemployment in rural counties," "lack of adequate child care," and the effects of uranium mining—were all ignored.[65] Finally, the state conference nominated four delegates to send to the national conference in Los Angeles. All, according to observers, were white and members of the anti-abortion movement.[66] "What was supposed to be a conference," explained a reporter, "became a one-sided power play."[67]

The policy recommendations that came from the conference focused on the state-protected, idealized traditional family. While white social conservatives argued that the government needed to "get out" of the family, most of their policy recommendations advocated using the long arm of the state for conservative ends.[68] They called for a constitutional amendment banning abortion, state laws that mandated teaching pro-life ideology in public schools, and a federal agency overseeing the protection of the (heterosexual) family. They added demands for state and federal programs that gave hiring preference to heads of household, as well as laws that prohibited the media from discussing any sexuality other than heterosexuality.[69] To social conservatives, these were less government invasions than familial protections. White social conservatives added familial "rights" to their "civil rights movement" for fetuses. At New Mexico's conference, conservatives envisioned a nuclear family unit that protected the rights and morals of its members but that could not survive without state support. Rather than protecting individual liberty or funding programs for people in need, white conservatives contended, the state was dutybound to protect this familial model.

What happened in New Mexico happened elsewhere. Arizona, for instance, witnessed similar outcomes. A phone survey showed that Arizonans were worried about a range of issues, and only ranked abortion as their twenty-third most important issue. At the state's Conference on Families, however, social conservatives dominated the meetings and ranked "moral issues" high in the state's list of priorities. They voted abortion their number two issue of concern, after child abuse and neglect. As in New Mexico, conference participants were not representative of the state's population. They were more white, married, female, and middle class than the state at large.[70]

In Arizona, New Mexico, and elsewhere, a privileged minority—white social conservatives—silenced the majority with the battle cry of "civil rights." One New Mexico journalist explained: "The smaller and less organized voices in Spanish, and in the Pueblo tongues and those who speak for the dispersed and disadvantaged or for the unique ethnic traditions within New Mexico were time after time outmanned, outnumbered, outmaneuvered."[71] Another journalist protested: "And suddenly our state, with or without your or my support, is going to that national conference sounding like we have never moved beyond the level of the Scopes monkey trial in Tennessee."[72] Ultimately the report sent to Washington from New Mexico was deeply conflicted—but it also perfectly encapsulated the racial politics of the anti-abortion movement. The cover letter was written in Spanish, English, Tewa (a Pueblo language), and Navajo, but the document as a whole held only the views of an increasingly powerful and organized conservative, white minority.

The 1980 Conference on Families in New Mexico was an important moment for white social-conservative mobilization around the fetus-focused traditional family. In the New Mexico conference, conservative activists made clear that legalized abortion was the biggest threat to the family and that opposition to abortion was the most essential family value. The conference also showed how successful anti-abortion activists were at mobilizing other white conservatives around this vision. They were building a base, and at the same time, deploying this conservative politics of family to drown out a lot of other familial concerns, often those expressed by nonwhite and poor people. A group supposedly in solidarity with civil rights movements refused to prioritize child abuse, pollution, and access to health care and public education as serious problems. Conservatives even sidelined many problems originating with the federal government, like the effects of Cold War uranium mining. They could not conceive of familial concerns outside of abortion and those supposedly threatening the heterosexual traditional family. Thus, in this instance, and in many other cultural and political arenas in the late twentieth century, the roar of outrage from "family values" conservatives silenced the economic, social, and health concerns of a host of others.

The tenor of state conferences did not bode well for the three national conferences. They, too, showed how differently Americans defined the family, its problems and solutions. Liberals had gotten the word "family" in the conference's initial title changed to "families." Conservatives were irate at the suggestion that the government should support a variety of familial forms—especially those without an abortion averted. Observers at the time and historians since have called the resulting national conferences in Los Angeles, Minneapolis, and Baltimore "angry," "bitter," and political "hornet's nest[s]."[73] In Los Angeles, where New Mexico's delegates attended, fifty conference participants protested legal abortion by tearing up their ballots for a family planning resolution and depositing them under an American flag.[74] Altogether, the national conferences put forward sixty-four potential solutions to familial problems. Thirty-four passed with a majority vote, but only seven got more than 90 percent support.[75] In all these conferences, white social conservatives demanded that legal abortion was a threat to the "traditional family" and the fetus was a core member of that family.

FOCUS ON THE FAMILY

In the last two decades of the twentieth century, pro-life activists worked in concert with other conservatives to influence policy, helping redefine the politics of the "traditional family." Alongside this political activism, purveyors in the Christian cultural products industry worked to market and sell this idealized family, which in turn helped make the conservative vision central to many individuals' sense of their own families. The Christian cultural products industry included music, films, books, toys, jewelry, bumper stickers, magazines, and tchotchkes sold through mail order, Christian and secular bookstores, and eventually the internet and major retail outlets like Walmart. Certain Christian businesses also added radio and television programs to their repertoire. One of the most important of these marketers was Focus on the Family, a nonprofit media empire run by evangelical psychologist James Dobson.

Born to an itinerant evangelical minister and a housewife in Louisiana, James Dobson moved west to attend a small Christian college in California, eventually getting his Ph.D. in psychology at the University of Southern California in 1967. While working at the Children's Hospital of Los Angeles, he said he witnessed the excesses of the sexual revolution. Dobson wrote that he "saw firsthand how divorce, abuse, and other forms of familial strife were tearing [children's] lives apart." His time there, Dobson stated, "only served to confirm my belief that the institution of the family was disintegrating."[76] In order to counter these social trends, Dobson wrote *Dare to Discipline,* his 1970 book which criticized "permissive" parenting and promoted a firm but loving familial hierarchy.[77] The book became an immediate bestseller. Dobson wrote later that he "had discovered that husbands and wives around the country were hungry for ways to restore broken marriages, raise well-adjusted children, and return to Judeo-Christian ethics."[78] Because of the overwhelming response to his book and to subsequent speaking engagements, Dobson created Focus on the Family in 1977.

In Focus on the Family's early years, Dobson organized parenting and family life presentations and seminars around Southern California, focusing on issues from adolescent psychology to the causes of depression in women. His brand of evangelical family management struck a chord. In 1981, he began a thirty-minute radio talk show that, by 1986, was broadcast on eight hundred radio stations nationwide.[79] In the midst of his success, Dobson moved his organization to Colorado Springs. By the mid-1990s, Focus on the Family had an enormous audience, drawing crowds of 15,000 to Dobson's speaking events, speaking to 2.4 million people monthly through newsletters, and reaching an estimated 8.9 million Americans (and 220 million worldwide) through Dobson's radio program.[80] The organization responded to 250,000 letters a month.[81] Jerry Falwell, head of the Moral Majority, called Dobson, a psychiatrist with no religious training, "the most influential minister in America today, second possibly only to Billy Graham."[82]

Dobson's congregation was made up of a very particular demographic: white women. They were mostly college educated, Protestant, and between the ages of 30 and 49. About half worked full time outside the home. They were also politically active: 90 percent voted in 1988.[83] Dobson explained his female audience this way: "No modern society can exceed the stability of its individual family units and women seem more aware of that fact than their husbands."[84] Religious studies scholar Ann Burlein argues that Dobson offered patriarchy as the solution to "the widespread devaluation of women and women's work."[85] Dobson and the rest of the pro-life movement also offered a socially conservative justice movement as the solution to the social devaluation of whiteness. Taping into deep reservoirs of gendered and racial angst, Dobson built an empire.

Dobson asserted that Focus on the Family was concerned strictly with families, not politics. Yet he regularly included fetuses (and anti-abortion politics) in his vision of the supposedly apolitical traditional family. Dobson's newsletters provided a list of the group's primary commitments, called "This We Believe." The column described what exactly the "traditional family" meant to Focus on the Family and, hopefully, to its readers. The family contained four essential parts: it was Christian, it was permanent, it was made to produce children, and it was committed to the "unborn" and all other human life.[86] In the Focus on the Family headquarters in Colorado Springs, Dobson even included fetuses in his own familial genealogy. In a room with family portraits going back four generations, one section focused on a maternal great grandmother who prayed for the entire family "including generations unborn."[87] Anti-abortion politics was no mere extension of Dobson's concern over the "traditional family." Fetuses were a central part of that family.

In his 1986 co-authored book on abortion, *The Decision of Life,* Dobson insisted that the Bible provided evidence that it was God's will to make the fetus a part of the family. Using quotes from the books of Genesis, Jeremiah, Luke, Matthew, and Psalms, Dobson argued that fetuses were known by God and formed by God. God made individuals in the womb to be a part of the family, and abortion severed that life and that familial connection. "If I am the last voice of protest on the face of this earth and am hated and hounded by the bloody industry that profits from the destruction of human life," he concluded, "I will continue to speak on this evil."[88] In Dobson's worldview, God, not people, made families and fetuses were simply unborn members of those families.

Dobson threw himself into abortion politics, despite his initial caution on most other political issues. He segregated formal politics into his magazine, *Citizen,* created in 1987. But not abortion. Because fetuses were a part of the family, legal abortion demanded a place in all Focus on the Family publications.[89] Outside of articles and news updates, Focus on the Family distributed pro-life pamphlets, letters, videos, and audiocassettes.[90] In the late 1980s and 1990s, articles on abortion even appeared in the magazines targeted at children. Two 1990 issues of *Brio,* the magazine geared toward eight- to twelve-year-olds, contained crosswords about abortion, for example.[91] In many of these forums, authors narrated fetuses as family members at risk. In a 1993 issue of *Focus on the Family* magazine, a woman told readers of her son's girlfriend's abortion. She had pleaded with the pregnant woman: "This baby is already part of our family."[92]

The villains of Focus on the Family's abortion stories were stock characters: careless men, socially brainwashed friends, and nefarious abortion providers. But now and again other, queerer adversaries exposed the fetus-focused family. In a May 1993 *Focus on the Family* magazine, one teen pro-life protestor recounted her experience with pro-choice activists: "Once I was in Houston at an abortion clinic, and a bunch of guys with the ACT-Up AIDS activist group had a 'kiss-in.' That's where they walk up to you and start French-kissing each other for five minutes or so ... Sometimes lesbians will chant and say nasty things to me." Legal abortion's attack on the family was made stark by the gay men and lesbians who supported it. To conservatives, these people embodied a rejection of the family; it was in their queer French-kissing and unladylike "nasty" invective, all while AIDS hovered in the air. Of course, this teen was not the only anti-abortion activist to use anti-gay hysteria to signal abortion's threat to the family. Radical activist Norman Weslin claimed that only four types of people worked for Planned Parenthood: "homosexuals, drug addicts, satan worshippers, and 'deathscorts.'" Weslin also claimed that pro-choice activists had poured "AIDS-infected urine" on his group.[93]

This anti-gay rhetoric had real political consequences. In 1992, James Dobson and Focus on the Family helped pass a referendum in Colorado banning laws that protected gays and lesbians from discrimination. The referendum would never have received the required signatures to get on the ballot without the support of Focus on the Family. This effort was born, in part, from Dobson's belief that "homosexual activists" led the movement to "redefine the family."[94] Over the years, pro-life and family values conservatives—most especially Focus on the Family—would connect abortion and gay rights over and over again.[95] Gay supporters of legal abortion secured the fetus's place in the traditional family, while the fetus proved the "perversity" of families that could not reproduce.

While Dobson openly and angrily opposed gay people and their families, he was marginally comfortable with single motherhood. Though Focus on the Family criticized the rising rates of single parenthood, the organization preferred single mothers to aborted fetuses. As with Unwed Parents Anonymous, Focus on the Family stories about abortion often ended with a woman realizing the truth of fetal life, not with the redemption of adoption or marriage. Focus on the Family authors suggested that single pregnant women should consider keeping their babies. "God will assume the role of father to the fatherless," one article explained. Adoption was often offered as a possible solution but was not privileged over single motherhood. Some Focus on the Family contributors noted that God would convey to the woman which option was better for her.[96]

Dobson gave material aid to crisis pregnancy centers, institutions in the business of convincing young women to become single mothers. In the 1980s and 1990s, he helped CPCs around the country solicit donations and also alerted them to the possibility they could obtain government funding.[97] In the early 2000s, Focus on the Family began a fundraising program to help buy ultrasound equipment for CPCs, which within ten years garnered upward of $900,000.[98] Dobson in these years put much effort and many resources toward single motherhood, even as he denounced its presence in American society. Ultimately, stopping abortions superseded all of Focus on the Family's other political concerns.

Dobson's pro-life stance did not go unnoticed. When Dobson would go out in public, one of his right-hand men recounted, "people would hug him and tell him how much they'd appreciate[d] his stand on abortion."[99] When anthropologist Susan Ridgeley studied how Dobson listeners applied his principles in the 1990s and 2000s, she found that family values politics "mainly seemed to mean" an opposition to legal abortion. Moreover, partly as a result of Dobson's advocacy, these people were likely to talk to friends and neighbors about their pro-life beliefs.[100] Dobson's clarion call resonated with white evangelicals across the country, partly because they were already primed by decades of pro-life activism to hear him.

Dobson eventually became more comfortable intervening in electoral politics. He created the Family Research Council in 1983 as his lobbying arm, but by the mid-1990s, that was not enough. He began using his stage at Focus on the Family to speak directly to the Republican Party. In 1995, he sent a letter to 2.1 million Americans as well as 8,000 local and national politicians, criticizing the Republican Party's stance on abortion. He said he was worried that after opposing abortion for two decades, the party was going to "build a 'big tent' under which the great moral issues of the day can be skirted." In his view, party leaders had been "intransigent and unsympathetic" to anti-abortion activists and he pledged "never again [to] vote for a politician who would kill one innocent baby."[101] Some criticized this missive as too explicitly political for a nonprofit group.[102]

Dobson's defenders, however, argued the letter was a part of a necessary moral crusade, whether it was explicitly political or not. One Coloradoan wrote his local newspaper that Dobson's abortion letter "was not about politics. It's about a war against God and the beliefs this nation was founded on."[103] Another wrote that "Abortion is without question the most important social issue of our time. . . . Dr. Dobson reminds me of Abraham Lincoln, who wasn't always popular with everyone either when he spoke out against social injustice."[104] Evangelical leader Ted Haggard likened Dobson to black race rebels: "Martin Luther King helped African Americans unlike anyone in a hundred years, and Jim Dobson is the leader for civil rights of people who can't speak for themselves: unborn babies."[105] Pro-life politics, in other words, constituted a moral human rights campaign, one with a deep history that was separate from the spin and compromise of partisan politics.

With the blessing of his followers, James Dobson continued to intervene in electoral politics, becoming one of the Religious Right's kingmakers. By the late 1990s, Dobson, along with others like Pat Robertson of the Christian Coalition and Gary Bauer of the Family Research Council, declared they would no longer be "good soldiers" for the Republican Party. They had suffered moderate candidates who said the right things about "life" during campaigns and then ignored socially conservative policy while in office. Dobson demanded that Republicans prioritize abortion, family values, and sexual morality. Republican candidates and elected officials—from Newt Gingrich to John Ashcroft to George W. Bush—lined up to be anointed by these men.[106] Once elected, many made good on their promises.

By the late twentieth century, Focus on the Family had helped integrate the ideology of the "traditional family" into the lives of many Americans. Dobson argued that this fetus-focused family was essential to personal success, community stability, and societal morality. He directed his listeners to vote on pro-life issues and for pro-life candidates, and he pushed the Republican Party to be rigidly and radically pro-life. Dobson made the fetus-focused family both a political rallying cry and a part of an essential personal identity for many white conservative Americans. The "timeless" traditional family had both a new member and a new purpose.

. . .

By the twenty-first century, American politics had been transformed by family values politics and the anti-abortion movement. Small conservative support groups, like Unwed Parents Anonymous, touched a variety of people in their time of need. UPA helped transform a personal crisis into an opportunity for moral transformation, and transform the ideal family from the breadwinner-focused nuclear family to a fetus-focused "traditional" family. Experienced activists and nascent social conservatives took these "values" into local and national political forums, reframing the political imperatives of "the family" and the Republican Party. The New Mexico Conference on Families demonstrates that even in a state where social conservatives were a minority, they were able to dominate political forums and shout down the concerns of feminists, people of color, and poor people at essential moments. In the 1980s and 1990s, empowered by their vision of moral decline and a nation at risk, family values conservatives reached increasingly large national audiences through proliferating conservative media outlets. None were more important than Focus on the Family. This media conglomerate, like so many other socially conservative groups and businesses, found a special home in the American West, but Dobson's empire touched all parts of the country. Thus, in the last decades of the century, this fetus-focused traditional family reached a variety of Americans on personal, political, and cultural levels.

Through the work of pro-life and socially conservative activists, the fetus had become not only a member of the "traditional family," but its justification. The "unborn" proved that the nuclear, heterosexual, hierarchical family was ordained by God. The "unborn" redeemed the unfortunately pregnant woman, changing her from a selfish individualist into a chaste mother. Single mothers, if they had avoided abortion, could now be exemplars of the traditional family and family values. The "unborn" established that this family model was biologically driven, sanctified by nature. The "unborn" and the "abortion Holocaust" demonstrated that the federal government was secular and potentially genocidal, run by feminists, gay people, the radical Left, and atheists. These ideological building blocks became the backbone of the family values movement, as activists used them in a wide range of political campaigns, from movements against funding for the arts to gay rights. Together these ideals made modern American social conservatism.

Conclusion

On April 20, 1999, Eric Harris and Dylan Kiebold walked into their high school in Columbine, Colorado, and murdered twelve students and a teacher. It was the deadliest school shooting in American history up until that point. While the nation mourned and sought explanations for the massacre, anti-abortion activists offered theirs. This tragedy came to the Front Range because Colorado was the "first state to legalize some forms of abortion," Colorado Right to Life said. "Violence in the womb has begotten violence outside the womb." National conservative leaders echoed this claim. Tom Delay, then House Minority Whip, blamed the shootings on abortion culture and the "liberal relativism that has hallowed out too many souls in our society." Seven months later while running for president, George W. Bush alluded to Columbine when he was asked about his stance on abortion. "There is something so wrong with a society where life is so devalued that people . . . walk into a school and blow people away," he said. He sought a world where the "unborn" would be "protected in law."[1]

This may seem like an example of cynical activists exploiting a national calamity, and it was that. But it was also a compelling explanation for those social conservatives who saw abortion as the root of all violence, past and present. Even Brian Rohrbough, the father of one of the Columbine victims. embraced the movement's logic. When asked to comment on later school shootings, he said that the "country was in moral free fall . . . Abortion has diminished the value of children."[2] Rohrbough went on to become a full-time pro-life activist. The anti-abortion movement had offered this man a powerful explanation for the death of his son. It had made abortion personal to someone yet again.

Rohrbough and a host of others hoped that in the twenty-first century, abortion would finally become illegal. They, like the activists who came before them, tried to chip away at abortion access or ban the practice entirely. Using of all their rhetorical tools—especially the language of fetal personhood, slavery, genocide, women's rights, and civil rights—and the many victims they made, pro-life activists made abortion much more difficult to get in the years following the new millennium. At the national level, they helped pass laws prohibiting women on Medicaid from using federal money for abortions, granting an incredible amount of federal money to crisis pregnancy centers through abstinence education, and prohibiting a rare abortion procedure the movement dubbed "partial-birth abortion." At the state level, activists were even more successful—often with the help of the fetus dolls, Precious Feet pins, and gory photos that were the movement's mainstays. The laws they got passed ranged in method and scope. By the twenty-first century, a majority of states required that a minor involve her parents in her abortion decision, either through notification or consent; demanded that a woman wait a certain amount of time before an abortion; restricted abortion after a certain point in gestation (often twenty weeks); limited health care coverage for abortions; and dictated that a woman must be given "counseling"—often with inaccurate information—before an abortion. A host of other anti-abortion laws affected a minority of states.[3] The abortion law of any state was rarely static; anti-abortion activists kept coming up with new ways to stop women from accessing their constitutionally guaranteed rights.

All of this was done in the name of protecting rights: fetal rights first and foremost, but also those of women, children, and families. A white, socially conservative movement had staked out their own corner of the rights revolution. Activists successfully convinced many—from casual observers to Supreme Court justices—that legal abortion infringed upon Americans' rights, as opposed to preserving them. People of color and women of all races were some of the biggest victims of abortion, activists claimed. White anti-abortion activists had long ago used elements of feminism and racial justice movements to prove they knew what was best for the dispossessed. Such ideas motivated activists but also made it into state law. By 2019, eight states had bans for "sex-selective" or "race-selective" abortions, which claimed that abortion was a lethal form of discrimination. Arizona was the first state to pass such a law. The version of these bills proposed to Congress was called the "Susan B. Anthony and Frederick Douglass Prenatal Non-Discrimination Act." Loretta Ross, coordinator of a women of color reproductive justice group, explained: "We are now accused of 'lynching' our children in the womb and practicing white supremacy on ourselves."[4] For white anti-abortion

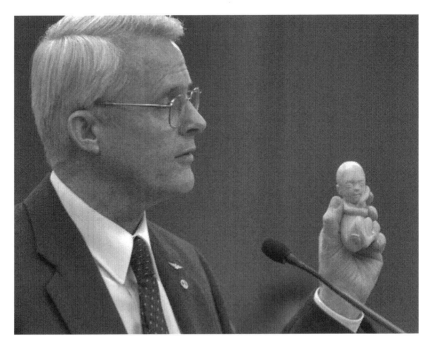

FIGURE 14. In 2005, Richard H. Black, then a member of the Virginia House of Delegates, showed a fetus doll while testifying in favor of a bill that would have required doctors to talk with women about fetal pain before an abortion. Two years earlier, Black sent similar dolls to all his colleagues in advance of a vote requiring parental consent before a minor's abortion. (Courtesy of AP Images)

activists, it was "the contraceptive mind"—it was legal abortion—that devalued the lives of women and people of color. Activists accordingly demanded that (white) children and families join the pantheon of society's "victims."

Because of the size of the socially conservative base and the power of Religious Right leaders, Republicans could only become more devout adherents to the pro-life movement. For many years, anti-abortion activists had to content themselves with politicians who still had a foot in an older Republican Party that had supported abortion reform. By the twenty-first century, the movement elected anti-abortion ideologues—people who could set the stage for overturning *Roe v. Wade*. Those GOP candidates could flout the social mores of both the Left and the Right in their personal lives and still claim the mantle of "morality"—as long as they opposed legal abortion and prioritized ending it. Nominating pro-life Supreme Court justices eventually became the political goal that superseded all others.

This movement did not transform all parts of the country uniformly. In states and regions with large numbers of white conservative Catholics, evangelicals, and Mormons, activists reshaped residents' daily lives in profound ways. While large parts of the Northeast and Pacific Coast remained insulated from the most serious effects of anti-abortion activism, those living in the South, the Plains, the Midwest, and the Mountain West were more likely to experience it keenly. Residents of these regions saw the effects of anti-abortion activism all around them. It changed their rituals of faith in their religious communities; it shifted what their children were taught in school; it created a perplexing maze of abortion law for those in search of reproductive health care; and it had changed many of their neighbors' sense of self. In these regions, especially, the movement helped elect a new breed of Republican who would extend and amplify those effects year after year.

The Mountain West was one of the regions most changed. The once solidly Democratic region had become reliably red by the 1980s. In fact, by the middle of the 1990s, Republicans had 83 percent of the region's delegation to the House of Representatives and 63 percent of the members of its state legislatures. Democrats won now and again but only when they were in the midst of a national-wave election. "How Republican is the Mountain West?" wondered a *High Country News* journalist in 1997. "That's sort of like asking, 'How wet is the ocean?'"[5] Social conservatives did more than just win elections in the region, in other words. Their politics were now so pervasive, so elemental, that it was as if their supremacy was too self-evident to be questioned.

Republican power did not affect all Mountain West states equally or consistently, to be sure. New Mexico, for example, retained more of its Democratic character than the other states, partly because of the relative power of people of color in the state.[6] The state's pro-life movement made very little headway within the state's legislature during the last three decades of the twentieth century. The movement's narrative of itself as the ultimate civil rights campaign never played well to the state's ethnic Mexican and Native American populations. The lesson was clear enough: because of its homogenization and its conservative racial politics, the pro-life movement was not able to adapt successfully in a place where people of color had relatively significant political power.

Anti-abortion activists reshaped all levels of American politics, from the schoolhouse to state legislatures to presidential elections. Indeed, the ways activists politicized people in intimate spaces allowed for the bigger regional and national political transformations. It was in homes, churches, schools, and crisis pregnancy centers, as well as on city sidewalks, where activists laid their groundwork and changed many Americans' relationships to fetal life. Indeed, it was in these spaces where activists asked Christians, women, children, and members of families to re-center their identities around the "defense of life." Over time, they politicized enough people to transform the Republican Party and conservative culture writ large.

In the twenty-first century, that culture helped restrict abortion access and kept Americans from truly addressing the many forms of violence afflicting the nation. If abortion was the origin of gun violence in America, there was no real need for gun reform. Guns were merely the scapegoat for an abortion-related problem. If abortion was at the root of racism, there was no real reason to oppose the gutting of civil rights measures. And if abortion was the source of women's oppression, then abortion restrictions were the only measures that could help. This was a conservative "civil rights movement" that had a single solution for the nation's many problems of discrimination and disenfranchisement, and one of its primary effects has been to undermine most efforts to do anything about them.

The movement's abortion-based explanation for all social ills also left conservatives unprepared and uninterested in dealing with the sexism, racism, and violence within their own ranks. When, in 2017, Trent Franks asked his staffers to be surrogates for him, and probably to have sex with him, the movement he had championed was silent. Neither could the movement explain the child molestation that afflicted pro-life conservative religious communities in the twentieth and twenty-first centuries. When white supremacists combined anti-abortion pleas with full-throated calls for a white nation free of people of color and Jews, the mainstream pro-life movement looked away. Various forms of violence within anti-abortion communities were simply aberrations. The movement certainly ignored the violence it perpetrated. Because of this movement, abortion providers had to risk their lives every day to provide health care for their patients. Some were murdered in the process. Outside abortion clinics women had to maneuver around aggressive protestors to get medical care; they also had to traverse an often hostile legal system that increasingly prioritized fetal lives over their own. Poor women and women of color were usually the ones who bore the brunt of these efforts. Those women were better off, the movement said. They were all helping the nation become truly "pro-life."

In the twenty-first century, pro-choice people worry about a future without *Roe v. Wade*. They worry whether women seeking abortions will again have to inhabit a world of coat hangers and back alleys. But the nation cannot return to the late 1960s. Too many Americans have been changed by the anti-abortion movement already. The world where religious leaders could convincingly claim that abortion was a moral good is gone. The world where increasing access to abortion, even in the narrow cases of incest and rape, was a bipartisan issue has been erased. The world where courts did not try women for murder in cases of illegal abortion is no longer logical. The anti-abortion movement has spent fifty years convincing many Americans that their lives are dependent on preserving fetal lives, and the greatest moral good would be to treat abortion just the same as murder. Americans will have to live with the legacy of that work.

NOTES

INTRODUCTION

1. For mortality rates in Uravan, see Boice, Mumma, and Blot, "Cancer and Noncancer Mortality in Populations Living Near Uranium and Vanadium Mining and Milling Operations in Montrose County, Colorado, 1950–2000," pp. 711–26. For history of Uravan, see Amundson, *Yellowcake Towns.*

2. Katrina Trinko, "Trent Franks, Pro-Life Warrior," *National Review Online,* June 19, 2013, http://www.nationalreview.com/article/351426/trent-franks-pro-life-warrior-katrina-trinko/page/0/2?splash = (accessed July 22, 2013).

3. Sean Sullivan, "Who Is Trent Franks?" *Washington Post,* June 2, 2013.

4. Ibid.

5. "Republicans Hold Fast on Senate Control," *Mohave Daily Miner,* November 7, 1984; Ken Hedler, "Franks Seeks Widening of School Tax Credits," *Kingman Daily Miner,* December 18, 2002; "Abortion Ruling Bodes Ill for Arizona," *Prescott Courier,* June 29, 1992.

6. Adam Serwer, "Republican Presiding Over VRA Hearing Once Claimed Abortion Worse than Slavery," MSNBC, July 7, 2013, http://tv.msnbc.com/2013/07/17/trent-franks-once-claimed-blacks-better-off-under-slavery/ (accessed July 20, 2013); Dana Milbank, "A New Civil Rights Movement?" *Harrisonburg Daily News Record,* December 9, 2011.

7. The abortion rate for black women's unintended pregnancies is only slightly more than the national average of 42 percent. "Unintended Pregnancy in the United States," Guttmacher Institute, January 2019, https://www.guttmacher.org/fact-sheet/unintended-pregnancy-united-states (accessed June 17, 2019).

8. E. J. Montini, "Franks Equates Abortion with Slavery," *Arizona Republic,* March 7, 2010. See also "Top 10 Craziest Tea Party Quotes of All Time," *New Jersey Today,* October 12, 2010; Tim Forkes, "GOP Knuckleheads Continue to Speak," *Baltimore Post-Examiner,* July 1, 2013.

9. "Trent Franks: Withdrawal of Abortion Ban 'One of the Greatest Disappointments of My Life,'" *U.S. Official News,* February 6, 2015.

10. The exception here is post-abortion counseling, which was implemented in crisis pregnancy centers around the country beginning in the 1980s. There activists did try to politicize women's personal experiences with abortion. See chapter 4.

11. For activists' lack of experience with abortion, see Luker, *Abortion and the Politics of Motherhood,* p. 138. Of course, many women had experience with pregnancy but that experience did not simply turn into a belief that life began at conception.

12. For the origin of this phrase, see chapter 5.

13. My analysis has been influenced by Bill Brown's theorization of "things"; philosopher Cornelius Castoriadis's idea of a social imaginary; Lauren Berlant's analysis of late-twentieth-century politics; and Finn Enke's understanding of the role of space in the feminist movement. See Brown, "Thing Theory"; Castoriadis, *The Imaginary Institution of Society;* Berlant, *The Queen of America Goes to Washington City;* Enke, *Finding the Movement.*

14. Seth Dowland argues that the family values movement used the language of liberty in its campaigns, often alienating people of color who otherwise might have been sympathetic. Anti-abortion rhetoric is the outlier to this general trend, however. See Dowland, *Family Values and the Rise of the Christian Right.*

15. Political scientist Joel Olson identifies this new racial formation in the conservative movement as a whole. See Olson, "Whiteness and the Polarization of American Politics," pp. 704–18.

16. For works that highlight the liberal origins of the anti-abortion movement, see Hughes, "The Civil Rights Movement of the 1990s?" pp. 1–23; Ziegler, *After Roe;* Williams, *Defending the Unborn;* Haugeberg, *Women Against Abortion.*

17. Two recent books have analyzed women's role in the anti-abortion movement. See Haugeberg, *Women Against Abortion* and Taranto, *Kitchen Table Politics.* They both build on pioneering work done by sociologists, especially Luker, *Abortion and the Politics of Motherhood* and Ginsburg, *Contested Lives.*

18. Shermer, ed., *Barry Goldwater and the Remaking of the American Political Landscape.* For more on Barry Goldwater and his supporters, see Goldberg, *Barry Goldwater;* Iverson, *Barry Goldwater;* Perlstein, *Before the Storm;* Middendorf, *Glorious Disaster;* Nickerson, *Mothers of Conservatism;* Shermer, *Sunbelt Capitalism;* McGirr, *Suburban Warriors.*

19. Goldwater did not hold to his promise once elected. He quickly reverted to his pro-choice position. See Edwards, *Goldwater,* pp. 404–5. See also interview with John Jakubczyk, March 16, 2010. For more on the divergence of Goldwater conservatism and the Religious Right, see William A. Link, "Time Is an Elusive Companion: Jesse Helms, Barry Goldwater, and the Dynamic of Modern Conservatism," in Shermer, ed., *Barry Goldwater and the Remaking of the Political Landscape,* pp. 238–58.

20. In 1975, journalist Kirpatrick Sale argued that that political power had shifted from the "eastern establishment" to the Sunbelt. He also argued this region's politics was dominated by the three Rs: rightism, racism, and repression. See Sale, *Power Shift.*

21. Robert E. Lang, Mark Muro, and Andrea Sarzynski, "Mountain Megas: America's Newest Metropolitan Places and a Federal Partnership to Help Them Prosper," Brookings Institution, July 20, 2008, p. 11.

22. Silk and Walsh, *One Nation, Divisible,* pp. 157–80 (quotes on p. 157).

23. See, for example, Deutsch, *No Separate Refuge;* Gutiérrez, *When Jesus Came, the Corn Mothers Went Away;* Wilson, *The Myth of Santa Fe;* Brooks, *Captives and Cousins;* Montoya, *Translating Property;* Neito-Phillips, *The Language of Blood;* Mitchell, *Coyote Nation;* Blackhawk, *Violence Over the Land.*

24. See, for example, Sheridan, *Los Tucsonenses* and *Arizona;* Luckingham, *Minorities in Phoenix;* Whitaker, *Race Work;* Jacoby, *Shadows at Dawn;* Benton-Cohen, *Borderline Americans.*

25. See, for example, Arrington, *Great Basin Kingdom;* Shipps, *Mormonism;* Bigler, *Forgotten Kingdom;* Peck, *Reinventing Free Labor;* Gordon, *The Mormon Question;* Blackhawk, *Violence Over the Land;* Mueller, *Race and the Making of the Mormon People.*

26. See, for example, West, *The Contested Plains;* Jameson, *All That Glitters;* Brosnan, *Uniting Mountain and Plain;* Andrews, *Killing for Coal;* Kelman, *A Misplaced Massacre.*

27. Stern, *Eugenic Nation;* Gutiérrez, *Fertile Matters;* Pascoe, *What Comes Naturally;* Torpy, "Native American Women and Coerced Sterilization," pp. 1–22; Lawrence, "The Indian Health Service and the Sterilization of Native American Women," pp. 400–19; Stern and Lira, "Mexican Americans and Eugenic Sterilization," pp. 9–34; Theobald, *Reproduction on the Reservation;* Lira, "Of Low Grade Mexican Parentage."

28. Myra Rich, *A History of Planned Parenthood of the Rocky Mountains* (Denver: Planned Parenthood, 1994), p. 1, folder RMPP, Associations, Committee Minutes, box 1, Rocky Mountain Planned Parenthood Collection, Western History and Genealogy Department, Denver Public Library, Denver, CO; Melcher, *Pregnancy, Motherhood, and Choice in 20th Century Arizona,* pp. 57–76; Davis, *Sacred Work,* p. 105; Schackel, *Social Housekeepers,* pp. 104–6.

29. LDS leaders had made statements over the years regarding fertility control but it was not until 1918, in the face of a rising birth control movement, that the hierarchy issued what amounted to an official statement against birth control. That is not to say Mormons did not practice birth control. Like the rest of the country, Mormon birth rates dipped during the Great Depression, and in the 1950s and 1960s, Mormons were usually having families of five or six children, rather than the ten suggested in earlier years. Bush, "Birth Control Among the Mormons," pp. 12–44 (quote on p. 21).

30. For more on anti-communist, free market, and pro-military conservatism in the Sunbelt, see Markusen et al., *The Rise of the Gunbelt;* Fernlund, ed., *The Cold War American West;* Hevly and Findlay, eds., *The Atomic West;* McGirr, *Suburban Warriors;* Self, *American Babylon;* Avila, *Popular Culture in the Age of White Flight;* Kruse, *White Flight;* Lassiter, *The Silent Majority;* Dochuk, *From Bible Belt to Sunbelt;* Nickerson and Dochuk, eds., *Sunbelt Rising;* Nickerson, *Mothers of Conservatism.* For one

excellent study of late-twentieth-century social conservatism in the region, see Moreton, *To Serve God and Wal-Mart*.

31. Marchant-Shapiro and Patterson, "Partisan Change in the Mountain West," pp. 359–78 (quotes on p. 369).

32. Hartmann, *A War for the Soul of America*, epilogue. For broad works on the culture wars, see Hunter, *Culture Wars;* Martin, *With God on Our Side;* Goldberg, *Kingdom Coming;* Wilcox, *Onward Christian Soldiers?;* Self, *All in the Family;* Williams, *God's Own Party;* Dowland, *Family Values and the Rise of the Christian Right;* Young, *We Gather Together*.

33. Scholars have also done extensive work on the nineteenth-century anti-abortion movement. Most who have studied it argue that, in the mid-nineteenth century, doctors, a previously unregulated group, advocated restrictive state laws on abortion in order to claim superior medical and legal authority over a variety of other healers. By 1900, all states had laws forbidding abortion at any stage of pregnancy, with the exception that doctors could perform therapeutic abortions at their discretion as long as they in some way preserved the life of the mother. See Mohr, *Abortion in America;* Luker, *Abortion and the Politics of Motherhood*, pp. 12–37; Smith-Rosenberg, "The Abortion Movement and the AMA, 1850–1880," in her *Disorderly Conduct*, pp. 217–45; Stormer, *Articulating Life's Memory;* Beisel and Kay, "Abortion, Race and Gender in Nineteenth-Century America," pp. 498–518.

34. Linda Greenhouse and Riva Siegel have recently (and convincingly) overturned common wisdom that pro-life activists had little success slowing abortion liberalization before *Roe*. Previous lines of academic and public thought argued that *Roe*'s radical change motivated an anti-abortion backlash that would not have existed if liberalization had proceeded on the state level. See Greenhouse and Siegel, *Before Roe v. Wade*. For more on pre-*Roe* anti-abortion activism, see Williams, *Defending the Unborn;* Frank, "The Colour of the Unborn," pp. 351–78.

35. National Abortion Federation, "NAF Violence and Disruption Statistics: Incidents of Violence and Disruption Against Abortion Providers in U.S. & Canada," 2009, http://www.prochoice.org/pubs_research/publications/downloads/about_abortion/violence_stats.pdf (accessed June 7, 2012).

36. Haugeberg, *Women Against Abortion;* Risen and Thomas, *Wrath of Angels*.

37. Mason, *Killing for Life*. Dallas Blanchard and Terry Prewitt, in their book on the murders of abortion doctors in Pensacola, Florida, offer a more psychological argument, suggesting that anti-abortion radicals, like many others who perpetuate violence, have a rigid worldview and a deep personal insecurity. See Blanchard and Prewitt, *Religious Violence and Abortion*, p. 274.

38. For other important analyses of abortion politics, see Solinger, ed., *Abortion Wars;* Gorney, *Articles of Faith;* Critchlow, *Intended Consequences;* Munson, *The Making of Pro-Life Activists*.

39. Abortion clinics in Pensacola, Florida, were the targets of anti-abortion violence in the 1980s and 1990s. In the 1980s, at least three abortion clinics were bombed. In the 1990s, pro-life activists murdered three in the city: abortion pro-

vider Dr. David Gunn in 1993 and abortion provider Dr. John Britton and his escort James Barrett in 1994. Wichita, Kansas, was the target of Operation Rescue Summer of Mercy in 1991, when thousands of activists blockaded Dr. George Tiller's abortion clinic over the course of six weeks. Tiller's clinic had been firebombed in 1986 and, in 1993, he was shot in both arms by a radical activist. He went back to work the next day. In 2009, Tiller was murdered in his church by an anti-abortion activist. For books that focus at least in part on one of these two places, see Frank, *What's the Matter with Kansas?;* Blanchard and Prewitt, *Religious Violence and Abortion;* Mason, *Killing for Life;* Risen and Thomas, *Wrath of Angels;* Baird-Windle and Bader, *Targets of Hatred;* Jeffris, *Armed for Life;* Singular, *The Wichita Divide.*

40. See, for example, Maynard-Moody, *The Dilemma of the Fetus;* Haraway, "Fetus," in her *Modest-Witness@Second_Millennium_ FemaleMan_Meets_Onco-Mouse,* pp. 173–213; Introduction to Morgan and Michaels, eds., *Fetal Subjects, Feminist Positions;* Duden, *Disembodying Woman;* Newman, *Fetal Positions;* Casper, *The Making of the Unborn Patient;* Taylor, *The Public Life of the Fetal Sonogram;* Morgan, *Icons of Life.*

41. Dubow, *Ourselves Unborn;* Schoen, *Abortion After Roe.* See also Daniels, *At Women's Expense.*

42. I did an additional three interviews: two with pro-choice activists and one with an abortion provider.

1. ROLLING ACROSS PARTY LINES

1. Interview with Margaret Sebesta (pseudonym), August 8, 2011.

2. Obituary for [Margaret Sebesta], https://www.findagrave.com/cgi-bin/fg .cgi?page = gr&GRid = 126772025&FLid = 74658702&FLgrid = 126772025& (accessed March 6, 2017).

3. Ibid.

4. The early pro-life activists that Kristin Luker interviewed also felt that legal abortion was like a "bolt out of the blue." Luker, *Abortion and the Politics of Motherhood,* p. 126.

5. Williams, *Defending the Unborn,* p. 4.

6. Ziegler, *After Roe.*

7. These activists include Margaret Sebesta (pseudonym), Benedict Urbish, Mary Ford, Marge Wilson, Charles John (Chuck) Onofrio, Elena Onofrio, John Archibold, Marie Hazlitt (Colorado Joint Council on Medical and Social Legislation); Ruth Dolan (Colorado Right to Life); Norman Weslin (Colorado Springs Right to Life); Helen Seader, Phil Seader, Veronica (Lanie) Pawloski, Ora DeConcini, Carey Womble, John Gillette, William A. Riordan, William A. Reese, Bernadine Haag, Adriana Huppenthal, Jack T. Arnold, Nancy Cousins, Doris C. Storms, Libby Ruiz, Nancy Comeau (Tucson Committee for Conservation for Human Life); Carolyn Gerster, Neil and Virginia Clements, William L. Martin, Velma Flowers, Marilyn Giedraitis, Earl J. Baker, Marion A. Jabczenski, Wallace

McWhirter (Arizona Right to Life); Emanuel A. Floor, Helen Struble, Rev. Robert Servatorious (Utah Right to Life League); Bruce Bangerter (American Independence Party, UT); Dennis Ray Dunn, Mrs. Richard Johnson, Bliss Hoover (Utah Anti-Abortion League); Julia Roth, Kathleen (Kathi) Betz (Cache Valley Right to Life, UT); Mrs. Pat Simpson, Janet Carroll, Joan Niernberger (Utah Right to Life); Randall Paz (Las Cruces Right to Life, NM); Ronald V. Dorn, Dorothy Gaeto, Muriel James, Emma Gomez, Harold L. Trott, Thomas G. Glennon, Shirley Hellwig, Mary Seeley, Mr. and Mrs. Leo A. Dunn (New Mexico Right to Life).

8. DeConcini and August, *Senator Dennis DeConcini*, pp. 24–25. For more on conquest of Arizona, see Sheridan, *Arizona,* ch. 5; Jacoby, *Shadows at Dawn.* For Mormon pioneers to the state, see Sheridan, *Arizona,* ch. 10.

9. For Libby Ruiz's father (Nicolas Garcia), see Year: 1930; Census Place: Tucson, Pima, Arizona; Roll: 61; Page: 2B; Enumeration District: 0029; Image: 384.0; FHL microfilm: 2339796 (accessed on Ancestry.com, *1930 United States Federal Census* [database online]; Provo, UT, 2002). For the origin of Libby Ruiz's name, see "Hopefuls' Background Varies," *Tucson Daily Citizen,* September 19, 1977.

10. Carolyn Gerster obituary, *Arizona Republic,* February 3, 2016.

11. Findlay, *Magic Lands,* p. 18. For more on postwar development in this region, see Abbott, *The New Urban America;* Fernlund, ed., *The Cold War American West;* Hevly and Findlay, eds., *The Atomic West;* Luckingham, *Phoenix,* pp. 136–220, and *The Urban Southwest;* Hunner, *Inventing Los Alamos;* Shermer, *Sunbelt Capitalism.*

12. "L. Gillette Dies at 71," *Tucson Daily Citizen,* January 28, 1964.

13. "ABWA Focusing on Visiting Nurses," *Albuquerque Journal,* July 26, 1970.

14. Douglas J. Kreutz, "A Dead Issue?" *Tucson Daily Citizen,* November 2, 1974. Virginia Clements's husband (Neil Clements) was a pediatric surgeon and anti-abortion activist: "Pima County Medical Society Announcement," *Tucson Daily Citizen,* March 31, 1966. Earl J. Baker was a thoracic surgeon: "Drive to Beat 3 Diseases Making Headway in State," *Arizona Republic,* October 15, 1967. Carolyn Gerster was a cardiologist: Carolyn Gerster obituary, *Arizona Republic,* February 3, 2016. Marion Jabczenski was an oncologist: Marion A. Jabczenski obituary, *Arizona Republic,* December 19, 2012.

15. Casper, *The Making of the Unborn Patient;* Morgan, *Icons of Life;* Dubow, *Ourselves Unborn.*

16. Kreutz, "A Dead Issue?"

17. Ibid.

18. Williams, *Defending the Unborn,* pp. 29–36.

19. Nash, *The Federal Landscape,* pp. 77–100.

20. McGirr, *Suburban Warriors,* p. 26.

21. For William Reese's personal history, see William A. Reese, letter to the editor, "Why We Are in Vietnam," *Tucson Daily Citizen,* January 29, 1970; Paul Allen, "D-M Office Opens to Deal with Drug, Race Problems," *Tucson Daily Citizen,* October 16, 1971; Maj. William A. Reese III, letter to the editor, "An Appeal to Nixon," *Tucson Daily Citizen,* February 22, 1973. For William Riordan's personal

history, see "Ex D-M Airman in Law Firm," *Tucson Daily Citizen,* January 29, 1964. For Jack Arnold's personal history, see Jack T. Arnold obituary, *Arizona Daily Star,* October 31, 2013.

22. For Leo Dunn, see Ken Wilkinson, "Issues Should Be Stressed, Not Personalities: Dunn," *Albuquerque Journal,* March 21, 1966. For the importance of the Sandia Corporation in the state, see Wood, *The Postwar Transformation of Albuquerque, New Mexico.*

23. It is not clear which denomination McWhirter was a member of, but given his birthplace, it is likely that he was an evangelical of some stripe. For McWhirter's personal history, see "In Memoriam: Wallace W. McWhirter M.D., 1919–1979," *Arizona Lifeline,* September 1979, University of Arizona Library Special Collections, University of Arizona, Tucson, AZ. Velma Flowers and Carey Womble also hailed from the South and the Plains.

24. Dochuk, *From Bible Belt to Sunbelt,* p. xx. For "southernization" of the U.S. West (especially California), see Gregory, *American Exodus* and *The Southern Diaspora.* For "southernization" of American politics, see Egerton, *The Americanization of Dixie;* Carter, *The Politics of Rage,* pp. 324–70; Schulman, *The Seventies;* Applebome, *Dixie Rising;* Feldman, *The Great Melding.*

25. "In Memoriam," *Arizona Lifeline,* September 1979.

26. Dudley, *Broken Words,* pp. 43–44. For more on this conference, see Flipse, "Below-the-Belt Politics," in *Conservative Sixties,* pp. 127–41.

27. Williams, *God's Own Party,* p. 115.

28. Dudley, *Broken Words,* p. 43. For more on these successive resolutions, see Williams, *God's Own Party,* pp. 118–19.

29. Tentler, *Catholics and Contraception,* p. 79.

30. Bernice Maher Mooney, "The Catholic Church in Utah," in *Utah History Encyclopedia,* p. 78. See also Mooney and Fitzgerald, *Salt of the Earth;* Pehl, "Wherever They Mention His Name," in *Catholicism in the American West,* pp. 73–94.

31. Peter J. Scarlet, "Catholics Still Lead in Fight Against Abortion," *Salt Lake Tribune,* October 16, 1976. By 1976, the membership of Utah Right to Life had diversified to include Mormons, though Catholics still made up 50 percent of the group.

32. "Business Portrait: Executive Draws on Wide Experience," *Salt Lake Tribune,* June 1, 1975. For more on Floor, see "Major Tourist Push Lined Up by State," *Ogden Standard-Examiner,* June 10, 1965; "Travel Council of Utah Is Optimistic," *Logan Herald Journal,* February 16, 1966; "Tourist Aide Sought by Utah Panel," *Salt Lake Tribune,* November 14, 1966; "Floor Resigns USU Position," *Logan Herald Journal,* May 6, 1968; "Two Controversial Bills Debated," *Ogden Standard-Examiner,* January 24, 1969.

33. "Fast Action on Abortion Law Sought," *Provo Herald,* June 17, 1973; "President of the Anti-Abortion League Reports to the People," *Provo Herald,* April 10, 1974.

34. "Vatican Council II," *Encyclopedia of American Religious History,* vol. 1, p. 1021.

35. Maines and McCallion, *Transforming Catholicism*, p. 1.

36. Gillis, "Vatican II," in *Religion and American Cultures Encyclopedia*, pp. 94–96. For a sampling of the literature on the Vatican II reforms and their implications, see McDannell, *Spirit of Vatican II;* Faggioli, *Vatican II;* O'Malley, *Tradition and Transition;* Massa, *The American Catholic Revolution*.

37. Cuneo, *The Smoke of Satan*, p. 22.

38. For California activists, see Luker, *Abortion and the Politics of Motherhood*, p. 128.

39. Activists who were a part or leaders of the Council of Catholic Women include: Helen Seader, Mrs. Leo Dunn, Shirley Hellwig, Emma Gomez, Mary Ford, Elena (Helen) Onofrio, and Marie Hazlitt.

40. Dolan, *The American Catholic Experience*, p. 395. The Christian Family Movement was also created out of these concerns. For more on the CCW, see Petit, "Organized Catholic Womanhood," in *Remapping the History of American Catholicism in the United States*, pp. 49–70; Lindley, *You Have Stept Out of Your Place*, p. 361; Harmon, *There Were Also Many Women There*, pp. 57–58; Weaver, *New Catholic Women*, pp. 119–22; MacCarthy, "Catholic Women and War," pp. 23–32.

41. Historian Stacie Taranto argues that it was the combination of lay empowerment and the sexual conservatism of *Humanae Vitae* that primed so many Catholic women to become pro-life activists. Taranto, *Kitchen Table Politics*, pp. 35–58.

42. "Around Albuquerque with Martin," *New Mexico Register*, February 14, 1958, Center for Southwest Research, University of New Mexico, Albuquerque, NM.

43. Henold, "This Is Our Challenge! We Will Pursue It," in *Empowering the People of God*, pp. 197–221.

44. "ACCW to Study, Discuss Abortion Legislation," *New Mexico Catholic Renewal*, December 1, 1968, Center for Southwest Research. University of New Mexico, Albuquerque, NM.

45. Hellwig was not the only pro-life activist to attend such conferences. In 1969, Emma Gomez, along with Hellwig, represented their archdiocesan Council of Catholic Women at a Catholic conference on building social movements. See "Country Club Sponsoring Annual East Egg Hunt," *Albuquerque Journal*, April 3, 1969.

46. I included leaders at deanery and diocesan levels. The highest position in the state's CCWs for an ethnic Mexican woman was the president of Casa Grande Deanery CCW and the lowest was the point person for the mass at a Yuma conference. For CCW leaders in Arizona, see "Yuma Deanery NCCW Installs New Officers," *Yuma Daily Sun*, November 21, 1960; "Luncheon Schedule to Honor Officers," *Arizona Republic*, February 7, 1961; "Catholic Women Name Chairmen," *Tucson Daily Citizen*, November 18, 1961; "Discuss Intermediate Institution for Group," *Yuma Daily Sun*, July 30, 1962; "Catholic Women to Convene Here," *Yuma Daily Sun*, September 26, 1962; "Prayer Sent for Opening Legislature," *Tucson Daily Citizen*, January 6, 1962; "Catholic Women Honor IC Sister," *Yuma Daily Sun*, May 21, 1964; "Catholic Women to Hold Convention in Tucson," *Tucson Daily Citizen*, November 28, 1964; "Bishop Pays Tribute to Women," *Tucson Daily Citizen*, Decem-

ber 4, 1964; "Pemberton Services Tomorrow," *Arizona Republic,* December 10, 1964; "Bishop Pays Tribute to Women," *Tucson Daily Citizen,* December 4, 1964; "Pre-Holiday Party," *Yuma Daily Sun,* November 24, 1964; "2 to Represent Tucson Women," *Arizona Republic,* August 18, 1965; Bill Herman, "Panel Differs on Juvenile Crime Rise," *Phoenix Gazette,* June 5, 1965; "Judge Molloy to Speak at Deanery," *Tucson Daily Citizen,* February 11, 1966; "Keep Phoenix on Top" ad, *Arizona Republic,* November 8, 1966; "Catholic Women Hear New Policies," *Yuma Daily Sun,* February 10, 1967; "Bishop Approves Deanery Groups," *Casa Grande Dispatch,* October 4, 1967; "Catholic Council Meets," *Yuma Daily Sun,* October 13, 1967; "Newman Center Sustaining Board Slates Luncheon Meeting Monday," *Tucson Daily Citizen,* September 17, 1968; "Meeting Scheduled," *Tucson Daily Citizen,* June 15, 1968; "Diocesan Council Officers," *Tucson Daily Citizen,* October 9, 1968; "Mrs. L. Franco heads Heart Drive," *Miami (AZ) Silver Belt,* February 13, 1969; "Bishop Addresses Catholic Women's Council," *Arizona Republic,* June 12, 1970.

47. Luckingham, *Minorities in Phoenix,* p. 30.

48. Now and again, Catholic newspapers reported on white resistance to the integration of Catholic and non-Catholic spaces in the South, but almost never turned their gaze toward their own segregated spaces. For example, see the following sample of articles of the New Mexico Catholic press in 1963: Gerald E. Sherry, "Crisis Coming to a Head," *New Mexico Register,* July 5, 1963; "Equal Rights for Negro Alternative to 'Mockery,'" *New Mexico Register,* July 5, 1963; "Nuns Picket Segregated 'Catholic' Club," *New Mexico Register,* July 12, 1963; "A Young Catholic Mother Marches for Racial Justice," *New Mexico Register,* July 26, 1963; "Negro Student Describes Birmingham Events," *New Mexico Register,* July 26, 1963; "Catholic Church Nears Total Integration Pattern," *New Mexico Register,* August 2, 1963, all at the Center for Southwest Research, University of New Mexico, Albuquerque, NM.

49. "Catholic Womanhood," *New Mexico Register,* August 2, 1963, Center for Southwest Research, University of New Mexico, Albuquerque, NM.

50. Pascoe, *Relations of Rescue.* For a sample of work on turn-of-the-century reform movements, see Hall, *Revolt Against Chivalry;* Cott, *The Grounding of Modern Feminism;* Muncy, *Creating a Female Dominion in American Reform;* Higginbotham, *Righteous Discontent;* Odem, *Delinquent Daughters;* Newman, *White Women's Rights;* Wexler, *Tender Violence;* Hewitt, *Southern Discomfort;* Jacobs, *White Mother to a Dark Race;* Cahill, *Federal Mothers and Fathers.*

51. Shirley Hellwig, Ronald Dorn, and Jack Arnold (Illinois); Murial James and Marion A. Jabczenski (Missouri); Adriana Huppental (Indiana); John Gillette (Iowa); Norman Weslin (Michigan) were all midwesterners.

52. Weslin, *The Gathering of the Lambs,* pp. 47, 62.

53. Shermer, *Sunbelt Capitalism,* p. 169. Importantly, Shermer argues that midwesterners cannot be blamed for Arizona's conservative turn. Rather, it was a combination of migration and local political realignments.

54. Dunn and Woodard, *The Conservative Tradition in America,* p. 40. See also Bowen, *The Roots of Modern Conservatism.* Similarly, Matthew Lassiter claims that an influx of northerners coincided with a conservative turn in Cobb County,

Georgia. See Lassiter, "Big Government and Family Values," in *Sunbelt Rising,* ed. Nickerson and Dochuk, pp. 82–109.

55. Hellwig obituary. For Seader, see "Mom Finds Time for UCC Job," *Tucson Daily Citizen,* October 22, 1964. For Onofrio, see Chuck Onofrio obituary, *Denver Post,* October 11, 2016. Kristin Luker notes that female activists in California also frequently had four or more children. Luker, *Abortion and the Politics of Motherhood,* p. 139.

56. Sebesta interview.

57. "Medicine Is a Family Affair," *Arizona Republic,* December 18, 1960; Maggie Savoy, "Career Is a Jealous Mistress," *Arizona Republic,* April 21, 1961; Margaret Thomas, "Mmes. Are Drs., Too," *Arizona Republic,* January 21, 1963; Mary Dumond, "Vaccine Against Valley Fever in the Making," *Arizona Republic,* December 11, 1965; Frankie Manley, "Three Couples . . . Six Careers," *Arizona Republic,* May 18, 1969.

58. Manley, "Three Couples . . . Six Careers"; "My Favorite Recipe," *Scottsdale Daily Progress,* December 6, 1972.

59. "Women's Day Is Thursday at Tempe," *Arizona Republic,* April 22, 1961; "Scottsdale Woman Doctor Speaks at ASU Women's Day Assembly," *Scottsdale Daily Progress,* April 19, 1961; Savoy, "Career Is a Jealous Mistress."

60. Phyllis Schlafly, leader of the anti-ERA movement, is one of the best examples of this balancing act. For a sampling of work on New Right women, see Klatch, *Women of the New Right;* Mathews and De Hart, *Sex, Gender, and the Politics of ERA;* McGirr, *Suburban Warriors;* Critchlow, *Phyllis Schlafly and Grassroots Conservatism;* Rymph, *Republican Women;* Nickerson, *Mothers of Conservatism;* Haugeberg, *Women Against Abortion;* Taranto, *Kitchen Table Politics;* Johnson, *This is Our Message.*

61. Sebesta interview. Joan Sebesta Weber is also a pseudonym.

62. Chuck Onofrio obituary. For Helen Onofrio, see Helen G. Onofrio, *Denver City Directory,* 1960, 1961, 1964, 1966, 1968, 1972, U.S. City Directories Database, 1822–1995 (accessed on ancestry.com).

63. For more on the Christian Family Movement, see Burns, *American Catholics and the Family Crisis, 1930–1962.*

64. For Gomez, see "Officers Announced by Alter Society," *Albuquerque Journal,* October 10, 1956; "ACCW Fall Conference to Be Held at St. Francis," *Santa Fe New Mexican,* December 8, 1968; "ACCW Deanery Hears Needs for Revitalized Christianity," *New Mexico Catholic Renewal,* December 1, 1968, and Eileen Stanton, "Women Hold Santa Fe Gathering to Discuss Abortions and Law," *New Mexico Catholic Renewal,* December 15, 1968, both at Center for Southwest Research, University of New Mexico, Albuquerque, NM; "Activities Planned by CDA," *Belen News Bulletin,* January 25, 1971; "Lamy Awards Given to Four," *Albuquerque Tribune,* May 4, 1972; "Four Being Honored at Convention Today," *Albuquerque Journal,* May 3, 1972.

65. "Birchers Attack Sex Education," *Scottsdale Daily Progress,* May 22, 1969.

66. For quotes, see "Laos Unopposed; 2 Demos Challenge Castro in Ward 5 Primary," *Tucson Daily Citizen,* September 19, 1977; Thom Walker, "Three Ward 5

Democrats Split on Goals," *Tucson Daily Citizen,* September 15, 1977 and Libby Ruiz, letter to the editor, "Not 'Oppressed,'" *Tucson Daily Citizen,* April 5, 1977. See also "Hopefuls' Background Varies," *Tucson Daily Citizen,* September 19, 1977; "Laos Only Choice in Ward 5 Races," *Tucson Daily Citizen,* September 1, 1977; Librada "Libby" Ruiz obituary, *Arizona Daily Star,* January 10, 2007.

67. One exception to this was Arizona in the 1964 presidential election when local son Barry Goldwater was the Republican candidate.

68. Self, *All in the Family.*

69. "Demos' Chairman Advises Party to Cease Bickering," *Tucson Daily Citizen,* March 10, 1970. For more on Arnold's politics, see "Arizona Can Be Proud" ad, *Tucson Daily Citizen,* October 29, 1960; "Arizonans . . . Take Council of Your Courage!" ad for Johnson, *Tucson Daily Citizen,* October 29, 1964; Dick Casey, "Shorter Judicial Campaigns Urged," *Tucson Daily Citizen,* September 6, 1966; "Arnold Will Give Up Top Democratic Post," *Tucson Daily Citizen,* September 15, 1970.

70. "American Party Veep Candidate Tells Goals," *Provo Herald,* November 3, 1972.

71. Mrs. Albert Haag, letter to the editor, "The Democrats Should Wake Up!" *Tucson Daily Citizen,* October 15, 1969; "Awareness House Drive Attacked as 'Bleeding' Cash," *Tucson Daily Citizen,* November 20, 1970. See also Gil Mathews, "Housewife Forms Citizens Group to Combat Crime," *Tucson Daily Citizen,* September 20, 1967; "High Court's Critics Set Up Corporation," *Tucson Daily Citizen,* January 2, 1968; "Women Asked to Join Campaign," *Tucson Daily Citizen,* November 22, 1968; Mrs. Albert Haag, letter to the editor, "How Can We Allow This to Go On?" *Tucson Daily Citizen,* April 2, 1969; Mrs. Albert Haag, letter to the editor, "ACLU Defender of Our Freedoms?" *Tucson Daily Citizen,* February 25, 1970; Bernadine Haag, letter to the editor, "Want Legalized 'Pot'?" *Tucson Daily Citizen,* July 9, 1971; Mrs. Albert Haag, letter to the editor, "Udall Is Amusing," *Tucson Daily Citizen,* October 19, 1973.

72. Ruiz obituary.

73. Bailey, *Sex in the Heartland.*

74. For a sampling of work on these two movements and conceptions of sex in society, see Echols, *Daring to be Bad;* Kissack, "Freaking Fag Revolutionaries," pp. 105–34; D'Emilio and Freedman, *Intimate Matters,* pp. 301–44; Gerhard, *Desiring Revolution;* Nelson, *Women of Color and the Reproductive Rights Movement;* Enke, *Finding the Movement;* Brier, *Infectious Ideas;* Gould, *Moving Politics;* Kline, *Bodies of Knowledge.*

75. Carlson, *Godly Seed,* p. 35.

76. Colorado obscenity law changed in 1961, but unmarried, childless women did not get access to contraception until 1971. For change to obscenity law, see "History of Choice in Colorado," http://www.prochoicecolorado.org/in-our-state/historyofchoice.shtml (accessed August 8, 2017). For unmarried women's access, see Martha J. Bailey, Melanie Guldi, Allison Davido, and Erin Buzuvis, "Early Legal Access: Laws and Policies Governing Contraceptive Access, 1960–1980," http://www-personal.umich.edu/~baileymj/ELA_laws.pdf (accessed August 8, 2017).

77. "Birth Control Bill Faces House Test," *Greeley Daily Tribune,* March 19, 1963; "Senate Passes Bills Totaling $154 Million," *Greeley Daily Tribune,* April 6, 1963; "Welfare Birth Control Urgent Cause" (no newspaper), March 18, 1965, folder 13, box 1, John Bermingham Papers, Western History and Genealogy Department, Denver Public Library, Denver, CO (hereafter Bermingham Papers).

78. "Birth Control Bill Testimony Is Heard," *Rocky Mountain News,* March 13, 1965.

79. Grand Knight Tom Grenan to Senator John Bermingham, telegram, March 23, 1965, folder 13, box 1, Bermingham Papers.

80. "Hope for Birth Control Measures," editorial, *Greeley Daily Tribune,* March 20, 1965; Sen. Bermingham, "The Religious Consensus on Family Planning and Responsible Parenthood," folder 13, box 1, Bermingham Papers.

81. Martin Moran, "Colorado Senate Approves Birth Control Bill, 23 to 9," *Rocky Mountain News,* March 18, 1965.

82. Paul H. Hallett, "Sex and Responsibility," *Denver Catholic Register,* March 18, 1965.

83. Paul H. Hallett, "Harnessing Moral Energy," *Denver Catholic Register,* March 25, 1965.

84. "Help the Poor with Social Truth," *Pueblo Chieftain,* March 16, 1965; "Birth Control Bill Testimony Is Heard"; Bermingham, "The Religious Consensus on Family Planning and Responsible Parenthood."

85. "Birth Curb Laws Victimize the Poor, Clergyman Said," *Greeley Daily Tribune,* March 15, 1965.

86. Connelly, *Fatal Misconception;* Gutiérrez, *Fertile Matters;* Smith, *Conquest;* Kluchin, *Fit to Be Tied;* Watkins, *On the Pill;* Roberts, *Killing the Black Body.* For more on poor women's access to birth control early in the century, see Schoen, *Choice and Coercion.*

87. "Birth Curb Laws Victimize the Poor, Clergyman Said."

88. Moran, "Colorado Senate Approves Birth Control Bill."

89. Paul H. Hallett, "Illegitimacy without Illegitimates," *Denver Catholic Register,* March 25, 1965.

90. Bermingham, "The Religious Consensus on Family Planning and Responsible Parenthood."

91. Solinger, *Beggars and Choosers,* pp. 140–3. For more on how black people more generally become associated with poverty and welfare, see Quadagno, *Color of Welfare;* Lieberman, *Shifting the Color Line.*

92. Gilens, "How the Poor Became Black," in *Race and the Politics of Welfare Reform,* pp. 101–30.

93. The 1965 Moynihan Report is the best example of this connection. For recent literature on the report, see Patterson, *Freedom Is Not Enough;* Geary, *Beyond Civil Rights;* Greenbaum, *Blaming the Poor.*

94. "Welfare Birth Control Urgent Cause," Bermingham Papers; Moran, "Colorado Senate Approves Birth Control Bill."

95. Mrs. Lydia Bushenko, letter to the editor, "No Litter Baskets for Smut," *Denver Catholic Register,* April 29, 1965.

96. Hallett, "Sex and Responsibility."

97. This did not preclude social conservatives from seeking government solutions to their moral problems. For example, Mary Zeigler shows how in the 1960s and 1970s, pro-life activists hoped for judicial activism on the side of fetal rights. Zeigler, *After Roe,* ch. 1.

98. Hallett, "Harnessing Moral Energy."

99. Frank Morriss, "Tragedies Flow from 1865," *Denver Catholic Register,* April 15, 1965.

100. McGreevy, *Catholicism and American Freedom,* pp. 208–10.

101. Fred F. McCaffrey, "A Voice from the Pews," *New Mexico Catholic Renewal,* December 15, 1968, Center for Southwest Research, University of New Mexico, Albuquerque, NM. For discussion of *Humanae Vitae,* see August 1968 issues of *New Mexico Catholic Renewal.*

102. For *Denver Catholic Register* poaching, see Fred F. McCaffrey, "A Voice from the Pews," *New Mexico Catholic Renewal,* April 30, 1967, Center for Southwest Research, University of New Mexico, Albuquerque, NM. For an example of a reader jumping ship because of the newspaper's liberal politics, see Catherine Carnevale, letter to the editor, *New Mexico Catholic Renewal,* March 10, 1968, Center for Southwest Research, University of New Mexico, Albuquerque, NM.

103. A Rocky Mountain Planned Parenthood member remembered that during birth control debates in the 1960s, future pro-life activists Margaret Sebesta and Chuck Onofrio had both been "violently opposed to contraception." RMPP Board of Trustees meeting, March 9, 1985, Aurora, Colorado, folder Board and Committee Meetings (e) 1985, box 2, Rocky Mountain Planned Parenthood Collection, Western History and Genealogy Department, Denver Public Library, Denver, CO.

104. The essential reading on this movement is Strub, *Perversion for Profit.*

105. "Archbishop Urges Support in Fight Against Pornography at Rally Here," *Albuquerque Tribune,* January 14, 1957.

106. J. R. Walsh, "Communities Can Halt Smut," *Denver Catholic Register,* January 28, 1960. See also Jack Magee, "Pornography Compared to Marijuana," *Santa Fe New Mexican,* May 13, 1964.

107. Strub, *Perversion for Profit,* p. 88.

108. Michelle Nickerson offers another origin point for the conservative expert and conservative critiques of elite knowledge production: conservative women's attacks on the psychology and psychiatry in the late 1950s and early 1960s. See Nickerson, *Mothers of Conservatism,* pp. 103–35.

109. "'Smut Peddlers' Studies Moral Plague," *Denver Catholic Register,* November 17, 1960. For more on Kilpatrick, see Strub, "Pornography, Heteronormativity, and the Genealogy of New Right Sexual Citizenship in the United States," in *Inventing the Silent Majority in Western Europe and the United States,* p. 350.

110. "Film of Evils of Smut Shown," *Denver Catholic Register,* March 25, 1965.

111. Strub, *Perversion for Profit,* p. 113.

112. "Denver Citizens Organize for Anti-Pornography Drive," *Denver Catholic Register,* March 11, 1965; "Pornography Ban Drive Underway," *Farmington Daily Times,* April 17, 1966.

113. Kandel, *Collected Poems of Lenore Kandel,* pp. 35–36.

114. "Cargo, Crowd of 1500 Listen to Poem Readings," *Albuquerque Journal,* March 29, 1969.

115. Kanowitz, "Love Lust in New Mexico and the Emerging Law of Obscenity," pp. 339–52.

116. Such campaigns built upon conservative women's activism on local school issues. See McGirr, *Suburban Warriors,* pp. 54–110; Nickerson, *Mothers of Conservatism,* pp. 69–103.

117. "Businessman Tells Views on U. Poem," *Albuquerque Journal,* March 29, 1969. For more on "taxpayers," see "DA Investigates 'Obscene' Poetry," *Albuquerque Journal,* March 29, 1969; Dale Scriven, secretary of Northeast Lions Club, letter to the editor, "Lions Anti-Poem," *Albuquerque Journal,* March 30, 1969; "'That Poem' Gets 'Crude, Filth' Tag," *Farmington Daily Times,* April 1, 1969.

118. Helen Airy, letter to the editor, "Send 'Em to BYU," *Albuquerque Journal,* April 20, 1969.

119. "'Love Lust' a Rally Point," *Las Vegas Daily Optic,* May 19, 1969.

120. "Cargo, Crowd of 1500 Listen to Poem Readings."

121. "'That Poem' Gets 'Crude, Filth' Tag"; "Businessman Tells Views on U. Poem."

122. "UNM President Heady Issues Text on Suspensions," *Albuquerque Journal,* March 29, 1969; "Regents Given Con-Con Okay with Changes," *Clovis Daily Journal,* September 18, 1969.

123. "'Poem Distribution' Warning Is Issued," *Albuquerque Journal,* March 29, 1969.

124. "'That Poem' Gets 'Crude, Filth' Tag."

125. Leslie Bottorff, "Love-Lust, Medicaid, Con-Con; '69 was a Rough Year," *Santa Fe New Mexican,* January 4, 1970.

126. "Dirty Poem Stirs State's Emotions," *Las Vegas Optic,* April 1, 1969.

127. "'That Poem' Gets 'Crude, Filth' Tag."

128. Bottorff, "Love-Lust, Medicaid, Con-Con."

129. R.I.G., letter to the editor, *Denver Catholic Register,* December 1, 1960.

130. Libby Ruiz and Muriel James expressed anti-pornography stances in newspapers, while many more participated in Knights of Columbus and Councils of Catholic Women.

131. One example of the clear connections between these two movements is the 1972 legislative session in New Mexico when activists put forward anti-porn and pro-life bills together. See "Questions of Morality," editorial, *Farmington Daily Times,* September 29, 1972.

132. Willke, with Meyers, *Abortion and the Pro-Life Movement,* pp. 13–19.

133. Williams, *Defending the Unborn*, p. 37. For more on the rise of human rights rhetoric and politics, see Bradley, *The World Reimagined;* Iriye, Goedde, and Hitchcock, eds., *The Human Rights Revolution;* Hoffmann, ed., *Human Rights in the Twentieth Century;* Bradley and Petro, eds., *Truth Claims.*

134. For more on Finkbine, see Luker, *Abortion and the Politics of Motherhood,* pp. 62–65; Jacoby, *Souls, Bodies, and Spirits,* p. 4; Gorney, *Articles of Faith,* pp. 40–51; Clow, "An Illness of Nine Months' Duration," in *Women, Health, and Nation,* pp. 45–47; Solinger, *Pregnancy and Power,* pp. 179–81.

135. For a sample of local sympathetic press, see "Wife's Problem with Childbirth Centers Here," *Scottsdale Daily Progress,* July 26, 1962; "Finkbine Case," *Scottsdale Daily Progress,* July 27, 1962; Robert Musel, "Sherri Finkbine, in Sweden, Makes Plea for Abortion," *Tucson Daily Citizen,* August 6, 1962; Don Carson, "Finkbines Didn't Want Publicity," *Tucson Daily Citizen,* August 2, 1962; Ward Cannel, "Must Tell of Abortion, Scottsdale Wife Feels," *Yuma Daily Sun,* March 5, 1964. Finkbine was but one of a growing number of white, middle-class women dealing with reproductive tragedies portrayed in the media. For broader analysis of this cultural phenomenon and how it contributed to support for abortion reform, see Reagan, *Dangerous Pregnancies.*

136. "Sherri Leaves Sweden Hospital," *Scottsdale Daily Progress,* August 24, 1962.

137. "Catholic Abortion Stand Clarified by Spokesman," *Tucson Daily Citizen,* July 28, 1962.

138. Fermaglich, *American Dreams and Nazi Nightmares,* p. 18. Recent scholars, like Fermaglich, have pushed back against the common narrative that the Holocaust did not enter the American consciousness until the late 1960s. See, for example, Staub, "Negroes Are Not Jews," pp. 3–27 and *Torn at the Roots,* pp. 45–111; Baron, "The Holocaust and American Public Memory," pp. 62–88.

139. Father Ginder, "The Slaughter of Innocents," *Dallas Texas Catholic,* August 27, 1960. For a discussion of Hitler and the Finkbines, see Father Conroy, "Macbeth Doth Murder Sleep," *Dallas Texas Catholic,* September 9, 1962.

140. Mrs. W. Hughes, letter to the editor, "Medical Editor Is Criticized for Column on Birth Control," *Arizona Republic,* March 11, 1964.

141. Mrs. Marceline Boyer, letter to the editor, "Choose God or Satan, Kenoshan Declares," *Kenosha (WI) News,* May 3, 1963.

142. Doris Storms, letter to the editor, "Never Had a Chance," *Tucson Daily Citizen,* February 1, 1973.

143. "Pornography Program Slated," *Las Cruces Sun Times,* February 5, 1970; Hallett, "Sex and Responsibility."

144. Susan Elliott, letter to the editor, "Is Mac for Murder," *Hutchinson (KS) News,* April 10, 1963; Abigail Van Buren, "Dear Abby Presents Sex Education," *Las Cruces Sun-News,* January 12, 1970.

145. Haag, *SHAM,* p. 184; William A. Reese III, letter to the editor, "Polio Remains Vietnam Crippler," *Tucson Daily Citizen,* July 22, 1970; Nancy L. Cousins,

letter to the editor, "Man of Courage Rejected," *Tucson Daily Citizen,* September 29, 1973; "The Equal Rights Amendment IS A FRAUD!" ad, *Tucson Daily Citizen,* February 6, 1973.

146. Gil Johnson, "'Sincerity' Is Basis for Low-Key Campaign," *Scottsdale Daily Progress,* August 16, 1976.

147. Sebesta interview.

2. IMAGINING LIFE

1. Saving Lives and Serving Families, January 1999, p. 4, folder 3, box 1–3, HH1421, Heritage House '76, Inc/Precious Feet People, Hall Hoag Collection of Dissenting and Extremist Printed Propaganda, John Hay Library, Brown University, Providence RI (hereafter Hall Hoag Collection). See also interview with Virginia Evers, March 19, 2010; Boucher, "The Politics of Abortion and the Commodification of the Fetus," pp. 69–88; Condit, *Decoding Abortion Rhetoric,* pp. 88–89.

2. The Precious Feet People Catalog, September 1981, p. 2, folder 1, box 1–3, HH1421, Heritage House '76, Inc/Precious Feet People, Hall Hoag Collection.

3. "The Story of Heritage House '76," folder 1, box 1–3, HH1421, Heritage House '76, Inc/Precious Feet People, Hall Hoag Collection. For national and international reactions to the Precious Feet, see, for example, *Viva Life* newsletter, January 1986, folder 1, box 1–8, HH120, Right to Life, New Mexico, Hall Hoag Collection; Heritage House, '76 Inc., "Getting Out the Word," Heritage House Newsletter, Spring 1988, folder 1, box 1–3, HH1421, Heritage House '76, Inc/Precious Feet People, Hall Hoag Collection.

4. Philosopher Cornelius Castoriadis has called this a social imaginary. Castoriadis, *The Imaginary Institution of Society.* Castoriadis was not the first philosopher to articulate the idea of the imaginary. In fact, he was entering into a long philosophical conversation about the creation of the self. Philosopher John-Paul Sartre first noted the idea of the imaginary in his book, *The Imaginary.* In this work, Sartre narrated the relationship between imagination and human consciousness, contending that people are not passive recipients of images but active and creative participants in perception and imagination. Philosopher Jacques Lacan articulated the notion that the imaginary was one of three orders of psychoanalysis, joining the symbolic and the real. He contended that the imaginary was the realm beyond language where the self confronted its alter ego, and that only by breaking through this realm could one get to the symbolic, where language existed and dialogue could occur. Castoriadis refined and critiqued Lacan, suggesting that in the imaginary, ideology is conjoined with signification, and that the imaginary has wider social and political implications. For description of Sartre's theory of imaginary, see Detmer, *Sartre Explained,* pp. 47–48; for Lacan's theory, see Evans, *An Introductory Dictionary of Lacanian Psychoanalysis,* pp. 84–85, and Gallop, *Reading Lacan,* pp. 59–60.

5. The essential reading on abortion before 1973 is Reagan, *When Abortion Was a Crime.*

6. For "bodily slavery" quote, see Garrow, *Liberty and Sexuality*, p. 314. For the wide range of reformers' opinions between the mid-1950s and 1967, see pp. 270–335. The number of people, especially feminists, making this critique and calling abortion "a right" would growing exponentially after 1967.

7. Ibid., pp. 323–24; Olga Curtis, "How Colorado Changed Its Abortion Law," *Denver Post* (Empire Magazine), May 18, 1967; Gordon G. Gauss, "Changes Noted in Attitude about Abortion," *Colorado Springs Gazette,* April 10, 1967.

8. "Social Workers Favor Liberalized Abortion Law," *Colorado Springs Gazette Telegraph,* November 19, 1967; Richard D. Lamm, "Act Now on Population Explosion, Legislator Warns," November 19, 1967, reprinted in "Overpopulation: The Ultimate Environmental Problem" pamphlet, 1970, folder Colorado (1), box 1, National Abortion Rights Action League, Printed Materials Collection, Schlesinger Library, Radcliffe Institute, Harvard University, Cambridge MA (hereafter NARAL Printed Materials Collection).

9. Connelly, *Fatal Misconception,* pp. 115–236. Of course, those worried about overpopulation in the 1960s and 1970s were much less concerned than feminists with issues of consent and choice, and more concerned with the "public good." This led to coercive sterilizations of and reproductive experiments on people, primarily women, of color in the United States and around the world. In Colorado, Lamm along with a Republican representative introduced a measure to the Colorado House in 1971 that encouraged women on welfare to have fewer children. In their bill, welfare mothers would get fifty dollars every three months that they did not get pregnant after their first two children. While this was not strictly coercive (like the forced sterilizations going on around the country), the bill was unconcerned with individual women's desires and terribly concerned with limiting certain "undesirable" or burdensome groups from reproducing. See "Bonus for Welfare Mothers Who Stop at Two, Proposed," *Colorado Springs Gazette,* February 17, 1971.

10. Lamm, "Act Now on Population Explosion"; Curtis, "How Colorado Changed Its Abortion Law."

11. Kruse, "Beyond the Southern Cross," in *The Myth of Southern Exceptionalism,* pp. 300–301; Karrer, "The National Right to Life Committee," pp. 527–57.

12. "Church Joins Abortion Debate," *Denver Post,* April 1, 1967.

13. "Catholics Hear Plea Against Abortion," *Denver Post,* April 3, 1967; "Abortion Hearing," *Denver Post,* April 2, 1967.

14. Tom Gavin, "Crowd Jeers Bill to Revise Abortion Law," *Denver Post,* April 4, 1967.

15. Interview with Margaret Sebesta (pseudonym), August 8, 2011.

16. For Stewart's profession and professional ties, see Mike Nolan, "Colorado Shuns Future as Mecca for Abortions," *The Daily News* (Huntingdon and Mount Union, PA), May 2, 1967.

17. Reagan, *Dangerous Pregnancies,* pp. 57, 47. This epidemic, much more so than all those previously, gained national attention. Historian Leslie Reagan argues that

this was because the epidemic had followed closely on "the thalidomide tragedy" in Europe. Americans watched from afar through newspapers, which published pictures of deformed "thalidomide babies."

18. Dubow, *Ourselves Unborn*, p. 65.

19. Those concerned with mentally disabled children, perhaps motivated by this epidemic, had been some of the first advocates of abortion reform in Colorado. See Martin Moran, "Changes Urged in Colorado's Abortion Laws," *Rocky Mountain News,* December 25, 1965; "Social Workers Favor Liberalized Abortion Law."

20. In fact, an eminent rubella researcher put the rate of congenital abnormalities at approximately 74.4 percent if the disease was contracted in the first four months of pregnancy, and from 11.1 to 29.9 percent if contracted in the last five months. Reagan, *Dangerous Pregnancies*, pp. 45–6.

21. Hal Hall, letter to the editor, "Right to Be Born," *Denver Post,* April 5, 1967.

22. Sebesta interview.

23. Dubow, *Ourselves Unborn*, p. 43.

24. Of course, many women also viewed their own miscarried or aborted fetuses. For a historical analysis of women's experiences with miscarriage, see Withycombe, *Lost.*

25. Quigley, *Modern Mummies*, p. 127.

26. Willke, *Handbook on Abortion*, pp. 9, 15, 19.

27. "Gynecology: New Grounds for Abortion," *Time Magazine,* May 5, 1967. See also Garrow, *Liberty and Sexuality,* p. 323.

28. Greg Pinney, "Women Stage Brief Anti-Abortion Protest at Capitol," *Denver Post,* April 6, 1967.

29. "5 Women, 2 Children Picket at Mansion," *Denver Post,* April 10, 1967.

30. Rev. Frank Freeman, St. James Catholic Church, letter to the editor, *Denver Post,* April 12, 1967.

31. Colorado Joint Council on Medical and Social Legislation, "Abortion in Colorado" pamphlet, 1968 or 69, Laws, Abortion, 1960–1969 Clippings File, Western History and Genealogy Department, Denver Public Library, Denver, CO.

32. Sebesta interview.

33. Interview with Phil and Helen Seader, March 18, 2010. For a similar claim, see Willke, with Meyers, *Abortion and the Pro-Life Movement,* p. 23.

34. Lorette Svejar to Governor Bruce King, October 3, 1972, folder 220, box 12, Governor Bruce King Papers (1st Term), New Mexico State Records Center, Santa Fe, NM.

35. Colorado Joint Council on Medical and Social Legislation, "Abortion in Colorado"; John E. Archibold, "Re-examine State Abortion Law, Opponent Urges," *Denver Post,* July 7, 1968; Pat McGraw, "Abortion Foes Say Backers Playing God," *Denver Post,* December 27, 1971.

36. Sebesta interview; Pinney, "Women Stage Brief Anti-Abortion Protest at Capitol." For another 1967 protest made up of only women and children, see "5 Women, 2 Children Picket at Mansion."

37. Gavin, "Crowd Jeers Bill to Revise Abortion Law"; Cal Queal, "How Colorado Changed Its Abortion Law," *Denver Post,* June 18, 1967.

38. Paul H. Hallett, "Abortion and Illegitimacy," *Denver Catholic Register,* October 14, 1973.

39. Olga Curtis, "How Many Abortions Are Too Many," *Denver Post* (Empire Magazine), January 18, 1970.

40. "Rush Seen: Abortions in Colorado," *Hartford Courant* (CT), April 30, 1967.

41. John Willke de-jarred a fetus on the "Phil Donahue Show" in 1979; Operation Rescue activists tried to hand one to Bill Clinton at the 1992 Democratic National Convention. See Willke, with Meyers, *Abortion and the Pro-Life Movement,* pp. 180–81; Ronald Sullivan, "Four Surrender in Use of Fetus Against Clinton," *New York Times,* July 17, 1992.

42. For a sampling of works on the subject, see Furniss, *The Mormon Conflict;* Bigler, *Forgotten Kingdom;* Gordon, *The Mormon Question;* Bagley, *Blood of Prophets;* Bigler and Bagley, *The Mormon Rebellion;* Rogers, *Unpopular Sovereignty.*

43. Quinn, "Exporting Utah's Theocracy since 1975," in *God and Country,* pp. 129–68 (quote on p. 130).

44. Alexander, *Utah, the Right Place,* p. 404.

45. Szasz, *Religion in the Modern American West,* pp. 107–8. For more on Mormon assimilation, see Hansen, *Mormonism and the American Experience;* Shipps, *Mormonism;* Mauss, *The Angel and the Beehive;* Alexander, *Mormonism in Transition;* Prince and Wright, *David O. McKay and the Rise of Modern Mormonism;* Givens, *The Latter-Day Saint Experience in America* and *People of Paradox;* LoRusso, "The Puritan Ethic on High," in *Out of Obscurity.*

46. Reeve, *Religion of a Different Color,* esp. pp. 247–59. See also Bush and Mauss, *Neither White nor Black;* Bringhurst and Smith, eds., *Black and Mormon;* Pierce, *Making the White Man's West,* pp. 179–208; Mueller, *Race and the Making of Mormon People.*

47. Garrow, *Liberty and Sexuality,* p. 598. In *Roe v. Wade,* Supreme Court justices ruled that state abortion bans were unconstitutional because they violated a woman's right to privacy. *Griswold v. Connecticut,* the 1965 Supreme Court case that overturned state laws prohibiting the use of contraceptives, had been the first case to rule officially that the Constitution protected the right to privacy. This right, the justices contended, was implied in the Bill of Rights and applied to the states through the due process clause of the Fourteenth Amendment. In *Roe,* however, this right was not absolute. The justices contended that it must be balanced by the state's interest in promoting public health, which increased over the course of the pregnancy, leading to the trimester-based decision. See Garrow, *Liberty and Sexuality;* Greenhouse, *Becoming Justice Blackmun;* Greenhouse and Seigel, eds., *Before Roe v. Wade;* Stein, *Sexual Injustice.*

48. Freemen Institute, "Let States Decide," *Rights of the Unborn,* April 1973, folder 14, box 23, Wayne Owens Papers, J. Willard Marriott Library Archives, University of Utah, Salt Lake City, UT (hereafter Owens Papers); Joan E. Christensen

to Wayne Owens, April 4, 1973, folder 13, box 23, Owens Papers; "Petition to Congress Concerning Abortion," undated, received May 29, 1973, folder 16, box 23, Owens Papers; Mrs. Hilda Wilson to Sir, May 30, 1973, folder 16, box 23, Owens Papers; Mr. and Mrs. Garth Pratt (City Councilman-Stake Presidency) to Rep. Wayne Owens, April 23, 1973, folder 15, box 23, Owens Papers; Mrs. Marie H. Russon to Honorable Wayne Owens, March 19, 1973, folder 13, box 23, Owens Papers; Charles E. Fournier to Congressman, undated, received October 1, 1975, folder 3, box 36, Allan Turner Howe Collection, J. Willard Marriott Library Archives, University of Utah, Salt Lake City, UT (hereafter Howe Collection).

49. See, for example, Mrs. Dorthella Baker and Richard D. Baker, April 22, 1973, folder 12, box 23, Owens Papers; Ruth F. Stewart to Mr. Owens, April 3, 1973, folder 14, box 23, Owens Papers; Mrs. Robert S. Grover to Sir, May 6, 1973, folder 15, box 23, Owens Papers.

50. "Petition to Congress Concerning Abortion."

51. Utah Right to Life League, "Do You Want Unrestricted Abortion at This Stage?" ad, *Salt Lake Tribune,* March 4, 1973.

52. Willke, *Handbook on Abortion.*

53. "'Baby Doe' Dominates Convention," *Tyrone Daily Herald* (PA), April 19, 1982; Costa, *Abortion,* p. 23; Hudson, *Onward Christian Soldiers,* p. 139. Some Right to Life groups also bought exhibits of these photos from Cincinnati Right to Life, the Willkes' home pro-life group. See, for example, *Arizona Lifeline,* February-March 1972, University of Arizona Library Special Collections, University of Arizona, Tucson, AZ.

54. Gorney, *Articles of Faith,* p. 100.

55. Lisa Cornwell, "Retirement Won't Slow Down Anti-Abortion Leader's Struggle," *Daily Sentinel* (Pomeroy and Middleport, OH), April 21, 1999.

56. Gorney, *Articles of Faith,* pp. 100–5.

57. Willke, *Handbook on Abortion,* pp. iv-v; Hudson, *Onward Christian Soldiers,* p. 139.

58. Stabile, "The Traffic in Fetuses," in *Fetal Subjects, Feminist Positions,* pp. 133–59 (quote on p. 145).

59. "Speakers Listed: Clergy Lunch on Schedule," *Salt Lake Tribune,* September 29, 1973. Constitutional lawyer and law professor Laurence Tribe credited the Willkes' pictures (in brochure form) with helping defeat liberalization referendums in Michigan and North Dakota in 1972. See Tribe, *Abortion,* p. 50.

60. Barbara Springer, "Family Physicians Meet in S.L., Hear Discussions on Abortion, Sex Education," *Salt Lake Tribune,* March 18, 1972; "Anti-Abortion Speeches Set," *Provo Herald,* October 7, 1973; "Topic of Abortion Sparks Inquiries," *Salt Lake Tribune,* October 10, 1973; "Session to Air 'Right to Life,'" *Salt Lake Tribune,* June 19, 1974.

61. "Topic of Abortion Sparks Inquiries," *Salt Lake Tribune,* October 10, 1973.

62. The second edition of the *Handbook on Abortion,* published in 1972, included a picture of a black infant born premature. But such images were not the ones most often used by the movement.

63. Young, *We Gather Together,* p. 124.

64. Margaret Fitzgerald to Congressman McKay, February 13, 1974, folder 20, box 161, Papers of Congressman Gunn McKay, Merill-Cazier Library Special Collections and Archives, Utah State University, Logan, UT (hereafter McKay Papers); Mr. and Mrs. Ralph E. Keller to Honorable Wayne Owens, undated (received March 11, 1974), folder 2, box 39, Owens Papers; Marguerite H. McGuire to Representatives of this Our America and Utah, January 23, 1976, folder 1, box 43, Howe Collection; Mrs. Judy Prince to Rep. Wayne Owens, undated (recorded April 9, 1973), folder 14, box 23, Owens Papers.

65. Ms. Lee Anne Walker to Congressman Howe, April 12, 1975, folder 1, box 19, Howe Collection.

66. For a statement on this topic by David O. McKay, then a member of the First Presidency and later the church's president, see David O. McKay to Tiena Nate, October 31, 1934, folder 1, box 26, Lester E. Bush Collection, J. Willard Marriott Library Archives, University of Utah, Salt Lake City, UT. Nineteenth-century LDS leaders were more likely to claim that life began at conception. See Young, *We Gather Together,* p. 101.

67. Crapo, "Grass-Roots Deviance from Official Doctrine," pp. 465–85 (statistics on p. 476).

68. Novick, *The Holocaust in American Life,* p. 13.

69. For examples of this argument, see Christopher Smith, "Foes, Backers of Abortion Law Change Detail Views," *Denver Post,* March 7, 1971; "Abortion Ruling Called Threat to the Old and Infirm," *Arizona Republic,* January 30, 1973; "How Far Will It Go?" *Freemen Institute,* April 1973, folder 14, box 23, Owens Papers; "Anti-Abortion Group to Host Zoo Visitors," *Arizona Republic,* January 20, 1977; "Anti-Abortion Proposal Advances Over Outcry," *Phoenix Gazette,* March 5, 1980; Linda Perry, "Abortion Nightmare Update," Speech to the New Mexico Right to Life State Convention, April 1985, folder 1, Linda E. J. Perry Collection, Schlesinger Library, Radcliffe Institute, Harvard University, Cambridge, MA; New Mexico Right to Life, *Viva Life,* September 1986 and July 1986, folder 1, box 1–8, HH120, Right to Life, New Mexico, Hall Hoag Collection.

70. James J. Rotter to Congressman Owens, January 22, 1973, folder 1, box 39, Owens Papers.

71. In fact, agitation for legalized abortion in Germany long preceded the rise of the Third Reich. German social reformers, radical feminists, socialists, and communists had pushed for reform since the beginning of the twentieth century to help women control the conditions of their existence, while Nazis pushed abortion only for the "unworthy." See Ferree et al., *Shaping Abortion Discourse;* Koonz, *Mothers in the Fatherland;* Stephenson, *Women in Nazi Germany.* For quote from Freemen Institute, see "How Far Will It Go?" Owens Papers. For more on the Freemen Institute, see White, "A Review and Commentary on the Prospects of a Mormon New Christian Right Coalition," pp. 180–88; Bradley, *Pedestals and Podiums,* p. 118.

72. Robert A. Hill to Congressman Allan Howe, March 31, 1976, folder 1, box 29, Howe Collection.

73. Willke, *Handbook on Abortion,* inside front cover, and pp. 87–88.

74. Rev. Robert L. Breunig, letter to the editor, *Denver Post,* March 7, 1971. See also Daniel Cummings to Wayne Owens, February 23, 1973, folder 11, box 23, Owens Papers.

75. Novick, *The Holocaust in American Life,* p. 13.

76. The Willkes were not the first to make this comparison. They drew on materials developed by a group called Women for the Unborn. See Willke, *Handbook on Abortion,* p. 115. See also Mason, *Killing for Life,* pp. 120–23. Also in 1973, William F. Buckley wrote an article about the *Roe* decision called "The Dred Scott Decision of the Twentieth Century." In February 1973, this article was discussed at an open forum in Salt Lake City. See "Abortion Issue," *Salt Lake Tribune,* February 10, 1973.

77. Frank Morriss, "To End the Obscenity of Abortion," *The Wanderer,* December 27, 1973.

78. For Utah comparisons, see Mary Lee Walton, Gary Walton, Roberta Hackett, and Ted Hackett, letter to the editor, "Thing[s] Must Change," *Salt Lake Tribune,* February 27, 1973; "Law Giving Fetus Rights Supported," *Ogden Standard-Examiner,* March 19, 1977; "Anti-Abortion Groups Eye Petition Drive," *Provo Herald,* March 21, 1977. For other slavery, Dred Scott, or abolitionist comparisons in the region, see "Physicians and Abortion," letter to the editor, *Tucson Daily Citizen,* February 7, 1973; Morriss, "To End the Obscenity of Abortion"; Frank Morriss, "Doctor Faces Prosecution in Anti-Abortion Effort," *The Wanderer,* December 27, 1973; Jack Crowe, "10,000 March to Protest Abortions," *Arizona Republic,* January 28, 1974.

79. See, for example, Jones, *The Trial of Don Pedro León Luján;* Knack, *Boundaries Between,* pp. 55–59; Blackhawk, *Violence Over the Land,* pp. 239–42.

80. Mrs. Nancy Berg, of Sandy, Utah, to Mr. Owens, February 17, 1973, folder 10, box 23, Owens Papers; Mrs. Clifton Painter to Wayne Owens, February 22, 1973, folder 12, box 23, Owens Papers.

81. See, for example, Paul and Beverly Lombardi to Representative Owens, February 21, 1973, folder 11, box 23, Owens Papers.

82. Keller to Owens, March 11, 1974.

83. Haines, *Against Capital Punishment,* pp. 22, 39. The majority opinion of *Furman v. Georgia* did not claim that capital punishment was inherently cruel and unusual, though two justices who joined the majority did make that argument. Within a few years of the decision, many states had adapted their laws to fit the guidelines put forth in the *Furman* decision. In 1976, because of these adjustments, the Supreme Court reinstated the death penalty in their *Gregg v. Georgia* decision.

84. Mrs. John Lyman to Wayne Owens, no date (probably spring 1973), folder 12, box 23, Owens Papers; Laura G. Hendrick to Sirs, March 1, 1973, folder 12, box 23, Owens Papers. For other discussions of abortion and the death penalty by Utahns, see Jon Robinson to Congressman Wayne Owens, January 19, 1974, folder 1, box 39, Owens Papers; Nancy Sluder to Rep. Owens, January 23, 1973, folder 10, box 4, Owens Papers; E. B. Carter to Honorable Wayne Owens, March 1, 1973, folder 12, box 23, Owens Papers.

85. For the civil rights movement in Utah, see Hornsby, *Black America*, pp. 851–52.

86. Young, *We Gather Together*, p. 124.

87. Others have discussed the deployment of civil rights rhetoric by pro-life activists but most focus on its use in the 1990s by Operation Rescue. See Hughes, "The Civil Rights Movement of the 1990s?" pp. 1–23; Marley, "Riding in the Back of the Bus," in *The Civil Rights Movement in American Memory*, pp. 346–62; Nelson, *More than Medicine*, pp. 146–54.

88. Mitchell, *Coyote Nation*, p. 207, n35.

89. For example, in a single year during the Great Depression, a school nurse in the Native American community of Nambe Pueblo, just north of Santa Fe, reported a number of abortions. See January 14–15, 1939, and February 15, 1939, entries, Maria Casias, School Nurse, 1938–39 Diary, diary 1, box 3, Nambe Community School Teachers' Diaries, 1935–1942 Collection, Center for Southwest Research, University of New Mexico, Albuquerque, NM. For one woman's account of attempting to get an illegal abortion in New Mexico, see Carol Thorman to Senator Bayh and Members of the Senate Subcommittee, May 15, 1974, folder New Mexico, 1969–1975, carton 4, National Abortion Rights Action League (NARAL) Collection, Schlesinger Library, Radcliffe Institute, Harvard University, Cambridge, MA (hereafter NARAL Collection).

90. Laurie McCord, "Legal Abortion—Becoming Routine?" *Albuquerque Tribune*, November 24, 1973; Keith Easthouse, Coleman Cornellus, and Robert Mayer, "Abortion and New Mexico," *Santa Fe Reporter*, May 3–9, 1989. For more on the 1969 legislation, see Helen Parsons to Mr. Footlick, January 26, 1969, folder New Mexico 1969–75, carton 4, NARAL Collection.

91. Because New Mexico's legislature never repealed its 1969 abortion law after *Roe v. Wade*, the state still technically has a parental consent law on the books. The 1969 law required the consent of a parent or guardian for a woman under the age of eighteen seeking an abortion. *Roe* made most of this law unconstitutional. But in 1992, the U.S. Supreme Court legalized parental consent laws in their *Planned Parenthood v. Casey* decision, putting the parental consent part of New Mexico's moribund abortion law under scrutiny. The New Mexico attorney general decided the parental consent section would never pass constitutional muster because it did not allow minors to bypass the law with a judge's consent. The state's parental consent law has not been used since 1973. New Mexico pro-life activists pushed constitutional parental consent and notification laws in the 1990s, but those bills never passed in the legislature. See New Mexico Attorney General, Opinion no. 90–19 (October 3, 1990); Arndorfer, Micheal, Moskowitz, Siebel, and Grant, *Who Decides?* p. 89; "NM Expects Abortion-Issue Debate," *The New Mexican*, August 24, 1992; "New Mexico, Restrictions on Young Women's Access to Abortion," NARAL Pro-Choice America, http://www.prochoiceamerica.org/government-and-you /state-governments/state-profiles/new-mexico.html?templateName = template-161602701&issueID = 6&ssumID = 2735 (accessed October 15, 2012).

92. As of 2012, forty-four states had passed exemption clauses. according to the Guttmacher Institute. See Guttmacher Institute, "State Policies in Brief, as of

September 2012," www.guttmacher.org/pubs/spib_RPHS.pdf (accessed September 27, 2012).

93. New Mexico is the only one of the twenty-one states having an equal rights amendment in their state constitution that interprets the amendment to include the right to abortion. For more on the court case, see Brief Amicus Curiae of the New Mexico Women's Bar Association and New Mexico Public Health Association in Support of Plaintiffs-Appellees, New Mexico Right to Choose, et al., vs. Dorothy Danfelser, Secretary of the New Mexico Human Services Department, Docket no. 23239 (1996), folder 19, box 1, Bruce Trigg Papers, Center for Southwest Research, University of New Mexico, Albuquerque, NM; "Supreme Court Considers Restrictions on Abortions in New Mexico," *Santa Fe New Mexican,* July 1, 1997; "State Must Pay for Abortions, High Court Rules," *Roswell Daily Record,* December 1, 1998; Mark Oswald, "High Court Rules Against State on Abortions for the Poor," *Santa Fe New Mexican,* December 1, 1998.

94. Moore and Costa, *Just the Facts,* New Mexico entry. NARAL has also regularly given New Mexico high grades for its support of reproductive rights. See Moore and Costa, New Mexico entry; "New Mexico, Political Info, Laws in Brief," NARAL Pro-Choice America, http://www.prochoiceamerica.org/government-and-you/state-governments/state-profiles/new-mexico.html (accessed October 15, 2012). Pro-life activists in the state acknowledged the state's generally pro-choice legislature. Interview with Dauneen Dolce, March 23, 2010.

95. Frank, "The Colour of the Unborn," pp. 351–78. There were, of course, anti-abortion activists who were overt white supremacists, and the white supremacist paramilitary movement was overtly anti-abortion. Belew, *Bring the War Home.*

96. Wilson, *The Myth of Santa Fe,* pp. 156, 148.

97. For discussions of national racial unrest, see, for example, "Businessmen Agree to Abide by Bill," *The New Mexican,* July 2, 1964; "Editors Visit Alabama on Governor's Invitation," *Clovis News-Journal,* June 16, 1965; "Nightriders Fire Churches in Louisiana," *Albuquerque Tribune,* August 3, 1965; Marquis Childs, "It Can Happen Anywhere," *The New Mexican,* July 31, 1967; "Fiery Talks Started Riots," *Las Vegas Daily Optic,* August 3, 1967; Bert Okuley, "Hit City Had Plan Ready," *Clovis News-Journal,* August 3, 1967; "Hoover Notes Racial Disharmony," *Las Cruces Sun-News,* January 7, 1971.

98. David Norvell, "Norvell Generous with Praise for Staff," *The New Mexican,* June 25, 1971.

99. For Women for the Unborn, see Taranto, *Kitchen Table Politics,* p. 79. For national march and quote, see Emmens, *The Abortion Controversy,* p. 71. For marches in New Mexico, see, for example, John Robertson, "Abortion Issue Spurs Demonstration at Capitol," *The New Mexican,* January 24, 1978; Dolce interview.

100. "Abortion Ruling to Be Marked," *Albuquerque Journal,* January 22, 1974; "Ruling Celebrated, Mourned," *Albuquerque Journal,* January 24, 1974.

101. "Pro-Life Week Held in State," *Las Vegas Daily Optic,* January 23, 1976.

102. "Right to Life Plans Funeral," *Albuquerque Tribune,* January 23, 1976. The Lutheran church in question, Redeemer Lutheran, was a part of the Missouri Synod, a politically conservative branch of the Lutheran denomination.

103. "Pro-Life Week Held in State." For quote, see "Committed for Life" ad, *Albuquerque Journal,* January 14, 1977.

104. See Butler, *Women in the Church of God in Christ;* Stephenson, *Dismantling the Dualisms for American Pentecostal Women in Ministry,* pp. 34–35.

105. Mason, "Bishop C.H. Mason, Church of God in Christ," in *African American Religious History,* p. 314.

106. "To Honor Rev. Griffin," *Albuquerque Tribune,* November 30, 1974. For black neighborhoods, see Dick McAlipin, "South Broadway—Albuquerque Ghetto?" *Albuquerque Journal,* May 12, 1968; "Team Policing South Broadway," *Albuquerque Tribune,* October 28, 1977; Michael Ann Sullivan, "Albuquerque's First African American Neighborhood," http://newmexicohistory.org/2014/03/24 /albuquerques-first-african-american-neighborhood/ (accessed October 13, 2019).

107. "Group Schedules Mock Funeral," *Albuquerque Tribune,* January 21, 1976; "A Blob or a Baby" ad, *Albuquerque Journal,* January 18, 1976. There were 5,090 abortions reported in New Mexico in 1975; see Ellen Sullivan, Christopher Tietze, and Joy G. Dryfoos, "Legal Abortion in the United States, 1975–1976," *Family Planning Perspectives* 9, no. 3 (June 1977): 116.

108. "Group Schedules Mock Funeral."

109. Gonzales, "Historical Poverty, Restructuring Effects, and Integrative Ties," in *In the Barrios,* p. 158–59 (quote on p. 159). Not long before, the neighborhood had also faced the challenges of urban renewal. The city had been working on a plan to renew downtown, which included a large educational complex that could accommodate ten to twelve thousand students, slated to go into the Martineztown neighborhood. This complex would have required the demolition of many existing residences. The city eventually scaled down their plans just to replacing Albuquerque High School. Though the new plan was an improvement, some Martineztown residents still faced eviction to make way for the new school. Eventually those protesting the evictions won, and the city stopped buying land in the area and began looking for an alternative location. See Wood, "The Transformation of Albuquerque, 1945–1972," pp. 285, 429–30. See also Leary, "Urban Homeland"; Aurelio Sanchez, "Martineztown Memories Linger in the City," *Albuquerque Journal,* December 24, 2005. For more on urban renewal in Albuquerque, see Fairbanks, "The Failure of Urban Renewal in the Southwest," pp. 303–26; Logan, *Fighting Sprawl and City Hall,* pp. 95–166.

110. "Mount Calvary Cemetery, Albuquerque, Bernalillo County, New Mexico," Interment Cemetery Records Online, www.interment.net/data/us/nm/bernalillo /mtcalvary/index.htm (accessed October 8, 2012).

111. "Martineztown Park Wins OK," *Albuquerque Tribune,* November 3, 1977. For more on the lack of a public park, see Martha Buddecke, "Sta. Barbara-Martineztown Old City Area," *Albuquerque Journal,* December 23, 1968.

112. "A Blob or a Baby" ad.

113. "Committed for Life" ad, *Albuquerque Journal,* January 14, 1977.

114. Wittman, *The Tomb of the Unknown Soldier, Modern Mourning, and the Reinvention of the Mystical Body,* pp. 3, 10.

115. For a list, see http://abortionmemorials.com/sites.php (accessed September 18, 2017).

116. In her interview, Dauneen Dolce remembered that early groups in New Mexico were almost entirely Catholic. Dolce's assessment is born out in the letters to Governor David Cargo about the 1969 law; most letter writers opposing the bill wrote openly about or alluded to their Catholicism. See, for example, telegram from Father Donald Bean, San Miguel Church, Socorro, NM, to Governor David Cargo, no date, folder 241, box 6, Governor David F. Cargo Papers, New Mexico State Records Center, Santa Fe, NM (hereafter Cargo Papers); telegram from Mrs. Jerome Doherty to Governor Cargo, March 12, 1969, folder 241, box 6, Cargo Papers; telegram from Dave and Frances Holmes to Gov. David Cargo, March 13, 1969, folder 241, box 6, Cargo Papers; Rev. Edward M. Gallagher to Governor David Cargo, March 26, 1969, folder 241, box 6, Cargo Papers; Reverend Ralph Weishaar to Governor Cargo, April 1, 1969, folder 241, box 6, Cargo Papers; Eileen Durjer to Governor Cargo, February 23, 1969, folder 241, box 6, Cargo Papers.

117. Dolce interview.

118. "The Theft of Life," folder 20, box 17, Robert E. Robideau American Indian Movement Papers, Center for Southwest Research, University of New Mexico, Albuquerque, NM (hereafter Robideau Papers).

119. "Alerta! Cuidado con las 'Esterelizaciones Forzadas,'" November 14, 1974, folder 20, box 20, Frank I. Sanchez Papers, Center for Southwest Research, University of New Mexico, Albuquerque, NM. For more on the sterilizations in LA, see Gutiérrez, *Fertile Matters.*

120. "The Theft of Life"; Coalition for Medical Rights of Women, *Coalition News,* August 1977, folder 40, box 27, National Indian Youth Council Records, Center for Southwest Research, University of New Mexico, Albuquerque, NM (hereafter Youth Council Records); "Women Didn't Realize," November 1978, folder 38, box 27, Youth Council Records. For the percentage of Indian women sterilized, see Lawrence, "The Indian Health Service and the Sterilization of Native American Women," pp. 400–19 (number on p. 400).

121. "Medicine Talk for the Indian Family" Seminar, Northwest Indian Women's Circle, Annual Report 1981, folder 21, box 21, Robideau Papers.

122. National Indian Health Board, "Abortion and Sterilization," folder 9, box 3, Roger A. Finzel American Indian Movement Papers, Center for Southwest Research, University of New Mexico, Albuquerque; "Fight the Abortion Cuts—No Forced Sterilizations" (probably 1978), folder 40, box 27, Youth Council Records.

123. *Viva Life* newsletter, February 1986 and March 1986, folder 1, box 1–8, HH120, Right to Life, New Mexico, Hall Hoag Collection; Dolce interview. For more civil rights rhetoric in the Four Corners states, see *Arizona Right to Life News-*

letter, April-May 1990 and March 1983, both at University of Arizona Library Special Collections, University of Arizona, Tucson, AZ.

124. For more on Mildred Jefferson, see Williams, *Defending the Unborn,* pp. 171–74; Haugeberg, *Women Against Abortion,* pp. 13–16.

125. Many black women, even those in the same movements as these individuals, opposed this link. By the late 1970s, such comparisons became much less common. See, for example, Roberts, *Killing the Black Body,* pp. 99–102.

126. On the other hand, Coretta Scott King, Martin Luther King's widow, has supported abortion rights and gay marriage and argued that her husband would have shared her beliefs. One central piece of evidence in Coretta Scott King's favor is that her husband had been a member of Planned Parenthood since the mid-1950s and, in 1966, he accepted the Planned Parenthood Margaret Sanger Award. In his acceptance speech, King said, "Our sure beginning in the struggle for equality by non-violent direct action may not have been so resolute without the tradition established by Margaret Sanger and people like her." See Davis, *Sacred Work,* p. 27. For Coretta Scott King's support of abortion rights, see "Thousands Retrace King's March," *Times-News* (Burlington, NC), August 29, 1993. For Alveda King's activism and claims about Martin Luther King, see for example "King Niece Advocates Right-Wing Standards," *Austin American-Statesman,* January 18, 1998; "King's Niece Campaigns for the Unborn 'Life Was Very Important to Him,' She Says," *Boston Globe,* January 17, 2000; Hilary White, "One Quarter of Black Population Missing from Abortion Genocide Says Dr. Alveda King," *LifeSiteNews,* August 24, 2007, at http://www.lifesitenews.com/news/archive//ldn/2007/aug/07082406 (accessed October 5, 2012); Jessica Greene, "Life Is a Civil Right, King Niece Says," *Ocala Star-Banner* (FL), January 12, 2008; King, *How Can the Dream Survive if We Murder Children?;* King, foreword to Howard, *Almost Wasn't,* pp. 9–10; Blumenthal, *Republican Gommorah,* pp. 147–49.

127. *Arizona Right to Life News,* August 2000, University of Arizona Library Special Collections, University of Arizona, Tucson, AZ.

128. Tobias, *Jews in New Mexico since World War II,* pp. 112–13.

129. This particular protest backfired, however. Fifty clergy from various denominations, including some staunchly pro-life ones, condemned the protest.

130. Sebesta interview.

3. CLAIMING RELIGION

1. Interview with Ruth Dolan, August 8, 2011.

2. This was not the case with birth control. Some Protestant and Jewish denominations had supported the birth control movement since the 1930s. See Davis, *Sacred Work.*

3. Dr. Carlton C. Allen, "The Population Explosion," sermon delivered at First United Presbyterian Church, Albuquerque, January 26, 1969, enclosed in Laurie K.

Bowen to Governor David Cargo, March 3, 1969, folder 241, box 6, Governor David F. Cargo Papers, New Mexico State Records Center, Santa Fe, NM (hereafter Cargo Papers).

4. Rykken Johnson, "Minister Calls State Law Repressive," *Rocky Mountain News,* November 10, 1969. The group had been founded in 1969 in New York. That same year, Rabbi Lewis Bogage, one of the founding members of the CCS in New York, helped start the group in Denver. For more on CCS in Colorado, see Olga Curtis, "Clergymen Who Offer Abortion Aid," *Denver Post,* January 25, 1970; interview with Rev. Jerry Kolb, November 7, 2011; Joan McCoy, "Abortion Group's Name Is a Misnomer," *Rocky Mountain News,* July 10, 1972. Other Clergy Consultation Service groups existed quietly or completely underground in the other Four Corner states. For a single mention of a CCS in Arizona, see Eileen Hulse, "Abortion Is a Fact," folder 8, box 35, Planned Parenthood of Northern and Central Arizona Collection, Arizona Historical Foundation, Hayden Library, Arizona State University, Tempe, AZ (hereafter Planned Parenthood AZ Collection). One New York member of CCS moved to Utah and, after *Roe,* spoke to the *Salt Lake Tribune* about his experience. It is possible that this minister provided religious counseling and recommendations in Utah before it was legal as well. See Rev. Ronald E. Clark, "Sex Education or . . . Abortion," *Salt Lake Tribune,* February 11, 1973. An Episcopal rector in Salt Lake City also noted he sent women to Los Angeles for abortions before *Roe.* See Szasz, *Religion in the Modern American West,* p. 134.

5. Greenhouse and Siegel, eds., *Before Roe v. Wade,* p. 29.

6. For United Methodist and Southern Baptist statements supporting abortion reform, see ibid., pp. 70–72. Other national religious associations and organizations that supported abortion reform before *Roe v. Wade* include: American Baptist Convention, American Ethical Union, American Humanist Association, American Jewish Congress, American Protestant Hospital Association, B'nai B'rith Women, Church Women United (Board of Managers), Episcopal Church, Moravian Church (Northern Province Synod), National Council of Jewish Women, United Church of Canada (General Council), United Church of Christ, United Methodist Church, United Presbyterian Church in the USA, United Universalist Church, Women's Division of the United Methodist Church, and the Young Women's Christian Association of the USA. See Tatalovich and Daynes, *The Politics of Abortion,* pp. 66–67.

7. For a few accounts of dueling amendments, Tribe, *Abortion,* pp. 162–63; Miller, *Good Catholics,* pp. 94–99; Ziegler, *After Roe,* pp. 148–49.

8. In 1969, when the Diocese of Phoenix was formed, it contained over 185,000 Catholics and fifty parishes. By 1975, those numbers had probably grown significantly. See "Cincinnati Man Is Named Bishop," *Tucson Daily Citizen,* September 3, 1969.

9. G. A. (Jack) Bradley to Reverend Monsignor Robert J. Donohoe, January 15, 1976, with attached statement from Bishop Edward A. McCarthy and recommendations, folder 4, box 22, Robert J. Donohoe Papers, Arizona Collection, Hayden Library, Arizona State University, Tempe, AZ (hereafter Donohoe Papers). These services were a part of a Respect Life Week, initially conceived of by American bishops in 1972. See United States Catholic Conference, *Respect Life!*

10. Sociologist Christel J. Manning argues this was a condition unique to Catholics. Jews and Protestants could more easily separate themselves into congregations of like-minded people. See Manning, "Women in a Divided Church," pp. 375–90.

11. Interview with Mike Berger, March 18, 2010.

12. Robert N. Lynch, "'Abortion' and 1976 Politics," *America,* March 6, 1976. Monsignor Robert Donohoe, Dean of Maricopa County and ecumenical pro-life organizer for the diocese, kept this particular article. See folder 2, box 21, Donohoe Papers.

13. Miller, *Good Catholics,* p. 63.

14. Interview with Margaret Sebesta (pseudonym), August 8, 2011.

15. Virgil C. Blum, "Public Policy Making: Why the Churches Strike Out," *America,* March 6, 1971. For an extended conversation about abortion arguments made in Catholic magazine *America* in the 1960s, see Tatalovich and Daynes, *The Politics of Abortion,* pp. 86–100.

16. O'Neil, *Church Lobbying in a Western State,* pp. 38–39.

17. Interview with John Jakubczyk, March 16, 2010.

18. Interview with Laurie Futch, March 16, 2010.

19. Interview with Phil and Helen Seader, March 18, 2010.

20. "Catholics Shown Abortion Slides," *Arizona Republic,* February 26, 1973.

21. James E. Palmer to Congressman Wayne Owens, March 4, 1974, folder 2, box 39, Wayne Owens Papers, Special Collections, J. Willard Marriott Library, University of Utah, Salt Lake City, UT (hereafter Owens Papers). For another example of pro-life petitions in church, see Jane Kay, "City Council to Consider Anti-Abortion Proposal," *Arizona Daily Star,* November 12, 1973.

22. Mrs. Amalia L. Santallanes to Governor King, August 26, 1979, folder 3140, 3141, 3142, box 101, Governor Bruce King Papers (2nd Term), New Mexico State Records Center, Santa Fe, NM (hereafter 2nd Term King Papers). For hundreds of similar letters, see folder 3140, 3141, 3142, box 101, 2nd Term King Papers. For an example of a letter-writing campaign directed at young adults, see letters from Gabriel Valdez, Richard Stanley, Paul Fratto, Gene Alberico, Frieda Vallejos, Rosalinsa Rocha, Mary Johnson, Fidel Giscumbo, Penny Lee Nichols, Pat Santistevan, Jaren Badovinatz, Bobby Sandoval, Kathy Martinez, David Valdez, Gerald A. Kramer, Kelly Bailey, Julie Johnson, Diane Sandoval, Melody Fithen, Brenda Manganares, Trudy Miller, Stephanie Grochowski, and Liz Geay, all to Congressman Wayne Owens, folder 17, box 23, Owens Papers.

23. "Abortion," *Newsweek,* June 5, 1978.

24. For example, see telegram from Dave and Frances Holmes, Albuquerque, to Gov. David Cargo, March 13, 1969, folder 241, box 6, Cargo Papers; telegram from Mrs. Jerome Doherty, to Governor Cargo, March 12, 1969, folder 241, box 6, Cargo Papers.

25. Eileen Duryer to Governor Cargo, February 23, 1969, folder 241, box 6, Cargo Papers.

26. Richard E. Villamana to Governor Cargo, March 24, 1969, folder 241, box 6, Cargo Papers. For another similar letters, see Reverend Ralph Weishaar to

Governor Cargo, April 1, 1969, folder 241, box 6, Cargo Papers; Rev. Raymond Amiro to Governor Cargo, March 28, 1969, folder 241, box 6, Cargo Papers.

27. Aldona S. Jameson to Governor Apodaca, August 23, 1977, folder 2024, box 85, Governor Jerry Apodaca Papers, New Mexico State Records Center, Santa Fe, NM.

28. Weslin, *The Gathering of the Lambs,* pp. 154–55.

29. National Conference of Catholic Bishops, "Pastoral Plan for Pro-Life Activities," November 20, 1975, folder 3, box 21, Donohoe Papers.

30. Jakubczyk interview.

31. Seader interview.

32. Ibid. For another example of the use of bulletins, see Taranto, *Kitchen·Table Politics,* p. 69.

33. Weslin, *The Gathering of the Lambs,* p. 83.

34. Virginia Culver, "Rector Says Women's Liberty, License Confused," *Denver Post,* March 6, 1971. For parish defection, see "State Working on Secession's Legality Decision," *Greeley Daily Tribune,* December 8, 1976; "Dissident Priest Expects Rebellion," *Colorado Springs Telegraph Gazette,* December 3, 1976; Dennis Hevesi, "Bishop James O. Mote, 84, Dies; Led Revolt Against Episcopal Church," *New York Times,* May 29, 2006.

35. Pascoe, *Relations of Rescue,* p. 22; Gordon, *The Mormon Question,* pp. 55–83.

36. John Taylor, Journal of Discourses, March 5, 1882, folder 1, box 26, Lester E. Bush Collection, Special Collections, J. Willard Marriott Library, University of Utah, Salt Lake City, UT (hereafter Bush Collection). For the escalation of government opposition to polygamy, see Gordon, *The Mormon Question,* pp. 183–220.

37. John Taylor, Journal of Discourses, October 19, 1884, folder 1, box 26, Bush Collection. See also John Taylor, Journal of Discourses, April 9, 1882, folder 1, box 26, Bush Collection. Six years earlier, John Taylor and George Q. Cannon used similar rhetoric about easterners bringing abortion to Utah. See John Taylor and George Q. Cannon, Journal of Discourses, July 21, 1878, folder 1, box 26, Bush Collection.

38. Quoted in Daynes and Tatalovich, "Mormons and Abortion Politics in the United States," p. 4.

39. Meanwhile, anti-polygamists argued that, in order to keep plural marriage a secret in the 1830s and 1840s, Joseph Smith had forced his wives, after his first one, to have abortions. See A. T. Schroeder, *Lucifer's Lantern,* no. 7 (September 1898): 184–88, folder 1, box 26, Bush Collection. Protestants and Mormons in the nineteenth and twentieth centuries levied similar accusations at Catholic nuns, arguing they were secretly having sex with men (usually priests) and terminating pregnancies to cover it up. In these stories, abortion acts as a potent signifier for sexual and religious deviance. For examples of folk tales about nuns and abortion, see Eileen Black, Provo UT, Fall 1970, writing about her childhood growing up in Long Beach, CA, folder 17, box 13, Human Condition Legends, Fife Folklore Collection, Special Collections and Archives, Merrill-Cazier Library, Utah State University, Logan, UT (hereafter Fife Collection); Nancy Lubeck, Pleasant Hill, CA, Winter 1975, writing

about Jerry Wright of Pleasant Hill, CA, folder 17, box 13, Human Condition Legends, Fife Collection.

40. Gottlieb and Wiley, *America's Saints,* p. 130. For more on the international church, see pp. 129–56.

41. For the ERA debate in Utah, see Holland, "Salt Lake City Is Our Selma"; Bradley, *Pedestals and Podiums;* Quinn, "The LDS Church's Campaign Against the Equal Rights Amendment," pp. 85–155, and "Exporting Utah's Theocracy since 1975," in *God and Country,* pp. 129–68; Gottlieb and Wiley, *America's Saints,* pp. 187–213.

42. Hunter, "A Religious Rhetoric of Abortion," p. 67. Hunter argues that abortion was only discussed indirectly through opposition to birth control between 1919 and 1971.

43. Arrington, *Great Basin Kingdom,* p. 32.

44. James E. Faust, "The Sanctity of Life," April 1975, General Conferences, The Church of Jesus Christ of Latter-day Saints website, https://www.lds.org/general-conference/1975/04/the-sanctity-of-life?lang = eng (accessed September 24, 2017).

45. Kerns, *The Speaker's Guide to 40 Years of General Conference,* Abortion entry. For the full text of these remarks, see General Conferences, The Church of Jesus Christ of Latter-day Saints website, https://www.lds.org/general-conference/1975/04/the-sanctity-of-life?lang = eng (accessed September 24, 2017).

46. Ben Tullis, "LDS General Conference Marks 90th, 65th Broadcast Anniversaries," *Deseret News,* September 29, 2014; Prince and Wright, *David O. McKay and the Rise of Modern Mormonism,* p. 124.

47. "LDS World Conference, Oct. 2–4," *Provo Daily Herald,* September 20, 1970.

48. Shepherd and Shepherd, *Binding Earth and Heaven,* pp. 112–14.

49. Ruth F. Stewart to Mr. Owens, April 3, 1973, folder 14, box 23, Owens Papers; Ruth F. Stewart to Rep. McKay, April 4, 1973, folder 14, box 147, Congressman Gunn McKay Papers, Special Collections and Archives, Merrill-Cazier Library, Utah State University, Logan, UT (hereafter McKay Papers).

50. Barbara B. Smith, "Life—The Essential," January 22, 1977, folder 1, box 4, Martha Sonntag Bradley Research Collection, L. Tom Perry Special Collections, Harold B. Lee Library, Brigham Young University, Provo, UT (hereafter Bradley Collection).

51. Letters for Life, Associated Students of BYU, no date (likely 1979), folder 6, box 3, Associated Students of Brigham Young University Women's Office History Collection, L. Tom Perry Special Collections, Harold B. Lee Library, Brigham Young University, Provo, UT (hereafter ASBYU Collection); "BYU Students Support 'Right to Life' Bills," no newspaper, 1979, folder 6, box 3, ASBYU Collection.

52. John L. Carpenter, "Anti-Abortion Group Illegally Fund Raising," *Phoenix Gazette,* April 30, 1974.

53. July 1, 1977 entry, June-Nov., 1977 Journal, folder 33, box 5, Sandra Allen Collection, Center for Southwest Research, University of New Mexico, Albuquerque, NM (hereafter Allen Collection).

54. July 24, 1977 entry, June-Nov., 1977 Journal, folder 33, box 5, Allen Collection.

55. July 11, 1977 entry, June-Nov., 1977 Journal, folder 33, box 5, Allen Collection. For more discussions of dark spirits or darkness when encountering non-Mormons, see August 2, 1977 and September 23, 1977 entries.

56. January 22, 1978 entry, Dec. 1977-May 1979 Journal, folder 34, box 5, Allen Collection.

57. January 15, 1978 entry, Dec. 1977-May 1979 Journal, folder 34, box 5, Allen Collection.

58. "An Important Introduction," folder 32, box 5, Allen Collection.

59. February 1978 entry, Dec. 1977-May 1979 Journal, folder 34, box 5, Allen Collection.

60. A 1973 poll contended that 85 percent of Mormon women opposed making abortions available to women who wanted them. See Lois Gogarty, "LDS Women Unaffected by Women's Lib," *Ensign,* August 1973, folder 9, box 10, Bradley Collection.

61. Futch interview; interview with Kay Allen, March 16, 2010. For examples of Mormon participation, see Right to Life of Utah newsletter, September 1977, folder 1, box 4, Bradley Collection; interview with Mary LeQuiu, March 22, 2010.

62. Interview with Dauneen Dolce, March 23, 2010. Political scientists Byron Daynes and Raymond Tatalovich offer an alternative explanation: Mormons focused more on state and regional abortion policy, which the church hierarchy could affect in more direct ways than public protest. See Daynes and Tatalovich, "Mormons and Abortion Politics," pp. 1–13.

63. Young, *We Gather Together,* p. 124.

64. Crapo, "Grass-Roots Deviance from Official Doctrine," pp. 473–74.

65. This was true of "personhood" laws and amendments, popular in the early twenty-first century, that sought to define personhood from the moment of conception and ban all abortions. See interview with Leslie Hanks, August 5, 2011.

66. For arguments on Mormon influence on the ERA, see Mathews and De Hart, *Sex, Gender, and the Politics of ERA;* Quinn, "The LDS Church's Campaign Against the Equal Rights Amendment"; Holland, "Salt Lake City Is Our Selma"; Bradley, *Pedestals and Podiums.* For Mormon influence on gay marriage campaigns in 2000 and 2008, see, for example, Don Lattin, "Mormon Church: The Powerful Force Behind Proposition 22," *San Francisco Chronicle,* February 6, 2000; Reed Cowan and Steven Greenstreet, directors, *8: The Mormon Proposition* (David V. Goliath Films, 2010); Perry and Cronin, *Mormons and American Politics,* pp. 95–99; Peggy Fletcher Stack, "Prop 8 Involvement a P.R. Fiasco for LDS Church," *Salt Lake Tribune,* November 22, 2008; Nicolas Riccardi, "Mormon Church Feels Heat Over Proposition 8," *Los Angeles Times,* November 17, 2008; Stephanie Mencimer, "Mormon Church Abandons Its Crusade Against Gay Marriage," *Mother Jones,* April 12, 2013.

67. Szasz, *Religion in the Modern American West,* pp. 139–141.

68. See chapter 1.

69. For more on evangelicals' positions on abortion in the 1960s, see Williams, *God's Own Party,* pp. 114–17; Young, *We Gather Together,* pp. 101–4; Flipse, "Below-the-Belt Politics," in *Conservative Sixties,* pp. 127–41; Williams, "Sex and Evangelicals," in *American Evangelicals in the 1960s,* pp. 97–120; Miller, *The Age of Evangelicalism,* p. 54.

70. For Holbrook's engagement with pro-life groups, see *Arizona Lifeline,* February 1975, University of Arizona Library Special Collections. For his work within the Southern Baptist Convention, see Williams, *God's Own Party,* pp. 118–19.

71. Heltzel, *Jesus and Justice,* pp. 102–3; Dudley, *Broken Words,* pp. 48–49; Williams, *God's Own Party,* pp. 155–56; Domenico and Hanley, eds., *Encyclopedia of Modern Religious Politics,* p. 490; Dowland, *Family Values and the Rise of the Christian Right,* pp. 120–21; Noll, *God and Race in American Politics,* p. 159; Risen and Thomas, *Wrath of Angels,* pp. 124–26.

72. Risen and Thomas, *Wrath of Angels,* p. 125.

73. Marsden, *Reforming Fundamentalism,* pp. 277–98; Young, *We Gather Together,* pp. 143–48.

74. Williams, "Sex and Evangelicals."

75. Garcia, "Roundtable on the Religious Right and Communities of Color," p. 15. The anti-abortion movement made more effort to organize in the African American community in the twenty-first century.

76. Baer and Singer, *African American Religion in the Twentieth Century,* pp. 88–99; Brown, "Racial Differences in Congregation-based Political Activism," pp. 1581–1604; Evans, "Polarization in Abortion Attitudes in U.S. Religious Traditions," pp. 397–422; Abramowitz, "It's Abortion, Stupid," p. 181; Robinson, "From Every Tribe and Nation?" pp. 591–601.

77. Harding, *The Book of Jerry Falwell,* p. 194.

78. Fletcher, *Preaching to Convert,* p. 187. See also Roberts, *The Hell House Outreach Manual;* Ratliff, director, *Hell House* documentary; Pellegrini, "Signaling Through the Flames," pp. 911–35.

79. Grainger, *In the World but Not of It,* p. 65; Bivins, *Religion of Fear,* p. 143.

80. Wilcox, "Evangelicals and Abortion," in *A Public Faith,* p. 106.

81. See for example, Ebaugh and Haney, "Church Attendance and Attitudes Towards Abortion," pp. 407–13; McIntosh, Alston, and Alston, "The Differential Impact of Religious Preference and Church Attendance on Attitudes Towards Abortion," pp. 195–213; Coughlin, "The Economic Person in Sociological Context," in *Socio-Economics,* ; Wilcox, "Evangelicals and Abortion," p. 111.

82. Gary Potter, Catholics for Christian Political Action, to Colleagues (American Conservative Union in AZ), undated (probably October 1978), box 51, Register of American Conservative Union, L. Tom Perry Special Collections, Harold B. Lee Library, Brigham Young University, Provo, UT.

83. Judie Glave, "Survey Finds Hispanics Agree with Church," *Alamogordo Daily News,* February 10, 1986. "Changing Faiths: Latinos and the Transformation of American Religion," Hispanic Trends, Pew Research Center, 2007, http://www.pewhispanic.org/2007/04/25/viii-ideology-and-policy-issues/ (accessed August 5,

2016). Most of these surveys covered the entire Latino community, often including ethnic Mexicans, Cubans, Puerto Ricans, and others.

84. Matovina, *Guadalupe and Her Faithful,* pp. 136–37.

85. Stevens-Arroyo, "The Latino Religious Resurgence," pp. 163–77.

86. Miller, *Good Catholics,* pp. 131–269, 80. For contemporary observers noting this shift, see "Abortion," *Newsweek,* June 5, 1978; Diane Lee, letter to the editor, *Denver Catholic Register,* October 31, 1974.

87. Barnhouse, *Northwest Denver,* pp. 55, 8.

88. "Out of the Pulpit, Into the Streets: Church Activists Are on the March," *U.S. News and World Report,* April 21, 1986; "Turning Weapons in Pledges," *New York Times,* December 11, 1988; Christopher Lopez, "Priest Ends Peace Fast: Concerned Parishioners Express Relief," *Denver Post,* August 5, 1993; Virginia Culver, "City's Voices Lifted in Prayer: All Faiths Seek an End to Violence," *Denver Post,* December 6, 1993; Stacey Baca, "Hispanics Tackle AIDs: Community Uniting to Bring the Fight Home," *Denver Post,* April 28, 1996; Jeffrey Leib, "Activists Ask Support for Strawberry Pickers, United Farm Workers Say Field Conditions Appalling," *Denver Post,* August 15, 1996.

89. Interview with Father Jose Lara, by Dana Echohawk, January 8, 2011, Center for Colorado and the West at Auraria Library, http://www.historycolorado.org /sites/default/files/files/Jose%20Lara.pdf (accessed July 18, 2016).

90. Vigil, *Crusade for Justice,* pp. 306–27. Our Lady of Guadalupe had also been the site of a funeral for a Crusade for Justice activist slain by police in 1973.

91. Robert Trujillo, letter to the editor, *Denver Catholic Register,* April 14, 1976. For more on the raid and the call for resignation, see "Vatican II Shock Waves Reach Denver," *Denver Catholic Register,* May 11, 1977.

92. Trujillo, letter to the editor.

93. Interview with Father Jose Lara.

94. Scott C. Frey of Boulder, letter to the editor, "Church's 'Haranguing' on Abortion Rejected," *Denver Catholic Register,* July 14, 1976.

95. Interview with Father Jose Lara.

96. Stevens-Arroyo, "Pious Colonialism," in *Mexican American Religions,* p. 60. For a theologian's take on Mexican everyday religion, see Espín, "Mexican Religious Practices, Popular Catholicism, and the Development of Doctrine," in *Horizons of the Sacred.*

97. Matovina, "Lay Initiatives in Worship on the Texas *Frontera,*" pp. 107–20 (quote on p. 120). While Matovina's source material is from Texas, historian Ann Butler agrees with Matovina that the power of the laity marks western Catholicism more generally. See Butler, "Western Spaces, Catholic Places," pp. 25–39, and *Across God's Frontiers.* The leadership of women in these communal rituals has led scholars to call this type of Catholicism institutionalized patriarchy with a "matriarchal core." See Diaz-Stevens, "The Saving Grace," pp. 60–78.

98. Stevens-Arroyo, "Pious Colonialism," pp. 66.

99. Rodriguez, *Our Lady of Guadalupe,* pp. 1–46.

100. For more on Latinas' relationship with the Virgin of Guadalupe, see Rodriguez, *Our Lady of Guadalupe*. Of course, some ethnic Mexicans used Guadalupe and the broader concept of *familia* to misogynistic ends. See Rodríguez, *Next of Kin*. Recent studies have shown that Latinas. seek abortions at higher rates than white women, but lower than black women. See Matovina, *Latino Catholicism,* pp. 217.

101. Interview with Father Jose Lara.

102. Colleen O'Connor, "Our Lady of Guadalupe: Immaculate Icon, Symbol of Piety, or Pop Culture Decoration," *Denver Post,* December 5, 2004.

103. Electra Draper, "Church Wall Causing Division," *Denver Post,* November 24, 2010.

104. Tina Greigo, "Church Wall Hiding Our Lady of Guadalupe Mural Brings Protest," *Denver Post,* July 2, 2010.

105. Stevens-Arroyo, "Pious Colonialism," pp. 66–9.

106. Throughout the last few decades of the century, a handful of ethnic Mexicans, usually either recent immigrants from Mexico or elite *Hispanos,* did participate. For example, in the early 2000s, a recent immigrant from Aguas Calientes led one of the few pro-life groups for ethnic Mexicans in the region. See interview with Socorro Gallegos, August 2, 2011.

107. Quoted in Matovina, *Latino Catholicism,* p. 212.

108. Stevens-Arroyo, "Pious Colonialism," p. 5. See also Díaz-Stevens and Stevens-Arroyo, *Recognizing the Latino Resurgence in U.S. Religion.*

109. Seader interview.

110. Silk, "Notes on the Judeo-Christian Tradition in America," pp. 65–85 (quotes on pp. 67–68). For more on religious pluralism in this period, see Moore, *GI Jews;* Mart, "The 'Christianization' of Israel and Jews in 1950s America," pp. 109–47; Schultz, *Tri-Faith America.*

111. Young, *We Gather Together,* pp. 9–37.

112. Interview with Mary Menicucci, March 26, 2010. These religious divisions were not present in all towns and cities but they were relatively common. See Ianora, *Crisis Pregnancy Centers,* introduction. For more on these tensions in the Four Corners states, see Allen interview; LeQuiu interview.

113. Dolan interview.

114. Jakubczyk interview.

115. For one example of ecumenical presentation at a local rally, see Judith Van Luchene and Jackie Rothenberg, "Women Voters Endorse Right to Choose Abortion," *Arizona Republic,* January 23, 1983.

116. Silk, "Notes on the Judeo-Christian Tradition," p. 83.

117. Maxwell, "A More Determined Discipleship." At the time of the lecture, Maxwell was a member of the Quorum of Seventy, though he would soon after join the Quorum of Twelve. These are the most important governing bodies of the LDS Church, right behind the First Presidency (which includes the President and his top two counselors). *Christianity Today,* a major evangelical periodical, and Catholic theology magazines both used the language of Judeo-Christian values to explain

their opposition to abortion in the aftermath of *Roe v. Wade*. See Young, *We Gather Together*, p. 113.

118. For a sample of primary source material on Judeo-Christian values, abortion, and the nation, see "Black Monday Decision" ad, *Clovis News-Journal,* March 30, 1970; Pat McGraw, "Abortion Foes Says Backers Playing God," *Denver Post,* December 27, 1971; Lorette Svejcar to Governor King, (received) October 3, 1972, folder 220, box 12, Governor Bruce King Papers (1st Term), New Mexico State Records Center, Santa Fe, NM; "Euthanasia on Its Way, Priest Says," *Arizona Republic,* October 19, 1973; Virginia Culver, "Catholic Hospitals Reject Abortions—Rule or No," *Denver Post,* January 31, 1973; *Arizona Lifeline,* February 1975, University of Arizona Library Special Collections, University of Arizona, Tucson, AZ; Joseph Cusack, "Moral Decay Imperils 'Nation Under God,'" *Scottsdale Daily Progress,* August 24, 1976; Colorado Pro-Family Coalition, "Articles of Incorporation," 1980, box 14, Equality Colorado Collection, Western History and Genealogy Department, Denver Public Library, Denver, CO.

119. Michael Romero Taylor, "Protestors Infringing on Others' Rights," letter to the editor, *Santa Fe New Mexican,* November 19, 1983.

120. Diane Woelfel, "Antiabortion Demonstration Continues at Boulder Clinic," *Boulder Daily Camera,* January 18, 1976.

121. Bill Conti, "Antiabortionists Conclude Novena at Free Clinic Here," *Boulder Daily Camera,* January 4, 1976.

122. Interview with Phil Leahy, March 23, 2010.

123. Interview with Laura Bowman, March 24, 2010.

124. Tonia Twitchell, "Anti-Abortion Protestors Rally in Effort to Close Tempe Clinic," no newspaper, no date, folder 64, box 30, Planned Parenthood AZ Collection.

125. For candles, see Tom Sharpe, "St. Vincent Medical Staff Oks Abortion," *Santa Fe New Mexican,* October 26, 1977. For hymns, see interview with Kayrene Pearson, by Molly Lauridsen, Oct. 17, 2003, folder 16, box 2, Anne Marie Pois Oral History Project Collection, University of Colorado-Boulder Archives, Boulder, CO (hereafter Pois Collection); Twitchell, "Anti-Abortion Protestors Rally in Effort to Close Tempe Clinic"; Lina Cornett, "Clinic Survives 20 Years of Conflict," no newspaper, Sept. 26, 1993, folder 1, box 2, Pois Collection.

126. "Gantlet," *Tempe Daily News* (?), June 23, 1984, folder 66, box 30, Planned Parenthood AZ Collection.

127. Leahy interview. For another protestor hoping for conversion of abortion providers, see "Abortion Protest," no newspaper, November 9, 1975, folder 1, box 2, Pois Collection.

128. Interview with Tom Longua, August 4, 2011.

129. Pam Izakowitz, "Birthright: Anti-abortion Group Pickets on Mother's Day," *Mesa Tribune,* May 8, 1983.

130. Jakubczyk interview.

131. Leahy interview.

132. Ibid.

133. Interview with Pearson, Pois Collection.

134. Activists in the pro-life rescue movement of the 1980s and the 1990s worked to extend this religious political space to more of the city. Thousands descended on a chosen city to protest abortion and tie up the city's jails. In so doing, they demanded that residents rethink the moral geography of their city.

135. Interview with Steven Imbarrato, March 23, 2010.

136. "Evangelicals: Emphasis Is on Ministry Work," *Colorado Springs Gazette-Telegraph,* November 24, 1991; "Battleground: Springs Considered a Divine Magnet," *Colorado Springs Gazette Telegraph,* September 25, 1993.

4. REDEFINING WOMEN'S RIGHTS

1. Interview with Angela Schnieder, March 17, 2010. For a newspaper description of Reachout, see Carla McClain, "Pregnant? Reachout Advises, But with a 'Pro-Life' View," *Tucson Daily Citizen,* August 14, 1981.

2. On the other activities of Conservation for Human Life, see interview with Helen and Phil Seader, March 18, 2010; "Abortion—The Destruction of Defenseless Human Life Is a Matter of Vital Public Concern!" *Tucson Daily Citizen,* February 16, 1971; "Protecting Human Life," letters to the editor, *Tucson Daily Citizen,* March 4, 1971; "Murder? Legal Abortion Examined," *Tucson Daily Citizen,* March 31, 1971; "Abortion Kickback Denied," *Tucson Daily Citizen,* August 15, 1972; letters to the editor, *Tucson Daily Citizen,* November 7, 1972; Conservation for Human Life, "Abortion Dehumanizes, Degrades, Destroys" ad, *Tucson Daily Citizen,* October 31, 1972.

3. Munson, *The Making of Pro-Life Activists,* p. 113. A couple of scholars have recently explored CPCs in depth while many others have addressed crisis pregnancy centers as a small part of their larger projects. See Kelly, "In the Name of the Mother," pp. 203–30; Haugeberg, *Women Against Abortion,* pp. 9–55; Ginsburg, *Contested Lives,* pp. 73–75, 114–22; Taylor, *The Public Life of the Fetal Sonogram,* pp. 144–68; Schoen, *Abortion After Roe,* pp. 180–86.

4. Though Robert Pearson's 1984 manual, *How to Start and Operate Your Own Pro-Life Outreach Crisis Pregnancy Center,* was used by many CPCs, his initial center resembled a traditional home for unwed mothers more than a modern CPC. For more on the first Pearson center, see Steinhoff and Diamond, *Abortion Politics,* p. 187.

5. Interview with Margaret Sebesta (pseudonym), August 8, 2011.

6. For the founding of these Birthrights, see Ianora, *Crisis Pregnancy Centers,* pp. 30–31; interview with Laurie Futch, March 16, 2010; Emma Gomez to Bruce King, March 18, 1972, folder 220, box 12, Governor Bruce King Papers (1st Term), New Mexico State Records Center, Santa Fe, NM; "Birthright Movement Launched," *Las Cruces Sun Times* (NM), May 5, 1972; "Birthright Chapter to Explain Program Aim at Orientation," *Salt Lake Tribune,* November 16, 1974.

7. While there were CPCs in all Four Corners states, Utah had the fewest. This was in large part because Mormons could rely on LDS Social Services for help with an unplanned pregnancy. While LDS Social Services probably counseled almost always to carry a pregnancy to term, the structure, employees, and expectations of LDS Social Services were different from CPCs. See LDS Social Services Unwed Parent Outreach Program, folder 9, box 6, Jaynann Payne Records and Papers, L. Tom Perry Special Collections, Harold B. Lee Library, Brigham Young University, Provo, UT.

8. Summerhill, *The Story of Birthright*.

9. Seader interview.

10. For the donation, see "'Reachout' Offers Problem Pregnancy Counseling," *Arizona Lifeline*, February 1975, University of Arizona Library Special Collections, University of Arizona, Tucson, AZ. For the status and occupation of James Doran, see "Initiative Given Boost," picture, *Tucson Daily Citizen*, June 1, 1962; "Civic Unity Council Elects," *Tucson Daily Citizen*, January 3, 1963; "TCC Agencies Make Requests," *Tucson Daily Citizen*, January 7, 1966.

11. For CPC started in spare bedroom, see Sebesta interview. For CPC started in ambulance garage, see interview with Mary LeQuiu, March 22, 2010.

12. Sebesta interview.

13. In the 1920 census, there were 419 African Americans in Pima County, or 1.2 percent of the population. By 1930, there were 1,251 or 2.2 percent of the population. In 1940 the numbers increased to 2,083 or 2.85 percent of the population. Percentages jumped significantly in the 1950 census with 5.017 African Americans in Pima County or 3.55 percent of the population. See Historical Census Browser, retrieved July 8, 2011, from the University of Virginia, Geospatial and Statistical Data Center, http://fisher.lib.virginia.edu/collections/stats/histcensus/index.html. For black neighborhoods of Tucson, see Getty, *Interethnic Relationships in the Community of Tucson*, pp. 138–39. For geographic and social divisions in Tucson, see Sheridan, *Los Tucsonenses* and *Arizona;* Otero, *La Calle*.

14. See Taylor, *In Search of the Racial Frontier;* Sheridan, *Arizona;* Whitaker, *Race Work*.

15. For more on this crisis, see "Project Would Cut Negro Ratio, Judge Says," *Tucson Daily Citizen*, April 16, 1968; "'Turnkey' Job Can Go Ahead," *Tucson Daily Citizen*, March 26, 1968; "New 'Turnkey' Hearing Demanded of Council," *Tucson Daily Citizen*, May 22, 1968; "Council Again Trying North Side Housing," *Tucson Daily Citizen*, July 8, 1969; "Fire Bombs Hit Four Units of El Capitan Apartments," *Tucson Daily Citizen*, April 10, 1969; "Home Near El Capitan Hit By Bottle Firebomb," *Tucson Daily Citizen*, April 11, 1969; "Police Lauded for Work During Fire Bomb Case," *Tucson Daily Citizen*, May 27, 1969; "Report on El Capitan Criticized by Students," *Tucson Daily Citizen*, May 29, 1969; Mrs. C.M. Hitchcock, "Clearing Up Some Confusion," letter to the editor, *Tucson Daily Citizen*, July 15, 1969; "Police Chief Seeks Meeting on Mansfield Park Issues," *Tucson Daily Citizen*, June 16, 1972; "Defense Starts for Police Accused in Search-Arrest," *Tucson Daily Citizen*, May 9, 1975. For increasing class tensions between African Americans in the postwar period, see Sugrue, *The Origins of the Urban Crisis*, pp. 181–207.

16. The director of Reachout in 2010, Angela Schneider, believed that the center moved from Linden St. to another, larger location around 1992. See Schneider interview.

17. Interview with Mary Menicucci, March 26, 2010.

18. "Clothing Donations," *Denver Catholic Register,* December 13, 1973.

19. See, for example, *Arizona Lifeline,* March 1973; *Arizona Lifeline,* February 1975; *Arizona Lifeline,* March-April 1975, all at University of Arizona Library Special Collections.

20. Sebesta interview.

21. Historian Karissa Haugeberg has argued that early CPCs were often started as a critique of Right to Life activism by women who were alienated by the mainstream movement and wanted to focus on women's needs. The activists in the Four Corners states tell a different story. Haugeberg, *Women Against Abortion,* pp. 18–19.

22. Jerry Montgomery, "17 and Pregnant? Birthright's Ear Just for Listening," *The New Mexican,* March 31, 1977. Some of the earliest CPCs have changed their names since they were founded.

23. "Crisis Pregnancy Centers" fact sheet, National Abortion Federation, 2006 (http://www.prochoice.org/about_abortion/facts/cpc.html#n1).

24. Seader interview. For one activist's published account of CPC counseling, see Curro, *Caring Enough to Help.*

25. "'Reachout' Offers Problem Pregnancy Counseling"; "Birthright Asks for Your Help!" *Arizona Lifeline,* March–April 1975, University of Arizona Library Special Collections.

26. Futch interview. See also Joan Rosley, "New Center to Offer Abortion Alternatives," *Tempe Daily News,* October 1, 1982.

27. "Helping a 14-Year-Old Girl Tell Her Mother, Principal," *National Right to Life News,* April 1976, p. 15.

28. "Anti-Abortion Group Formed; To Meet Monday," *Albuquerque Journal,* December 5, 1971; Menicucci interview.

29. See for example McClain, "Pregnant? Reachout Advises, But with a 'Pro-Life' View," and "Report from Reachout," *Arizona Right to Life-Tucson Chapter Newsletter,* November 1986, University of Arizona Library Special Collections.

30. *Matter of Choice;* Dabner, director, *The Silent Scream.* For a couple of examples of CPCs' use of films, see *Arizona Right to Life Newsletter,* Spring 1985, University of Arizona Library Special Collections; Jeanie Kasindorf, "Abortion in New York," *New York Magazine,* Sept. 18, 1989; Schoen, *Abortion After Roe,* p. 290–91 n120.

31. Montgomery, "17 and Pregnant?"; Edelmann and Baufle, directors, *The First Days of Life.*

32. Dubow, *Ourselves Unborn,* p. 47. This postwar medical culture was the product of at least eighty years of interest in fetal development. For more on the history and cultural ramifications of embryology, see Morgan, *Icons of Life.*

33. Casper, *The Making of the Unborn Patient,* p. 60.

34. Edelmann, *The First Days of Life,* pp. 32, 48. Edelmann's book and his movie of the same title were both produced in 1971.

35. Dianne Monahan and Karen Sullivan-Ables, "What You Should Know Before You Choose . . . Abortion as Your Option" pamphlet, Heritage House '76, Inc/Precious Feet People, folder 1, box 1–3, HH1421, Hall Hoag Collection, John Hay Library, Brown University, Providence, RI.

36. Gail Maiorana, "Man Accused of Luring Patients to View Films," *Tempe Daily News*, February 5, 1986.

37. Schneider interview. For more on the use of ultrasounds at CPCs, see Taylor, *The Public Life of the Fetal Sonogram*, pp. 144–68.

38. "New Center to Offer Abortion Alternatives," *Tempe Daily News*, October 1, 1982.

39. Marlene J. Perrin, "Anti-Abortionists Masquerade as Clinics," *USA Today*, July 24, 1986.

40. Interview with Kay Allen, March 16, 2010.

41. "Helping a 14-year-old Girl Tell her Mother, Principal."

42. Interview with John Jakubcyzk, March 16, 2010.

43. Seader interview.

44. *Reachout News*, March 1986. Subsequent newsletters show similar numbers. See *Reachout News*, March 7, 1987, and August 1987. Later newsletters omitted success rates; one interpretation of this archival silence is that success rates actually went down in the late 1980s and 1990s. (All *Reachout News* issues in author's possession.)

45. For quotes, see David Cannella, "Abortion Foe Is Guilty of False Imprisonment," *Arizona Republic*, April 2, 1986. See also Pat Sabo, "Abortion Foe's 'Deceit' Earns Judge's Wrath," *Phoenix Gazette*, April 2, 1986; Maiorana, "Man Accused of Luring Patients to View Films."

46. Marlene J. Perrin, "Bogus Abortion 'Clinics' Draw Legal Fire," *USA Today*, July 24, 1986; Joseph Berger, "Centers' Abortion Ads Called Bogus," *New York Times*, July 16, 1986; Jane Gross, "Pregnancy Centers: Anti-Abortion Role Challenged," *New York Times*, January 23, 1987; Tamar Lewin, "Anti-Abortion Centers Ads Misleading," *New York Times*, April 24, 1994; see Ginsburg, *Contested Lives*, pp. 120–21.

47. "Anti-Abortion Clinics Focus of Hearing in the House Today," *New York Times*, December 17, 1986; "Congressional Inquiry Examines Reports of Bogus Abortion Clinics," *New York Times*, September 21, 1991.

48. "Consumer Protection and Patient Safety Issues Involving Bogus Abortion Clinics," Hearing before the Subcommittee on Regulation, Business Opportunities, and Energy of the Committee on Small Business, House of Representatives, 102nd Congress, First Session, September 20, 1991, pp. 8, 5, 11.

49. Joyce, *The Child Catchers*, p. 105.

50. "Report from Reachout."

51. For more on this concern over the "epidemic" in teen pregnancy, see Vinovskis, *An "Epidemic" of Adolescent Pregnancy?*; Petchesky, *Abortion and a Woman's Choice*; Nathanson, *Dangerous Passage*; and Luker, *Dubious Conceptions*.

52. Seader interview.

53. Ibid; LeQuiu interview.

54. Ehrlich, *Who Decides?* p. 73.

55. Faludi, *Backlash,* pp. 419–20.

56. Seader interview.

57. For examples of such arguments, see Pamela Zekman and Pamela Warrick, "Counseling the Patient: Buy This Abortion," *National Right to Life News,* February 1979; Micheal Lyons, "Taking It to the Streets," *Arizona Living Magazine,* April 1985, folder 4, box 35, Planned Parenthood of Northern and Central Arizona Collection, Arizona Historical Foundation, Hayden Library, Arizona State University, Tempe, AZ.

58. Allen interview. For more on twenty-first-century CPC efforts to address poverty, see Hussey, "Crisis Pregnancy Centers, Poverty, and the Expanding Frontiers of American Abortion Politics," pp. 985–1011.

59. Allen interview.

60. Seader interview.

61. Ibid.; Futch interview; LeQuiu interview.

62. LeQuiu interview.

63. For one in-depth analysis of this stereotype, see Hancock, *The Politics of Disgust.*

64. Futch interview.

65. *Reachout News,* March 7, 1987, March 1989, February 1990, April 1990, October 1990, and February 1992.

66. *Reachout News,* March 1989.

67. LeQuiu interview.

68. Dinah Monahan, "Earn While You Learn," At The Center: A Ministry of Life Matters Worldwide, October 2003, http://www.atcmag.com/Issues/ID/118/Earn-While-You-Learn (accessed November 15, 2017).

69. For a pro-life discussion of suicide as a complication of abortion, see *Arizona Right to Life News,* Winter 1995, University of Arizona Library Special Collections; Larry and Lynette Hieber, letter to the editor, "Abortions Not So Safe," *Yuma Daily Sun,* March 25, 1986.

70. Dubow, *Ourselves Unborn,* p. 161. See also Speckhard, *Post-Abortion Counseling,* p. 6.

71. Weslin, *The Gathering of the Lambs,* p. 154.

72. Some psychiatrists used this line of argument to get women access to therapeutic abortions and to argue for abortion law liberalization. For the use of psychological arguments in the 1950s, see Reagan, *When Abortion was a Crime,* pp. 181–90. For an example of a psychiatrist arguing that unwanted pregnancy causes psychological trauma and thus abortion should be legal, see Bernadine Prince to Manuel Lujan, October 17, 1974, folder New Mexico, 1969–75, carton 4, National Abortion Rights Action League Collection, Schlesinger Library, Radcliffe Institute, Harvard University, Cambridge, MA.

73. This is the wording in DSM-III-R, published by the American Psychiatric Association in 1987. Quoted in Hamburg, foreword in *Post-Traumatic Therapy and Victims of Violence,* p. 7.

74. Quoted in Lee, *Abortion, Motherhood, and Mental Health*, pp. 119, 120. See also Siegel, "The Right's Reasons," pp. 1641–92; Major, "Psychological Implications of Abortion—Highly Charged and Rife with Misleading Research," pp. 1257–58; Needle and Walter, "Is There a Post Abortion Syndrome?" in *Abortion Counseling;* Dubow, *Ourselves Unborn,* pp. 160–1; Reeves, "The Development of Post-Abortion Syndrome within the Crisis Pregnancy Center Movement in America."

75. Marie Dillon, "Crisis Center Tries to Offer an Alternative to Abortion," *Scottsdale Daily Progress,* October 30, 1982.

76. "We Care" Crisis Pregnancy Service pamphlet, folder 1, Heritage House '76 Inc/Precious Feet People, Hall Hoag Collection, John Hay Library, Brown University, Providence, RI.

77. Monahan, "Earn While You Learn."

78. Ibid.

79. LeQuiu interview; Schnieder interview; interview with Laura Bowman, March 24, 2010.

80. Monahan, "Earn While You Learn."

81. Bowman interview.

82. LeQuiu interview.

83. Ibid.

84. Emily Bazelon, "Is There a Post-Abortion Syndrome?" *New York Times,* January 21, 2007.

85. Allen interview; *Reachout News,* March 1989, p. 3, and August 1991, p. 3 (both in author's possession). For more on chapters of WEBA in the Four Corners states, see *Arizona Right to Life Newsletter,* Summer 1984, and Spring 1985, both in University of Arizona Library Special Collections. WEBA began in 1982 after Vincent Rue spoke to the National Right to Life conference. See Siegel, "The Right's Reasons," pp. 1658–9.

86. "WEBA News," *Arizona Right to Life Newsletter,* Spring 1985, University of Arizona Library Special Collections. For a similar group that didn't use the WEBA name, see "Tears Speak . . . "*Arizona Right to Life News,* August 1997, University of Arizona Library Special Collections.

87. Post-abortion stress syndrome was one manifestation of a larger transformation in American culture: the persistent search for psychological cures to personal and social problems. This trend often offered depoliticized explanations for personal problems. Feminist consciousness raising and post-abortion therapy were exceptions. For more on this cultural shift, see Moskowitz, *In Therapy We Trust.*

88. Interview with Meme Eckstein, August 5, 2010.

89. Speckhard, *Post-Abortion Counseling,* p. ii.

90. Banks, *Ministering to Abortion's Aftermath,* pp. 46–8 (quote on p. 48, emphasis in original). The use of this book is noted in "WEBA News," *Arizona Right to Life Newsletter,* Spring 1985, University of Arizona Library Special Collections.

91. Jakubczyk interview; LeQuiu interview.

92. Flippen, *Jimmy Carter, the Politics of Family, and the Religious Right,* p. 51.

93. Meme Eckstein articulated her concerns as a post-abortion counselor this way: "I realized that this was very sensitive and I didn't even realize the extent." Eckstein interview.

94. Speckhard, *Post-Abortion Counseling*, pp. 4–14.

95. Ibid., pp. 29, 32, 34.

96. Ibid., p. 24. For more on post-abortive group counseling, Eckstein interview.

97. For a similar use of dolls in a more religiously focused post-abortion group, see Bazelon, "Is There a Post-Abortion Syndrome?"

98. Speckhard, *Post-Abortion Counseling*, pp. 54–55, 58–60, 52.

99. Eckstein interview.

100. For more on post-traumatic therapy, see Ochberg, ed., *Post-Traumatic Therapy and Victims of Violence;* Goldstein, Krasner, and Garfield, eds., *Posttraumatic Stress Disorder;* Wilson and Raphael, eds., *International Handbook of Traumatic Stress Syndromes.*

101. In Anne Speckhard's 1986 study, women with "high-stress" abortion experiences, who affiliated themselves with conservative religious groups or pro-life groups, had "increased feelings of grief and guilt" but ultimately found solace through forgiveness of the sin and the critique of the social systems that allowed legal abortion. Speckhard, "The Psycho-Social Aspects of Stress Following Abortion," pp. 140, 142.

102. Seader interview.

103. Risen and Thomas, *Wrath of Angels,* pp. 101–32.

104. Aid to Women in Phoenix was one such CPC. See Maiorana, "Man Accused of Luring Patients to View Films"; Pat Sabo, "Abortion Foe's 'Deceit' Earns Judge's Wrath," *Phoenix Gazette,* April 2, 1986; David Cannella, "Abortion Foe Is Guilty of False Imprisonment," *Arizona Republic,* April 2, 1986.

105. Neither Carenet, one major umbrella organization for CPCs, nor Birthright condone the use of graphic photos and videos of dead fetuses. LeQuiu interview.

106. Micheal Webb, letter to the editor, "Abortion Foe Responds," *Sierra Vista Herald,* February 17, 1985.

107. "House Committee Endorses Abortion Information Bill," *Prescott Courier* (AZ), March 5, 1985; Rick Kornfeld, "2 Groups Present Opposing Views on Abortion at Press Conferences," *Arizona Daily Star,* May 17, 1985.

108. All the leaders noted in this chapter were white. I do not have a full list of all WEBA leaders in the region, so I cannot say with absolute certainty that all were white.

109. Reardon, *Aborted Women,* appendix. Anne Speckhard's 1985 PhD dissertation focused on thirty women who had "high-stress" abortion experiences, many of whom joined the pro-life movement. All of Speckhard's interviewees were white. Speckhard, "The Psycho-Social Aspects of Stress Following Abortion," p. 48.

110. This is not to say that all white women were receptive to pro-life activists' theories. Huge majorities of women who had abortions never experienced

post-abortion trauma. A team of psychologists followed over four hundred women after they had their abortions, charting their emotional reactions over two years. Only 1 percent claimed to have post-abortion stress. Major, Cozzarelli, Cooper, Zubek, Richards, Wilhite and Gramzow, "Psychological Responses of Women after First-Trimester Abortion," pp. 777–84.

111. Melissa Rigg, "Scars of Abortion," *Arizona Daily Star,* no date (probably 1984), folder 72, box 30, Planned Parenthood AZ Collection. "Helen" is a pseudonym.

112. Karen Ables, letter to the editor, "A Planned Parenthood Experience," *Arizona Republic,* October 5, 1987.

113. "WEBA News," *Arizona Right to Life Newsletter,* Spring 1985, University of Arizona Library Special Collections.

114. Allen interview.

115. Rigg, "Scars of Abortion." Also, LeQuiu interview.

116. "WEBA—The Voice of Experience," *Arizona Right to Life Newsletter,* Summer 1984, University of Arizona Library Special Collections. For more on Karen Sullivan's (later Sullivan-Ables's) post-abortion trauma, see Karen Sullivan-Ables, letter to the editor, "Planned Parenthood Failed to Give Choice in Abortion," *Chandler Arizonan,* August 1, 1986; Karen Ables, letter to the editor, "A Planned Parenthood Experience," *Arizona Republic,* October 5, 1987; *Arizona Right to Life News,* March 1998, University of Arizona Library Special Collections.

117. Jakubcyzk interview.

118. Rosemary Schabert, "Abortion Issue Brings Out Beast in State Leaders," *Mesa Tribune,* April 14, 1985.

119. Laurie Roberts, "Many Expected to Attend Panel Hearing on Abortion," *Arizona Republic,* February 19, 1985.

120. This woman-centered rhetoric, contend political scientists Paul Saurette and Kelly Gordon, became the "dominant" pro-life argument at the end of the twentieth century and represented "nothing less than a discursive tectonic shift." Saurette and Gordon, *The Changing Voice of the Anti-Abortion Movement,* p. 206. See also Siegel, "The Right's Reasons."

121. Haugeberg, *Women Against Abortion,* p. 52.

122. Patrick O'Driscoll, "Abortions in Rural West: A Long, Tough Road," *Denver Post,* June 2, 1991; "State Facts about Abortion: Arizona," "State Facts about Abortion: Colorado," "State Facts about Abortion: Utah," and "State Facts about Abortion: New Mexico," Guttmacher Institute, May 2018, https://www.guttmacher.org/fact-sheet/state-facts-about-abortion (accessed July 2018).

5. POLITICIZING THE YOUNG

1. Brett DelPorto, "Abortion Causing U.S. Malaise, Activist Tells 200 at Capitol Rally," *Deseret News,* January 23, 1988.

2. For more on panic and the use of child-protective logic in the late twentieth century, see Edelman, *No Future;* Lancaster, *Sex Panic and the Punitive State;* Sheldon, *The Child to Come.*

3. Graham, *Young Activists,* p. 12. For more on youth in the civil rights movement, see de Schweinitz, *If We Could Change the World;* Schumaker, *Troublemakers.* For more on religious youth cultures, see Luhr, *Witnessing Suburbia.*

4. Reese, *America's Public Schools,* pp. 6–9 (quote on p. 327).

5. Susan Smith to NARAL, December 16, 1971, folder Arizona Correspondence, carton 2, National Abortion Rights Action League Collection, Schlesinger Library, Radcliffe Institute, Harvard University, Cambridge, MA (hereafter NARAL Collection) (there are at least eight other letters in this folder from high school and college students requesting materials on abortion for a class); Cindy Sue Culver (eighth grade) to Governor Bruce King, April 12, 1972, folder 220, box 12, Bruce King Papers (1st Term), New Mexico State Records Center, Santa Fe, NM. This type of education also extended to young adults' college years. See Diane Wilson to NARAL, March 17, 1972, folder Utah 1969–1975, carton 5, NARAL Collection; Jean Barnard to NARAL, September 18, 1972, folder Utah 1969–1975, carton 5, NARAL Collection; David Schoen to Lee Gidding, April 3, 1970, folder Campus, 1969–1970, carton 6, NARAL Collection; Cynthia L. Hathaway to Governor Cargo, March 26, 1969, folder 241, box 6, Governor David F. Cargo Papers, New Mexico State Records Center, Santa Fe (hereafter Cargo Papers).

6. See, for example, Cathy Janus, "Both Sides of Abortion Issue Explored at Independence High School," *Teen Gazette* (insert in the *Phoenix Gazette*), January 13, 1979.

7. Interview with Margaret Sebesta (pseudonym), August 8, 2011. For another example of activism in schools in another part of the country, see Taranto, *Kitchen Table Politics,* p. 71.

8. Joan McCoy, "Abortion Group's Name Is Misnomer," *Rocky Mountain News,* July 10, 1972.

9. For more school activism by invitation, see Janus, "Both Sides of the Issue Explored"; interview with John Jakubczyk, March 16, 2010.

10. Interview with Nancy Ellefson, March 24, 2010.

11. Ibid. The *Handbook on Abortion* is discussed in depth in chapter 2.

12. United Parents Under God, "That They May Live: A Presentation on Abortion," folder 1, United Parents Under God Ephemeral Materials, Wilcox Collection of Contemporary Political Movements, Kansas Collection, Kenneth Spencer Research Library, University of Kansas, Lawrence, KS (hereafter Wilcox Collection). The publication was probably created in the early to mid-1970s because the few citations in it are from between 1970 and 1973. Emphasis in original.

13. One journal article that looked at survival rates over a three-year period for infants born between 22 and 25 weeks' gestation found that only 56 percent of those born at these gestational ages lived longer than thirty minutes. None of those born at 22 weeks survived six months. See Allen, Donohue, and Dusman, "The Limit of Viability—Neonatal Outcome of Infants Born at 22 to 25 Weeks'

Gestation," pp. 1597–1601. Even when prenatal medical technologies improved in the twenty-first century, doctors continued to argue that survival before 22 weeks' gestation was highly unlikely because the fetus's lungs develop between 22 and 24 weeks. See Perignotti and Donzelli, "Perinatal Care at the Threshold of Viability," 193–98.

14. United Parents Under God, "That They May Live."

15. United Parents Under God, "Total Gov't Control of Public Education!" folder 1, United Parents Under God Ephemeral Materials, Wilcox Collection.

16. Interview with Meme Eckstein, August 5, 2011.

17. Interview with Dauneen Dolce, March 23, 2010.

18. *Arizona Right to Life Newsletter,* Spring 1985, University of Arizona Library Special Collections, Tucson, AZ.

19. "Saving Lives, Serving Families," Heritage House '76 Incorporated Catalog, January 1999, p. 89, folder 3, box 1–3, HH1421, Heritage House '76, Inc/Precious Feet People, Hall Hoag Collection, John Hay Library, Brown University, Providence, RI (hereafter Hall Hoag Collection)

20. *Matter of Choice.*

21. *Arizona Right to Life News,* April 1983, University of Arizona Library Special Collections.

22. Ibid.; *Arizona Right to Life News,* January 1983 and July 1983, University of Arizona Library Special Collections.

23. D. D. Wigley, President of New Mexico Right to Choose Education Fund to Supporter, no date (1988), folder 5, box 58, Louis E. and Carmen K. Freudenthal Family Papers, 1837–1990, New Mexico State University Special Collections and Archives, Las Cruces, NM.

24. Jakubczyk interview; interview with Angela Schneider, March 17, 2010; Dolce interview.

25. *Arizona Right to Life-Tucson Chapter Newsletter,* November 1988, University of Arizona Library Special Collections. For similar responses, see *Arizona Right to Life News,* January 1983, University of Arizona Library Special Collections.

26. *Arizona Lifeline (Arizona Right to Life-* Southern Region *Newsletter*), May 1980, University of Arizona Library Special Collections.

27. *Arizona Right to Life News,* March 1983, University of Arizona Library Special Collections.

28. Ellefson interview; Wigley to Supporter.

29. *Arizona Right to Life-Tucson Chapter Newsletter,* June 1989.

30. Trudy Welsh, "Film Sparks Controversy at School," *Colorado Springs Telegraph Gazette,* May 21, 1993; Alan D. and Eva L. Lind, "Parents Back Science Teacher," letter to the editor, *Colorado Springs Gazette Telegraph,* May 30, 1993. For another letter to the editor arguing that the pro-life film provided a balance to the pro-choice media (that is, Hollywood), see James C. Furfarl, "Help Children Avoid the Choice," letter to the editor, *Colorado Springs Gazette Telegraph,* June 15, 1993. For more letters to the editor claiming that those opposing the film were censoring what the majority supported, see Douglas L. Lamborn, "Film's Foes Seek to Cen-

sor," letter to the editor, *Colorado Springs Gazette Telegraph,* May 29, 1993; Laura Davis, "Was Attack on Film Political?" letter to the editor, *Colorado Springs Telegraph Gazette,* June 14, 1993.

31. Irvine, *Talk About Sex,* pp. 88–90, 92–93.

32. Ibid., p. 100.

33. Moran, *Teaching Sex,* p. 214. See also Goodson and Edmundson, "The Problematic Promotion of Abstinence," pp. 205–10; Trudell and Whatley, "Sex Respect," pp. 125–40; Mayo, *Disputing the Subject of Sex.*

34. *Arizona Right to Life-Tucson Chapter Newsletter,* May/June 1988, University of Arizona Library Special Collections. For more discussion of sex education and Sex Respect in Tucson Right to Life, see *Arizona Right to Life*-Tucson Chapter *Newsletter,* November 1986, November 1987, Summer 1988, November 1988, March 1989, and June 1989, all in University of Arizona Library Special Collections.

35. Sonia L. Nazario, "Schools Teach the Virtues of Virginity," *Wall Street Journal,* February 20, 1992.

36. *Arizona Right to Life News,* June 1997, University of Arizona Library Special Collections.

37. *Arizona Right to Life News,* August 1997, University of Arizona Library Special Collections.

38. *Arizona Right to Life News,* June 1997, University of Arizona Library Special Collections.

39. *Arizona Right to Life News,* December 1998, University of Arizona Library Special Collections.

40. Ibid.; *Arizona Right to Life News,* March 1998, University of Arizona Library Special Collections. The Precious Feet pins are discussed in depth in chapter 2.

41. Susan Hope Everett, "A Palm-Size Pro-Life Message," *Columbia: Knights of Columbus Magazine,* January 1989, pp. 14–15 (quotes on p. 14), Project Young One Collection, Wisconsin Historical Society, Madison, WI (hereafter Project Young One Collection).

42. *National Right to Life News,* vol. 17, no. 12 (June 7, 1990), p. 22, folder 4, Pro-Life Action League Collection, Wisconsin Historical Society, Madison, WI.

43. For testimonials on the use of the Young One, see "What Pro-Lifers Are Saying," Young One promotional literature, Project Young One Collection.

44. Everett, "The Palm-Size Pro-life Message," p. 14.

45. *Taylor vs. Roswell Independent School District,* No. 11–2242, Tenth Circuit Court of Appeals, April 8, 2013.

46. For the classic study about children of color internalizing racial standards of beauty through dolls, see Clark and Clark, "Racial Identification and Preference in Negro Children," in *Readings of Social Psychology,* pp. 169–78. Thurgood Marshall cited the Clarks' study in *Brown v. Board of Education.*

47. For the turn to multiculturalism in the toy industry, see, for example, DuCille, *Skin Trade,* pp. 8–59; Chin, *Purchasing Power;* Magee, *Africa in the American Imagination,* pp. 95–114. For one important critique of multiculturalism, see Lowe, *Immigrant Acts.*

48. For the use of fetus dolls of color in school contexts, see Steven G. Vegh, "Anti-Abortion Fetus Dolls Handed Out to Norfolk Students," *Virginian-Pilot,* May 21, 2010; Rosemary Black, "Virginia School Principal Suspended After Employee Hands Out Pro-Life Fetus Dolls to Students," *New York Daily News,* May 28, 2010. For purveyors of fetus dolls of color, see Heritage House, http://www.hh76.org/default.aspx?GroupID = 135; Gods Little Ones, http://www.godslittleones.com/comfortdolls.html; Wee Bundles, http://www.weebundles.com/ (all accessed March 17, 2016).

49. *Arizona Right to Life News,* March 1998, University of Arizona Library Special Collections.

50. Interview with Mary LeQuiu, March 22, 2010. The director of Reachout in Tucson also noted one of their board members regularly did abstinence education. Schneider interview.

51. LeQuiu interview.

52. Goldberg, *Kingdom Coming,* p. 139.

53. Haffner and Wagoner, "Vast Majority of Americans Show Support for Sexuality Education," pp. 22–23. For other similar polls, see, for example, Reese, *America's Public Schools,* p. 327; "What Americans Think: Sex Education Survey Findings Compared," *Spectrum* 71, no. 2 (Spring 1998): 30; Welshimer and Harris, "A Survey of Rural Parents' Attitudes Towards Sexuality Education," pp. 347–52; "Poll Respondents Say Abortion Should be Legal," *Scottsdale Daily Progress,* November 11, 1987.

54. Irvine, *Talk About Sex,* p. 188.

55. Landy, Kaeser, and Richards, "Abstinence Information and the Provision of Information about Contraception in Public School District Sexuality Education Policies," pp. 280–86.

56. "You Are Special," 1986, Literature folder, Wisconsin Right to Life Collection, Wisconsin Historical Society, Madison, WI.

57. For a literary analysis of conservatism in various kinds of children's literature, see Abate, *Raising Your Kids Right.*

58. "Saving Lives, Serving Families," pp. 64–67, Hall Hoag Collection.

59. Ibid., p. 64.

60. Philosopher Judith Butler dubs this logical circle "the heterosexual matrix." See Butler, *Gender Trouble,* pp. 47–106.

61. "Saving Lives, Serving Families," p. 67, Hall Hoag Collection.

62. Ibid., pp. 74, 18. Bumper stickers made for girls included "Single, Special, Selective and Worth the Wait" and "Safe Sex Still Breaks the Heart."

63. "Saving Lives, Serving Families," p. 89, Hall Hoag Collection.

64. *Arizona Right to Life News,* December 1999, University of Arizona Library Special Collections; "What Pro-Lifers Are Saying."

65. Kathy Dobie, "With God on Their Side: Inside Operation Rescue," *Westward,* April 27, 1989.

66. Dolce interview.

67. Interview with June Maskell (pseudonym), November 19, 2018.

68. Bonnie Bartak, "Tots and Mothers Picket Abortion Clinic," *Arizona Republic,* July 14, 1973.

69. Jakubczyk interview.

70. "Rick Santorum Brings Dead Baby Home for Children," *Santa Rosa Press Democrat* (CA), January 6, 2012.

71. Gaither, *Homeschool.* Different states had different standards that homeschoolers had to meet. But these standards usually left an incredible amount of room for parents' own philosophies, which of course was the point of homeschooling.

72. For historiography on busing opposition, see Lassiter, *The Silent Majority;* Kruse, *White Flight;* Formisano, *Boston Against Busing;* Lucas, *Common Ground.*

73. Tucson and Denver had some form of mandatory busing program. As was true in many other parts of the country, students of color were more likely to be bused out of their neighborhoods or to have longer bus rides than Anglo students. See J. Hunter Halloway, "A Tale of Two Cities and Their Busing Problems," *Greeley Tribune,* September 24, 1971; "Bridging Three Centuries: The Desegregation Questions, 1968–1983," TUSD District History, http://www.tusd1.org/contents/distinfo/history/history9310.asp (accessed September 8, 2012). Phoenix, Salt Lake City, and Albuquerque did not have mandatory busing programs.

74. "Busing Started Five Years Ago; Controversy Still Undiminished," *Greeley Tribune,* October 9, 1969; J. Hunter Halloway, "A Tale of Two Cities and Their Busing Problems," *Greeley Tribune,* September 24, 1971; James Brooke, "Court Says Denver Can End Forced Busing," *New York Times,* September 17, 1995. For more on Denver debate, see "Busing Issue in Amendment 8 on Next Ballot," *Colorado Springs Gazette Telegraph,* October 31, 1974; Jeffrey St. John, "School Busing Issue Termed Child Cruelty," *Colorado Springs Gazette Telegraph,* November 17, 1971. For a broader perspective on school integration in Denver, see Romero, "Of Race and Rights," pp. 367–426.

75. Interview with Kevin Lundberg, August 7, 2011.

76. St. John, "School Busing Issue Termed Child Cruelty."

77. "The Crossing of Swords on Abortion" no newspaper, November 1980, folder 4, box 35, Planned Parenthood of Northern and Central Arizona, Arizona Historical Foundation, Hayden Library, Arizona State University, Tempe, AZ (hereafter Planned Parenthood AZ Collection).

78. Christian Coalition of Colorado, Merry Christmas letter, December 1996, folder 11, box 14, Equality Colorado Collection, Western History and Genealogy Department, Denver Public Library, Denver, CO (hereafter Equality Colorado Collection). For more conservative critiques in this vein, see White House Conference on Families, District 1 minutes, folder 22, box 30176, Governor Tony Anaya Papers, New Mexico State Records Center, Santa Fe, NM; 1997 Concerned Women of America, *Colorado News Digest,* Spring 1997, folder 34, box 15, Equality Colorado Collection; Christian Coalition of Colorado, *Colorado: A Supplement of the Christian American,* February 1995, folder 12, box 14, Equality Colorado Collection; Pro-Family Coalition of Colorado, 1991 Pro-Family Conference Program, folder 38, box 21, Equality Colorado Collection.

79. Stevens, *Kingdom of Children,* pp. 11–12; Mayberry et al., *Homeschooling.*

80. McDannell, "Creating the Christian Home," in *American Sacred Space,* p. 190.

81. Kunzman, "Homeschooling and Fundamentalism," p. 19. For the original, see Planty et al., *The Condition of Education 2009,* p. 135. When interviewees had to choose a single reason they homeschooled, "moral and religious instruction" again topped the list with 36 percent of the group.

82. Cheryl Wittenauer, "'Homeschoolers' Cite Morals, Religion Reasons for Choice," *The New Mexican,* April 30, 1989.

83. National Household Education Survey numbers and quote in Smith and Sikkink, "Is Private Schooling Privatizing?" pp. 16–20 (quote on p. 19). Emphasis in the original. For more on civic participation, see Sikkink, "Public Schooling and Its Discontents."

84. Lundberg interview. For an account of pro-life activism in an Illinois homeschooling group, see Stevens, *Kingdom of Children,* p. 152.

85. Maskell interview.

86. Weslin, *The Gathering of the Lambs,* p. 170.

87. Luhr, *Witnessing Suburbia,* pp. 176, 98, 137–38.

88. Weslin, *The Gathering of the Lambs,* p. 178.

89. *Arizona Right to Life News,* December 1999, University of Arizona Library Special Collections.

90. *Right to Life Newsletter of Colorado,* March 1991, folder 38, box 21, Equality Colorado Collection.

91. For pictures of children and young adults protesting in the 1980s and 1990s, see "God Is Pro-Life" photograph, July 12, 1986; "Stop Abortion" photograph, July 12, 1986; "Abortion Kills" photograph, no date, all in folder Photographs: Demonstrations R.M.P.P., box 2, Rocky Mountain Planned Parenthood Collection, Western History and Genealogy Department, Denver Public Library, Denver, CO (hereafter RMPP Collection). See also "Walkers Focus on Pro-Life Issues," *Sun Sentinel* (Fort Lauderdale, FL), May 21, 2006. Survivors of the Abortion Holocaust was a self-proclaimed "Christian pro-life group" founded in 1998 and made up of people born after 1973. The group claimed, "the Survivors feel that we are directly affected by this holocaust because it happened to us—we are the target. Abortion has claimed the lives of our classmates, friends, our brothers and sisters." See "Who Are the Survivors?" Survivors of the Abortion Holocaust website, http://www.survivors.la/who-are-the-survivors.asp. For use of this phrase by teens in the early 1990s, see Paul Solotaroff, "Surviving the Crusades," *Rolling Stone,* October 14, 1993.

92. "Overview of the National Right to Life Committee Convention, June 20–22, 1985," and "National Right to Life Committee Convention—An Overview," folder Board and Committee Meetings 1985, box 2, RMPP Collection. For efforts to engage youth in the Four Corners, see *Viva Life,* December-January 1994, folder 31, box 2, New Mexico Women's Political Caucus Papers, Center for Southwest Research, University of New Mexico, Albuquerque, NM; Eckstein interview; *Colo-*

rado Concerned Women for America Newsletter, January 1990, folder 35, box 15, Equality Colorado Collection.

93. The one item marketed explicitly to children was a "Love Life" T-shirt with a stylized fetus in a womb on the front. See The Precious Feet People Catalog, September 1981, folder 1, box 1–3, HH1421, Heritage House '76, Inc/Precious Feet People, Hall Hoag Collection.

94. "Saving Lives, Serving Families," pp. 20–21, 24–25, Hall Hoag Collection. For more on the marketing of evangelical products to children and young adults in the 1990s, see Hendershot, *Shaking the World for Jesus,* pp. 34–51; Luhr, *Witnessing Suburbia.*

95. "Saving Lives, Serving Families," Hall Hoag Collection.

96. McCallum, ed., *Death of Truth,* pp. 14–15.

97. Quoted in Adams, "Choice Ideology and the Parameters of Its Practice," p. 146.

98. Maskell interview.

99. Questioning of Joseph Scheidler, *Abortion Clinic Violence: Oversight Hearings Before the Subcommittee on Civil and Constitutional Rights of the Committee on the Judiciary, House of Representatives, Ninety-ninth Congress, First and Second Session, March 6, 12, and April 3, 1985; and December 17, 1986* (Washington, DC: U.S. Government Printing Office, 1987), p. 74.

100. Eight of the murders occurred between 1993 and 1998; a ninth was of Kansas abortion provider George Tiller in 2009. For more on these murders, see Baird-Windle and Bader, *Targets of Hatred,* esp. pp. 139–251; Jeffris, *Armed for Life;* Singular, *The Wichita Divide.*

101. For more on Operation Rescue, see Risen and Thomas, *Wrath of Angels;* Ginsburg, "Rescuing the Nation," in *Abortion Wars,* pp. 227–50, and "Saving America's Souls," in *Fundamentalisms and the State,* pp. 567–88; Diamond, *Road to Dominion,* pp. 229, 250–53, 291; Faludi, *Backlash,* pp. 407–12; Steiner, *The Rhetoric of Operation Rescue.*

102. Risen and Thomas, *Wrath of Angels,* p. 332.

103. Don Terry, "98 Are Arrested as Abortion Foes Defy Judge and Block Clinic," *New York Times,* August 10, 1991, p. 6.

104. "Operation Rescue Uses Children in Protests," *Morning Edition,* National Public Radio, Washington, DC, August 14, 1991.

105. In Wichita, the presence and radicalism of these children convinced local police officers that they had been too lenient with Operation Rescue, leading them to institute more forceful handling of the protesters. See Risen and Thomas, *Wrath of Angels,* pp. 326–32. For more on teenage activists and the rescue movement, see Karen M. Thomas, "Teenage Activists: Pawns or Free Choice?" *Chicago Tribune,* June 7, 1992; Jeff Gottlieb, "Teens Give New Life to Operation Rescue," *Los Angeles Times,* October 12, 1998. For outrage about Operation Rescue's youth activists, see "Endangering Kids for the Pro-Life Cause," editorial, *Milwaukee Journal Sentinel,* August 13, 1991.

106. Paul Solotaroff, "Surviving the Crusades," *Rolling Stone,* October 14, 1993, pp. 57–62. For more on this protest, see "Operation Rescue Runs Florida Training Camp," *Morning Edition,* National Public Radio, Washington, DC, April 12, 1993.

107. Pro-Life Action Network of Denver, "Pro-Life Action Calendar, 1994," folder 8, box 2, Denver Police Department Intelligence Files, Western History and Genealogy Department, Denver Public Library, Denver, CO.

108. Bill Scanlon, "Anti-Abortion Picketing Calm," *Rocky Mountain News,* March 5, 1997. For more on these protests, see Shelley Gonzales, "Operation Rescue Targets Schools," *Rocky Mountain News,* February 25, 1997; Shelley Gonzales, "Abortion Foes to Defy Schools' Request," *Rocky Mountain News,* February 26, 1997; "Students Hear Anti-Abortion Message," *Colorado Springs Gazette Telegraph,* March 4, 1997.

109. Colorado NARAL, "Operation Rescue Targets Students," *The Voice for Choice* newsletter, Spring 1997, Voice for Choice, Colorado National Abortion Rights Action League Serial, Western History and Genealogy Department, Denver Public Library, Denver, CO.

110. "Pro-Life Demonstrations at Local High Schools Stir a Storm of Reaction," letters to the editor, *Rocky Mountain News,* March 16, 1997; Bill Scanlon, "Fetus Photos Shake Up Middle-Schoolers," *Rocky Mountain News,* March 4, 1997; Shelley Gonzales, "Operation Rescue Targets Schools."

111. "Operation Rescue Uses Children in Protests."

112. For one local example of this, see "Protesters' Aggression Strengthens Resolve of One Volunteer Clinic Escort," *Rocky Mountain News,* April 23, 1992.

113. Sandler, *Righteous,* pp. 33–34.

114. Elizabeth Hayt, "Surprise, Mom: I'm Against Abortion," *New York Times,* March 30, 2003.

115. Dolce interview.

116. Eckstein interview.

117. *Arizona Right to Life News,* December 1998, University of Arizona Library Special Collections.

6. MAKING FAMILY VALUES

1. Interview with Phil and Helen Seader, March 18, 2010.

2. I use "abortion reform" here instead of "pro-choice" because many of these early activists used the benevolent language of reform rather than the more individualistic term "choice." Through the end of the century, after *Roe,* this argument about abuse and "unwantedness" persisted in pro-choice circles but it was not as prevalent as it had been earlier. See, for example, Beatrice Blair to Dawn I. Brett, December 1, 1974, Colorado 1974–75 folder, carton 2, National Abortion Rights Action League (NARAL) Collection, Schlesinger Library, Radcliffe Institute, Harvard University, Cambridge, MA (hereafter NARAL Collection).

3. For a sample of such arguments, see Telegram from Dave and Frances Holmes, Albuquerque, to Gov. David Cargo, March 13, 1969, folder 241, box 6, Governor David F. Cargo Papers, New Mexico State Records Center, Santa Fe, NM; "Com-

mitted for Life" ad, *Albuquerque Journal,* January 14, 1977; Margot Sheahan, guest editorial, "Compassion Needed," *Spectrum West,* September 14, 1977, folder 1, Margot Anne Meade Sheahan Papers, Schlesinger Library, Radcliffe Institute, Harvard University, Cambridge, MA (hereafter Sheahan Papers); Helen Epstein, "Abortion: An Issue that Won't Go Away," *New York Times Magazine,* March 30, 1980; New Mexico Right to Life, *Viva Life,* July 1986, folder 1, Right to Life, New Mexico, box 1–8, HH120, Hall Hoag Collection, John Hay Library, Brown University, Providence, RI (hereafter Hall Hoag Collection).

4. Coontz, *The Way We Never Were.* Historians have also taken to task the 1950s suburban family ideal, perhaps the model most important to late-twentieth-century conservative nostalgia. See for example Meyerowitz, ed., *Not June Cleaver;* Weiss, *To Have and to Hold.*

5. Dowland, *Family Values and the Rise of Christian Right.* Dowland ignores the importance of rights rhetoric to this part of the family values movement. For more on family values politics, see Taranto, *Kitchen Table Politics;* Self, *All in the Family;* Dochuk, *From Bible Belt to Sunbelt;* Martin, *With God on Our Side;* Wilcox, *Onward Christian Soldiers?;* Williams, *God's Own Party.*

6. For an extended analysis of Focus on the Family's use of white nostalgia, see Burlein, *Lift High on the Cross,* pp. 131–57.

7. "Questions and Answers about UPA," folder 1, Sheahan Papers.

8. Barbara Gallagher, "Margot Sheahan," folder 1, Sheahan Papers. For more on unwed pregnancy before 1973, see Solinger, *Wake Up Little Susie.*

9. Gallagher, "Margot Sheahan," Sheahan Papers.

10. Margot Sheahan to Eva S. Mosley, October 12, 1986, folder 1, Sheahan Papers.

11. Sheahan, *The Whole Parent,* pp. xiii, xv.

12. Margot Sheahan, "Unwed Parents Anonymous," *Heartbeat,* Spring 1982, folder 1, Sheahan Papers.

13. Sheahan, *Whole Parent,* pp. xx. For Sheahan's discussion of natural order, see Sheahan, *Whole Parent,* pp. 4, 71; Jude Peitzmeier, "Unwed Parents Find Support," *Scottsdale Daily Progress,* August 18, no year (probably 1983), folder 1, Sheahan Papers.

14. Sheahan, "Unwed Parents Anonymous," Sheahan Papers.

15. Sheahan, *Whole Parent,* pp. 5, 107.

16. Ibid., p. 114; "It's O.K. to Say No! You'll Like Yourself Better" pamphlet, folder 1, Sheahan Papers.

17. Sheahan, *Whole Parent,* p. 113.

18. Ibid., p. 107. For other descriptions of abortions in the book, see pp. 5, 7, 27, 41, 56–7, 59, 81.

19. Everett Craighead, "Unwed Parents Anonymous Helps Ease Distressful Situation," *Phoenix Gazette,* June 24, 1982.

20. For "solutions," see Sheahan, "Unwed Parents Anonymous," Sheahan Papers. For "cop-out" and "moral implications," see "Questions and Answers about UPA," Sheahan Papers.

21. J. J. Casserly, "Foundation of Love Helps Unwed Mothers Build New Lives," *Arizona Republic,* February 28, 1985.

22. "Testimonies from Unwed Parents Anonymous," folder 1, Sheahan Papers.

23. Casserly, "Foundation of Love."

24. Arizona Right to Life pamphlet, Northern Region, no date, folder 1, Sheahan Papers.

25. Solinger, *Wake Up Little Susie.*

26. Joyce, *The Child Catchers,* pp. 54, 104–117.

27. Sheahan, *The Whole Parent,* p. 104.

28. The author's personal observations at Women's Pregnancy Options CPC, run by Project Defending Life in Albuquerque.

29. Solinger, *Beggars and Choosers,* p. 197.

30. Peitzmeier, "Unwed Parents Find Support."

31. Sheahan, *Whole Parent,* p. xx.

32. "Pro-Life Unit Plans Protest," *Mesa Tribune,* June 5, 1980.

33. Shapiro, ed., *Abortion,* pp. 61, 228. See also McBride, *Abortion in the United States,* p. 45.

34. Liz Doup, "Abortion Bills Studied," *Scottsdale Daily Progress,* March 11, 1977; Laurie Asseo, "Husband Must Be Told Before Abortion, Under Proposal in House," *Tucson Daily Citizen,* March 26, 1985; "2 Abortion Bills Die in Committee," *Mohave Daily Miner,* April 3, 1985; Rosemary Schabert, "Senate Panel Rejects Restrictions on Abortion," *Tempe Daily News,* April 3, 1985; "In Utah, They Know How to Punish a Woman" ad, folder 18, box 4, Linda Sillitoe Collection, Special Collections, J. Willard Marriott Library, University of Utah, Salt Lake City, UT (hereafter Sillitoe Collection).

35. The conference committee formed the districts. Council on the New Mexico Conference on Families, "Statement of Purpose," folder 17, box 37, Bruce King Papers, University of New Mexico School of Law Library, Albuquerque, NM (hereafter King Papers).

36. David Gerke, "Families Stampede?" letter to the editor, *The New Mexican,* March 26, 1980.

37. Ramona Morales, Chairman, District Five, to Mrs. Alice King and Dr. George Goldstein, April 18, 1980, folder 18, box 35, King Papers. Of the three counties in district 5—Luna, Hidalgo, and Grant—only Grant seemed to have social conservatives present. See Topics Out of Grant County Families Forum, folder 18, box 35, King Papers. There is no record of Catron County's meeting.

38. Gómez, "Urban Imperialism in the Modern West," in *Essays in Twentieth-Century New Mexico History,* pp. 136–37.

39. Szasz, *Larger than Life,* p. 82. For more on uranium mining in the region, see for example Barry, "What Price Energy?" pp. 18–23; Eichstaedt, *If You Poison Us;* Brugge, Benally, and Yazzie-Lewis, eds., *The Navajo People and Uranium Mining;* Pasternak, *Yellow Dirt.*

40. White House Conference on Families, District 1, March 15, 1980, folder 22, box 30176, Governor Tony Anaya Papers, New Mexico State Records Center, Santa

Fe, NM (hereafter Anaya Papers). There was a translator present, who translated everyone's testimonies into English or Navajo. There was one person who spoke in a third language (probably either Zuni or Spanish).

41. Ibid. One English speaker, a teacher, did not hew quite as much to socially conservative rhetoric, though she did discuss the problems of discipline within schools.

42. O'Neill, *Working the Navajo Way,* pp. 82–84. For more thorough treatments of boarding schools, see Adams, *Education for Extinction;* Trennert, *The Phoenix Indian School;* Littlefield, "Indian Education and the World of Work, 1893–1933," in *Native Americans and Wage Labor.* For more on the specifics of Navajo education in the first half of the century, see Sánchez, "*The People,*" p. 25; Iverson, *Diné,* pp. 172–76; Bailey and Bailey, *A History of the Navajo,* p. 169.

43. Manuelito, "The Role of Education in American Indian Self-Determination," pp. 73–87; McPherson, *Navajo Land, Navajo Culture,* pp. 207–12. For more on Navajo education in the postwar period, see Roessel, *Navajo Education;* Thompson, *The Navajos' Long Walk for Education;* Deyhle and Margonis, "Navajo Mothers and Daughters," pp. 135–67; Iverson, *Diné,* pp. 190–98, 255–58; Reyhner and Eder, *American Indian Education,* pp. 271–78.

44. White House Conference on Families, District 1, March 15, 1980, Anaya Papers.

45. Ibid.

46. Anne Hillerman, "Conference Reviews Role of Families," *The New Mexican,* March 13, 1980.

47. White House Conference on Families, Los Alamos County, Issue Votes, folder 22, box 30176, Anaya Papers.

48. Hillerman, "Conference Reviews Role of Families." For an obituary for Silas García, see *Viva Life,* September 1986, folder 1, Right to Life, New Mexico, box 1–8, HH120, Hall Hoag Collection.

49. Rather than have one big district meeting, the district's leaders organized two meetings: one for Los Alamos, Rio Arriba, Taos, and Santa Fe counties, and another for Mora, Colfax, and San Miguel counties.

50. Gary Tietjen, "Majority Spoke Out at Meeting," letter to the editor, *The New Mexican,* April 1, 1980.

51. Gloria V. García, Joe Cortez, Dotti Montoya, Vicki Truot, Vera Valdez, Esta Diamond Gutiérrez, Linda Pedro, Judy Chaddick, Bertha Romero, and Debbie Barton, "Disputes Representative," letter to the editor, *The New Mexican,* April 9, 1980. See also [name illegible], San Juan Pueblo, to Fred Wilnkleman [*sic*], March 31, 1980, folder 22, box 30176, Anaya Papers.

52. Anne Poore, "Family Conferences Encounter Problems," *The New Mexican,* March 26, 1980.

53. García et al., "Disputes Representative," Anaya Papers.

54. Testimony Results from Los Alamos County, WHCOF District Hearing, March 15, 1980, folder 22, box 30176, Anaya Papers.

55. García et al., "Disputes Representative," Anaya Papers; Poore, "Family Conferences Encounter Problems." For Mary Bond's response to the controversy, see

"LA Favors 'Traditional Family,'" *The New Mexican,* March 14, 1980. For Mary Bond's pro-life affiliation and activism, see "SF Abortion Opponent Cites 'Personal' Example," *The New Mexican,* October 30, 1977; "Anti-Abortionists Call Veto 'Offense Against God,'" *The New Mexican,* March 22, 1978; Paul Sturiale, "Abortion Pros, Cons March at State Capitol," *The New Mexican,* January 22, 1979; María Puente, "Abortion Bills Fail in Senate as Time Expires," *The New Mexican,* March 18, 1979; District II (Contacts), folder 2, box 38, King Papers. District 3, which included Albuquerque, also elected New Mexico Right to Life president Charlotte Goodwin to be their representative. See New Mexico Conference on Families, District III Report, folder 18, box 37, King Papers.

56. Rep. Silas T. García and Lucy García, "Garcia Answers Criticism," *The New Mexican,* May 27, 1980.

57. For more on economic relationships with Los Alamos, see Trujillo, *Land of Disenchantment.*

58. In the early 1980s, Rio Arriba had a median family income of only $11,699. (The median in Los Alamos County was three times as much.) See Jon Bowman, "Census Shows LA County Income Higher than Others," *The New Mexican,* September 18, 1982.

59. For families in poverty, see "Figuring Out the Risks: Factors Show Likelihood of Child Turning Violent," *The New Mexican,* January 16, 1994. By the 1990s, poverty and social inequality in the region led, in part, to massive heroin addiction, and, by the early twentieth-first century, the county had the highest rate of drug fatalities in the country. See Erik Echolm, "A Grim Tradition, and a Long Struggle to End It," *New York Times,* April 2, 2008; Angela Garcia, "Land of Disenchantment," *High Country News,* April 3, 2006, http://www.hcn.org/issues/319/16202/print_view (accessed April 9, 2012). See also Glendinning, *Chiva.*

60. García et al., "Disputes Representative," Anaya Papers.

61. Poore, "Family Conferences Encounter Problems."

62. Fred McCoffrey, "Family Conference Close-Minded," *The New Mexican,* June 14, 1980; Poore, "Stacked Family Conference Ignored Issues."

63. David Baptiste, Herb Koffler, Cathy Topp, Lynne Johnson, Pally Turner, Shelley Koffler, Barbara Gray-Pendleton, Julian G. Bartlett, Margaret Vasquez-Geffrey, David K. Sallee, and Margaret G. Bartlett to Alice King and George Goldstein, May 28, 1980, folder 19, box 37, King Papers.

64. Minority Report for Family Crisis/Violence, folder 19, box 37, King Papers.

65. Poore, "Stacked Family Conference Ignored Issues." For other minority reports that discuss the dominance of socially conservative groups, see New Mexico Conference on Families, Minority Report on Child Care/Day Care, May 24, 1980; New Mexico Conference on Families, Government and Families Workshop Minority Report, May 24, 1980; A Minority Report on Sex Education from the New Mexico Conference on Families, May 24, 1980; A Minority Report on Abortion from the New Mexico Conference on Families, May 24, 1980, all in folder 19, box 37, King Papers.

66. Poore, "Stacked Family Conference Ignored Issues"; McCoffrey, "Family Conference Close-Minded."

67. McCoffrey, "Family Conference Close-Minded."

68. On certain issues, conservatives did recommend less government regulation. They argued for the elimination of the Department of Education, the elimination of state or federal funding for child care, the retraction of any legislation that infringed on parents' right to discipline children, and the elimination of a handful of taxes, for example. For elimination of the Department of Education, see Topic Family Values, State Issues Priority Form, New Mexico, White House Conference on Families, May 24, 1980, folder 20, King Papers. For elimination of funding for child care, see Topic Child Care/Day Care, State Issues Priority Form, New Mexico, White House Conference on Families, May 24, 1980, folder 20, King Papers. For parents' right to discipline, see Topic Family Crises/Violence, State Issues Priority Form, New Mexico, White House Conference on Families, May 24, 1980, folder 20, King Papers. For the elimination of certain taxes, see Topic Tax Policies/Economics, State Issues Priority Form, New Mexico, White House Conference on Families, May 24, 1980, folder 20, King Papers.

69. For constitutional amendment and mandated pro-life school policy, see Topic Abortion, State Issues Priority Form, New Mexico, White House Conference on Families, May 24, 1980, folder 20, King Papers. For heads of household policy and the federal agency, see Topic Government and Families, State Issues Priority Form, New Mexico, White House Conference on Families, May 24, 1980, folder 20, King Papers. For defining the family as heterosexual and laws against the media, see Topic Family Values, State Issues Priority Form. For creationism, see Topic Education/Parenting, State Issues Priority Form, New Mexico, White House Conference on Families, May 24, 1980, folder 20, King Papers.

70. O'Neil, "Public Hearings and Public Preferences," pp. 488–502.

71. Poore, "Stacked Family Conference Ignored Issues."

72. McCoffrey, "Family Conference Close-Minded."

73. For "angry," see Nadine Brozan, "2d Day of Family Conference: Workshops and a Walkout," *New York Times,* June 7, 1980. For "bitter," see Sharon Johnson, "After Heated Debates, Family Parley Ends Quietly," *New York Times,* July 14, 1980. For "hornet's nest," see Self, *All in the Family,* p. 335.

74. Balmer, *Redeemer,* p. 132.

75. Wisenale, "Family Policy at the End of the 20th Century," in *Redefining Family Policy,* p. 5.

76. Gilgoff, *The Jesus Machine,* pp. 18–21 (quote on p. 21).

77. Hulbert, *Raising America,* p. 335. See also Dobson, *Dare to Discipline.*

78. "Created to Meet a Need," *Focus on the Family* newsletter, no date (ca. 1987), Focus on the Family folder, Wilcox Collection of Contemporary Political Movements, Kansas Collection, Kenneth Spencer Research Library, University of Kansas, Lawrence, KS (hereafter Wilcox Collection).

79. Ibid; Gilgoff, *Jesus Machine,* p. 24. For more on evangelical family management, Johnson, "Dr. Dobson's Advice to Christian Women," pp. 55–82.

80. Rita Healey, "Is Dobson's Political Clout Fading?" *Time,* January 24, 2008.

81. For numbers of letters received, see Lesage, "Christian Media," in *Media, Culture and the Religious Right,* p. 31.

82. "Dobson's Ministry in Focus," *Colorado Springs Gazette Telegraph,* March 30, 1997.

83. "Focus: Book on Discipline Came First," *Colorado Springs Gazette Telegraph,* March 8, 1993; Burlein, *Lift High on the Cross,* p. 122.

84. Dr. James Dobson, "The Future of the Family," *Focus on the Family* newsletter (Special Introductory Issue), 1986, Focus on the Family folder, Wilcox Collection. See also Johnson, "Dr. Dobson's Advice to Christian Women."

85. Burlein, *Lift High on the Cross,* p. 123.

86. "This We Believe," *Focus on the Family* newsletter (Special Introductory Issue), 1986, Focus on the Family folder, Wilcox Collection. For another iteration of these core principles, see "Principles at Work in Your Family," *Helping You Build a Healthier Home* newsletter, no date (ca. 1990s), Focus on the Family folder, Wilcox Collection.

87. Gilgoff, *Jesus Machine,* p. 61.

88. Dobson and Bergel, *The Decision of Life.*

89. Ridgeley, *Practicing What the Doctor Preached,* p. 187. See also Focus on the Family Resource List, October 1986, Focus on the Family folder, Wilcox Collection.

90. For a sample of letters from Dobson with pro-life content, see, for example, James Dobson to Friend, August 1991, Focus on the Family folder, Wilcox Collection; James Dobson to Friends, March 1995, Focus on the Family folder, Wilcox Collection; James Dobson to Friend, April 1995, Focus on the Family folder, Wilcox Collection.

91. Ridgeley, *Practicing What the Doctor Preached,* p. 199. For a sample of articles in *Brio* magazine, the publication targeted at teen girls, see Katherine G. Bond, "Personal Choices," *Brio* magazine, February 1994; "God Said . . . I said," *Brio* magazine, January 2001.

92. Jean Fielder Ensley, "Popsicle Crosses," *Focus on the Family* magazine, May 1993.

93. "The Miracle Child," *Focus on the Family* magazine, May 1993; Weslin, *The Gathering of the Lambs,* p. 219. "Deathscorts" is a pro-life term for the pro-choice activists who escort women from their cars into clinics and thus serve as buffers from anti-abortion protestors.

94. Chet Hardin, "The Twisted Road from Amendment 2 to 'I Do,'" *Colorado Springs Independent,* May 1, 2013. For a sample of work on this referendum, entitled Amendment 2, see Schultze and Guilfoyle, "Facts Don't Hate; They Just Are," in Kintz and Lesage, eds., *Media, Culture, and the Religious Right,* pp. 327–44; Tymkovich, Dailey, and Farley, "A Tale of Three Theories: Reason and Prejudice in the Battle Over Amendment 2," *University of Colorado Law Review* 68 (Spring 1997): 287–333; Garfield, "Don't Box Me In: The Unconstitutionality of Amendment 2 and English-Only Amendments," *Northwestern University Law Review* 89 (Winter 1995): 690–740; Goldberg, "Gay Rights through the Looking Glass: Politics, Morality, and the

Trial of Colorado's Amendment 2," *Fordham Urban Law Review* 21 (Summer 1994): 1057–81; Ridgeley, *Practicing What the Doctor Preached,* pp. 186–87.

95. These two issues were so intertwined that a Colorado gay rights organization, Equality Colorado, began collecting information about local pro-life groups. See Equality Colorado Collection, Denver Public Library, Denver, CO.

96. "Reflections on the Single Mother," *Focus on the Family* magazine, September 1982. For example, see "Why I Chose Life," *Focus on the Family* magazine, May 1991; Katherine G. Bond, "Personal Choices," *Brio* Magazine, February 1994; Jody Reeves, "Life Is Worth Holding On To," *Focus on the Family* magazine, January 1996; "Dr. Dobson's Solid Answers," *Focus on the Family* magazine, January 1998; Tom Nevin, "The Sanctity of Life," *Focus on the Family* magazine, January 1998; "God Said . . . I said," *Brio* magazine, January 2001.

97. James Dobson to CPC Friend, February 11, 1987, folder 14, carton 95, National Organization for Women Records, 1959–2002, Schlesinger Library, Radcliffe Institute, Harvard University, Cambridge, MA.

98. Sofia Resnick, "Crisis Pregnancy Centers Push Anti-Abortion Agenda Nationally," *Colorado Independent,* February 23, 2012.

99. Gilgoff, *Jesus Machine,* p. 36.

100. Ridgeley, *Practicing What the Doctor Preached,* p. 195.

101. "GOP Candidates Come to Listen," *Colorado Springs Gazette Telegraph,* July 9, 1995; Joseph D. McInerney, letter to the editor, *Colorado Springs Gazette Telegraph,* March 14, 1995; Dobson to Friend, April 1995, Focus on the Family folder, Wilcox Collection.

102. "Abortion Foray Shows Ministry Is Political," letters to the editor, *Colorado Springs Gazette Telegraph,* March 14, 1995.

103. Kevin Coleman, letter to the editor, *Colorado Springs Gazette Telegraph,* March 18, 1995.

104. Jane Drew, "Uproar Unwarranted Over Abortion Missive," letter to the editor, *Colorado Springs Gazette Telegraph,* March 18, 1995.

105. Gilgoff, *Jesus Machine,* p. 3.

106. Laurie Goodstein, "Religious Right, Frustrated, Trying New Tactic on G.O.P.," *New York Times,* March 23, 1998. For kingmaker, see Michael Crowley, "James Dobson: The Religious Right's New Kingmaker," *Slate,* November 4, 2004. https://slate.com/news-and-politics/2004/11/james-dobson.html.

CONCLUSION

1. Mark Soraghan, "Letter's Abortion-Massacre Link 'Appalls' Senate after Tragedy," *Denver Post,* April 27, 1999; Cal Thomas, "Government Cannot Impose Morality from the Top," *Colorado Springs Gazette,* June 28, 1999; "Excerpts from Bush's Comments on Abortion," *New York Times,* November 22, 1999.

2. "Free-Speech: Brian Rohrbough," *CBS Evening News,* October 2, 2006, https://www.cbsnews.com/news/freespeech-brian-rohrbough/ (accessed June 13, 2019).

3. Guttmacher Institute, "An Overview of Abortion Laws," October 1, 2017, https://www.guttmacher.org/state-policy/explore/overview-abortion-laws (accessed November 30, 2017).

4. For quote and more on such bans, see Denbow, "Abortion as Genocide," quote on p. 611.

5. Ed Quillen, "Mountain West: A Republican Fabrication," *High Country News,* October 13, 1997. For more on limited Democratic victories in these states, see Silk and Walsh, *One Nation, Divisible,* p. 178.

6. For a breakdown of partisan affiliation by race in the state, see Frey and Teixeira, "America's New Swing Region: The Political Demography and Geography of the Mountain West," in *America's New Swing Region,* p. 55.

BIBLIOGRAPHY

ARCHIVES

Archdiocese of Denver Digital Repository, Denver, CO
    Denver Catholic Register
Arizona Collection, Hayden Library, Arizona State University, Tempe, AZ
    Robert J. Donohoe Papers
Arizona Historical Foundation, Hayden Library, Arizona State University, Tempe, AZ
    Planned Parenthood of Northern and Central Arizona Collection
Arizona State Library, Archives and Public Records, State of Arizona Research Library, Phoenix, AZ
    Arizona Register
Center for Colorado and the West, Auraria Library, Denver, CO
    Interview with Father Jose Lara
Center for Southwest Research, University of New Mexico, Albuquerque, NM
    Sandra Allen Collection
    Roger A. Finzel American Indian Movement Papers
    Nambe Community School Teachers' Diaries, 1935–1942 Collection
    National Indian Youth Council Records
    New Mexico Catholic Renewal
    New Mexico Register
    New Mexico Women's Political Caucus Papers
    Robert E. Robideau American Indian Movement Papers
    Frank I. Sanchez Papers
    Bruce Trigg Papers
J. Willard Marriott Library, University of Utah, Salt Lake City, UT
    American Civil Liberties Union of Utah Collection
    Lester E. Bush Collection
    Allan Turner Howe Collection
    Wayne Owens Papers

Linda Sillitoe Collection
John Hay Library, Brown University, Providence, RI
    Hall-Hoag Collection of Dissenting and Extremist Printed Propaganda
Kansas Collection, Kenneth Spencer Research Library, University of Kansas, Lawrence, KS
    Wilcox Collection of Contemporary Political Movements
L. Tom Perry Special Collections, Harold B. Lee Library, Brigham Young University, Provo, UT
    Associated Students of Brigham Young University Women's Office History Collection
    Martha Sonntag Bradley Research Collection
    Jaynann Payne Records and Papers
    Register of American Conservative Union
Merill-Cazier Library Special Collections and Archives, Utah State University, Logan, UT
    Fife Folklore Collection
    Congressman Gunn McKay Papers
New Mexico State Records Center, Santa Fe, NM
    Governor Tony Anaya Papers
    Governor Jerry Apodaca Papers
    Governor David F. Cargo Papers
    Governor Bruce King Papers (1st Term)
    Governor Bruce King Papers (2nd Term)
New Mexico State University Special Collections and Archives, Las Cruces, NM
    Louis E. and Carmen K. Freudenthal Family Papers, 1837–1990
Schlesinger Library, Radcliffe Institute, Harvard University, Cambridge, MA
    National Abortion Rights Action League (NARAL) Collection
    National Abortion Rights Action League, Printed Materials Collection
    National Organization for Women Records, 1959–2002
    Linda E. J. Perry Collection
    Margot Anne Meade Sheahan Papers
University of Arizona Library Special Collections, University of Arizona, Tucson, AZ
    Arizona Lifeline serial
    Arizona Right to Life News serial
    Arizona Right to Life Newsletter serial
    Arizona Right to Life-Southern Region Newsletter serial
    Arizona Right to Life-Tucson Chapter Newsletter serial
University of Colorado-Boulder Archives, Boulder, CO
    Anne Marie Pois Oral History Project Collection
University of New Mexico School of Law Library, Albuquerque, NM
    Bruce King Papers
Western History and Genealogy Department, Denver Public Library, Denver, CO
    John Bermingham Papers

Clippings File, Abortion, 1960–1969
Colorado National Abortion Rights Action League serial
Denver Police Department Intelligence Files
Equality Colorado Collection
Rocky Mountain Planned Parenthood Collection
Wisconsin Historical Society, Madison, WI
    Project Young One Collection
    Pro-Life Action League Collection
    Wisconsin Right to Life Collection

SELECTED NEWSPAPERS

Albuquerque Journal
Albuquerque Tribune
Arizona Daily Star
Arizona Daily Sun
Arizona Republic
Belen News Bulletin (NM)
Boulder Daily Camera (CO)
Casa Grande Dispatch (AZ)
Chandler Arizonan (AZ)
Clovis Daily Journal (NM)
Clovis News-Journal (NM)
Colorado Independent
Colorado Springs Gazette Telegraph
Dallas Texas Catholic
Denver Post
Deseret News (UT)
Farmington Daily Times (NM)
Fort Morgan Times (CO)
Gallup Independent (NM)
Greeley Daily Tribune (CO)
Greeley Tribune (CO)
High Country News (CO)
Hobbs Daily News-Sun (NM)
Kingman Daily Miner (AZ)
Las Cruces Sun-News (NM)
Las Vegas Daily Optic (NM)
Logan Herald Journal (UT)
Los Angeles Times
Mesa Tribune (AZ)
Mohave Daily Miner (AZ)
The New Mexican (NM)

New Mexico Aggie
New York Times
Ogden Standard-Examiner (UT)
Phoenix Gazette
Phoenix New Times
Prescott Courier (AZ)
Provo Herald (UT)
Pueblo Chieftain (CO)
Rocky Mountain News (CO)
Roswell Daily Record (NM)
Salt Lake Tribune
Santa Fe Reporter
Scottsdale Daily Progress (AZ)
Sierra Vista Herald (AZ)
Silver City Daily Press (NM)
Tempe Daily News (AZ)
Tucson Daily Citizen
Washington Post
Yuma Daily Sun (AZ)

INTERVIEWS

Kay Allen, March 16, 2010
Mike Berger, March 18, 2010
Laura Bowman, March 24, 2010
Dr. Curtis Boyd, August 10, 2011
Ruth Dolan, August 8, 2011
Dauneen Dolce, March 23, 2010
Meme Eckstein, August 5, 2011
Nancy Ellefson, March 24, 2010
Bob Enyart, August 7, 2011
Virginia Evers, March 19, 2010
Laurie Futch, March 16, 2010
Socorro Gallagos, August 2, 2011
Leslie Hanks, August 5, 2011
Steven Imbarrato, March 23, 2010
John Jakubczyk, March 16, 2010
Jerry Kolb, November 7, 2011
Phil Leahy, March 23, 2010
Mary LeQuiu, March 22, 2010
Tom Longua, August 4, 2011
Kevin Lundberg, August 7, 2011

June Maskell (pseudonym), November 18, 2018
Mary Menicucci, March 26, 2010
Angela Schnieder, March 17, 2010
Phil and Helen Seader, March 18, 2010
Margaret Sebesta (pseudonym), August 8, 2011
Edwin Sheperson, March 25, 2010
Barb Willis, March 15, 2010

SOURCES

Abate, Michelle Ann. *Raising Your Kids Right: Children's Literature and Political Conservatism.* New Brunswick, NJ: Rutgers University Press, 2011.

Abbott, Carl. *The New Urban America: Growth and Politics in Sunbelt Cities.* Chapel Hill: University of North Carolina Press, 1987.

Abortion Clinic Violence: Oversight Hearings Before the Subcommittee on Civil and Constitutional Rights of the Committee on the Judiciary, House of Representatives, Ninety-ninth Congress, First and Second Session, March 6, 12, and April 3, 1985; and December 17, 1986. Washington, DC: U.S. Government Printing Office, 1987.

Abramowitz, Alan I. "It's Abortion, Stupid: Policy Voting in the 1992 Presidential Election." *Journal of Politics* 57, no. 1 (Feb. 1995): 176–86.

Adams, Abigail Rae. "Choice Ideology and the Parameters of Its Practice: Alternative Abortion Narratives in New Mexico." PhD diss., University of New Mexico, 2009.

Adams, David Wallace. *Education for Extinction: American Indians and the Boarding School Experience, 1875–1928.* Lawrence: University Press of Kansas, 1995.

Alexander, Thomas G. *Mormonism in Transition: A History of Latter-day Saints, 1890–1930.* Urbana: University of Illinois Press, 1996.

———. *Utah, the Right Place: The Official Centennial History,* rev. ed. Layton, UT: Gibbs Smith, 1996.

Allen, Marilee C., Pamela K. Donohue, and Amy Dusman. "The Limit of Viability—Neonatal Outcome of Infants Born at 22 to 25 Weeks Gestation." *New England Journal of Medicine* 329, no. 22 (November 25, 1993): 1597–1601.

Allitt, Patrick. *Catholic Intellectuals and Conservative Politics in America, 1950–1985.* Ithaca, NY: Cornell University Press, 1993.

Amundson, Micheal A. *Yellowcake Towns: Uranium Mining Communities in the American West.* Boulder: University Press of Colorado, 2002.

Andrew, John A. *The Other Side of the Sixties: Young Americans for Freedom and the Rise of Conservative Politics.* New Brunswick, NJ: Rutgers University Press, 1997.

Andrews, Thomas G. *Killing for Coal: America's Deadliest Labor War.* Cambridge, MA: Harvard University Press, 2008.

Applebome, Peter. *Dixie Rising: How the South Is Shaping American Values, Politics, and Culture.* New York: Times Books, 1996.

Arndorfer, Elizabeth, Jodi Micheal, Laura Moskowitz, Liza Siebel, Juli A. Grant. *Who Decides? A State-by-State Review of Abortion and Reproductive Rights, 1998*. New York: NARAL Foundation, 1998.

Arrington, Leonard. *Great Basin Kingdom: An Economic History of the Latter-Day Saints, 1830–1900*. Cambridge, MA: Harvard University Press, 1958.

Avila, Eric. *Popular Culture in the Age of White Flight: Fear and Fantasy in Suburban Los Angeles*. Berkeley: University of California Press, 2004.

Baer, Hans A., and Merril Singer. *African American Religion in the Twentieth Century: Varieties of Protest and Accommodation*. Knoxville: University of Tennessee Press, 1992.

Bagley, Will. *Blood of Prophets: Brigham Young and the Massacre at Mountain Meadows*. Norman: University of Oklahoma Press, 2002.

Bailey, Beth. *Sex in the Heartland*. Cambridge, MA: Harvard University Press, 1999.

Bailey, Garrick Alan, and Roberta Glenn Bailey. *A History of the Navajo: The Reservation Years*. Santa Fe, NM: School of American Research Press, 1986.

Baird-Windle, Patricia, and Eleanor J. Bader. *Targets of Hatred: Anti-Abortion Terrorism*. New York: Palgrave, 2001.

Balmer, Randall. *Redeemer: The Life of Jimmy Carter*. New York: Basic Books, 2014.

Banks, Bill, and Sue Banks. *Ministering to Abortion's Aftermath*. Kirkwood, MS: Impact Books, 1982.

Barnhouse, Mark A. *Northwest Denver*. Charleston, SC: Arcadia Publishing, 2012.

Baron, Lawrence. "The Holocaust and American Public Memory, 1945–1960." *Holocaust and Genocide Studies* 17 (Spring 2003): 62–88.

Barry, Tom. "What Price Energy? Hazards of Uranium Mining in the Southwest." *American Indian Journal of the Institute for the Development of Indian Law* 5 (January 1979): 18–23.

Beisel, Nicola, and Tamara Kay. "Abortion, Race and Gender in Nineteenth-Century America." *American Sociological Review* 69, no. 4 (2004): 498–518.

Belew, Kathleen. *Bring the War Home: The White Power Movement and Paramilitary America*. Cambridge, MA: Harvard University Press, 2018.

Benton-Cohen, Katherine. *Borderline Americans: Racial Division and Labor War in the Arizona Borderlands*. Cambridge, MA: Harvard University Press, 2009.

Berlant, Lauren. *The Queen of America Goes to Washington City: Essays on Sex and Citizenship*. Durham, NC: Duke University Press, 1997.

Bigler, David L. *Forgotten Kingdom: The Mormon Theocracy in the American West, 1847–1896*. Logan: Utah State University Press, 1998.

Bigler, David L., and Will Bagley. *The Mormon Rebellion: America's First Civil War, 1857–1858*. Norman: University of Oklahoma Press, 2011.

Bivins, Jason C. *Religion of Fear: The Politics of Horror in American Evangelicalism*. New York: Oxford University Press, 2008.

Blackhawk, Ned. *Violence Over the Land: Indians and Empires in the Early American West*. Cambridge, MA: Harvard University Press, 2006.

Blanchard, Dallas A., and Terry J. Prewitt. *Religious Violence and Abortion: The Gideon Project*. Gainesville: University Press of Florida, 1993.

Blumenthal, Max. *Republican Gommorah: Inside the Movement that Shattered the Party*. New York: Nation Books, 2009.

Boice, John D., Jr., Micheal T. Mumma, and William J. Blot. "Cancer and Noncancer Mortality in Populations Living Near Uranium and Vanadium Mining and Milling Operations in Montrose County, Colorado, 1950–2000." *Radiation Research* 167, no. 6 (June 2007): 711–26.

Boucher, Joanne. "The Politics of Abortion and the Commodification of the Fetus." *Studies in Political Economy* 73 (Summer 2004): 69–88.

Bowen, Michael. *The Roots of Modern Conservatism: Dewey, Taft, and the Battle for the Soul of the Republican Party*. Chapel Hill: University of North Carolina Press, 2011.

Bradley, Mark Philip. *The World Reimagined: Americans and Human Rights in the Twentieth Century*. New York: Cambridge University Press, 2016.

Bradley, Mark Philip, and Patrice Petro, eds. *Truth Claims: Representation and Human Rights*. New Brunswick, NJ: Rutgers University Press, 2002.

Bradley, Martha Sonntag. *Pedestals and Podiums: Utah Women, Religious Authority, and Equal Rights*. Salt Lake City, UT: Signature Books, 2005.

Brier, Jennifer. *Infectious Ideas: U.S. Political Responses to the AIDS Crisis*. Chapel Hill: University of North Carolina Press, 2009.

Bringhurst, Newell G., and Darron T. Smith, eds. *Black and Mormon*. Bloomington: University of Illinois Press, 2004.

Brooks, James F. *Captives and Cousins: Slavery, Kinship, and Community in the Southwest Borderlands*. Chapel Hill: University of North Carolina, 2002.

Brosnan, Kathleen. *Uniting Mountain and Plain: Cities, Law, and Environmental Change Along the Front Range*. Albuquerque: University of New Mexico Press, 2002.

Brown, Bill. "Thing Theory." In *Things*, ed. Bill Brown. Chicago, IL: University of Chicago Press, 2004.

Brown, R. Khari. "Racial Differences in Congregation-based Political Activism." *Social Forces* 84, no. 3 (2006): 1581–1604.

Brugge, Doug, Timothy Benally, and Esther Yazzie-Lewis, eds. *The Navajo People and Uranium Mining*. Albuquerque: University of New Mexico Press, 2006.

Burlein, Ann. *Lift High on the Cross: Where White Supremacy and the Christian Right Converge*. Durham, NC: Duke University Press, 2002.

Burns, Jeffrey. *American Catholics and the Family Crisis, 1930–1962: An Ideological and Organizational Response*. New York: Garland Publishing, 1988.

Bush, Lester E., Jr. "Birth Control Among the Mormons: An Introduction to an Insistent Question." *Dialogue* 10 (Autumn 1976): 12–44.

Bush, Lester E., Jr., and Armand L. Mauss. *Neither White nor Black: Mormon Scholars Confront the Race Issue in a Universal Church*. Salt Lake City, UT: Signature Books, 1984.

Butler, Anne M. *Across God's Frontiers: Catholic Sisters in the American West, 1850–1920*. Chapel Hill: University of North Carolina Press, 2012.

———. "Western Spaces, Catholic Places." *U.S. Catholic Historian* 18, no. 4 (Fall 2000): 25–39.

Butler, Anthea D. *Women in the Church of God in Christ: Making a Sanctified World*. Chapel Hill: University of North Carolina Press, 2007.

Butler, Judith. *Gender Trouble: Feminism and the Subversion of Identity*. New York: Routledge, 1990.

Cahill, Cathleen D. *Federal Mothers and Fathers: A Social History of the United States Indian Service, 1869–1933*. Chapel Hill: University of North Carolina Press, 2011.

Carlson, Allan. *Godly Seed: American Evangelicals Confront Birth Control, 1873–1973*. New York: Routledge, 2017.

Carter, Dan T. *The Politics of Rage: George Wallace, the Origins of the New Conservatism, and the Transformation of U.S. Politics*, 2d ed. Baton Rouge: Louisiana State University Press, 2000.

Casper, Monica J. *The Making of the Unborn Patient: A Social Anatomy of Fetal Surgery*. New Brunswick, NJ: Rutgers University Press, 1998.

Castoriadis, Cornelius. *The Imaginary Institution of Society*, rev. ed. 1975; Cambridge, MA: MIT Press, 1998.

Chin, Elizabeth. *Purchasing Power: Black Kids and American Consumer Culture*. Minneapolis: University of Minnesota Press, 2001.

Clark, Kenneth B., and Mamie Clark. "Racial Identification and Preference in Negro Children." In *Readings of Social Psychology*, ed. Theodore M. Newcomb and Eugene L. Hartley. New York: Henry Holt and Co., 1947.

Clow, Barbara. "'An Illness of Nine Months' Duration': Pregnancy and Thalidomide Use in the United States and Canada." In *Women, Health, and Nation: Canada and the United States since 1945*, ed. Georgina D. Feldberg. Montreal: McGill-Queens University Press, 2003.

Condit, Celeste Michelle. *Decoding Abortion Rhetoric: Communicating Social Change*. Urbana: University of Illinois Press, 1990.

Connelly, Mathew. *Fatal Misconception: The Struggle to Control World Population*. Cambridge, MA: Harvard University Press, 2008.

Coontz, Stephanie. *The Way We Never Were: American Families and the Nostalgia Trap*. New York: Basic Books, 1992.

Costa, Marie. *Abortion: A Reference Handbook*. Santa Barbara, CA: ABC-CLIO, 1996.

Cott, Nancy F. *The Grounding of Modern Feminism*. New Haven, CT: Yale University Press, 1987.

Coughlin, Richard M. "The Economic Person in Sociological Context: Case Studies in the Mediation of Public Interest." In *Socio-Economics: Towards a New Synthesis*, ed. Amitai Etzioni and Paul R. Lawrence. London: Routledge, 1991.

Crapo, Richley H. "Grass-Roots Deviance from Official Doctrine: A Study of Latter-Day Saint (Mormon) Folk-Beliefs." *Journal for the Scientific Study of Religion* 26, no. 4 (1987): 465–85.

Critchlow, Donald T. *Intended Consequences: Birth Control, Abortion, and the Federal Government in Modern America*. New York: Oxford University Press, 1999.

———. *Phyllis Schlafly and Grassroots Conservatism: A Woman's Crusade*. Princeton, NJ: Princeton University Press, 2005.

Cuneo, Michael W. *The Smoke of Satan: Conservative and Traditionalist Dissent in Contemporary American Catholicism.* New York: Oxford University Press, 1997.

Curro, Ellen. *Caring Enough to Help: Counseling at a Crisis Pregnancy Center.* Grand Rapids, MI: Baker Book House, 1990.

Daniels, Cynthia R. *At Women's Expense: State Power and the Politics of Fetal Rights.* Cambridge, MA: Harvard University Press, 1996.

Davis, Tom. *Sacred Work: Planned Parenthood and Its Clergy Alliances.* New Brunswick, NJ: Rutgers University Press, 2005.

Daynes, Byron W., and Raymond Tatalovich. "Mormons and Abortion Politics in the United States." *International Review of History and Political Science* 23, no. 2 (1986): 1–13.

DeConcini, Dennis, and Jack L. August, Jr. *Senator Dennis DeConcini: From the Center of the Aisle.* Tucson: University of Arizona Press, 2006.

D'Emilio, John, and Estelle Freedman. *Intimate Matters: A History of Sexuality in America,* 2d ed. Chicago, IL: University of Chicago Press, 1997.

Denbow, Jennifer. "Abortion as Genocide: Race Genocide and Nation in Prenatal Nondiscrimination Bans." *Signs: Journal of Women in Culture and Society* 41, no. 3 (2016): 603–26.

de Schweinitz, Rebecca. *If We Could Change the World: Young People and America's Long Struggle for Racial Equality.* Chapel Hill: University of North Carolina, 2009.

Detmer, David. *Sartre Explained: From Bad Faith to Authenticity.* Peru, IL: Carus Publishing Co., 2008.

Deutsch, Sarah. *No Separate Refuge: Culture, Class, and Gender on an Anglo-Hispanic Frontier in the American Southwest, 1880–1940.* New York: Oxford University Press, 1987.

Deyhle, Dorothy, and Frank Margonis. "Navajo Mothers and Daughters: Schools, Jobs, and the Family." *Anthropology and Education Quarterly* 26, no. 2 (June 1995): 135–67.

Diamond, Sara. *Road to Dominion: Right Wing Movements and Political Power in the United States.* New York: Guilford Press, 1995.

Diaz-Stevens, Ana Maria. "The Saving Grace: The Matriarchal Core of Latino Catholicism." *Latino Studies Journal* 4, no. 3 (Sept. 1993): 60–78.

Diaz-Stevens, Ana Maria, and Anthony M. Stevens-Arroyo. *Recognizing the Latino Resurgence in U.S. Religion.* Boulder, CO: Westview Press, 1998.

Dobson, James. *Dare to Discipline.* Carol Stream, IL: Tyndale House, 1977.

Dobson, James, and Gary Bergel. *The Decision of Life.* Arcadia, CA: Focus on the Family, 1986.

Dochuk, Darren. *From Bible Belt to Sunbelt: Plain-folk Religion, Grassroots Politics, and the Rise of Evangelical Conservatism.* New York: W. W. Norton, 2011.

Dolan, Jay P. *The American Catholic Experience: A History from Colonial Times to the Present.* New York: Galilee Trade, 1987.

Domenico, Roy Palmer, and Mark Y. Hanley, eds. *Encyclopedia of Modern Religious Politics.* Westport, CT: Greenwood Press, 2006.

Dorsey, Bruce. *Reforming Men and Women: Gender in the Antebellum City*. Ithaca, NY: Cornell University Press, 2002.

Dowland, Seth. *Family Values and the Rise of the Christian Right*. Philadelphia: University of Pennsylvania Press, 2015.

Dubow, Sara. *Ourselves Unborn: The History of the Fetus in Modern America*. New York: Oxford University Press, 2011.

DuCille, Anne. *Skin Trade*. Cambridge, MA: Harvard University Press, 1996.

Duden, Barbara. *Disembodying Woman: Perspectives on Pregnancy and the Unborn*. Trans. Lee Hoinacki. Cambridge, MA: Harvard University Press, 1993.

Dudley, Jonathan. *Broken Words: The Abuse of Science and Faith in American Politics*. New York: Crown Publishers, 2011.

Dunn, Charles W., and J. David Woodard. *The Conservative Tradition in America*, rev. ed. Lanham, MD: Rowman and Littlefield Publishers, 2003.

Ebaugh, Helen Rose Fauchs, and C. Allen Haney. "Church Attendance and Attitudes Towards Abortion: Differentials in Liberal and Conservative Churches." *Journal of the Scientific Study of Religion* 17 (1978): 407–13.

Echols, Alice. *Daring to Be Bad: Radical Feminism in America, 1967–1975*. Minneapolis: University of Minnesota Press, 1989.

Edelman, Lee. *No Future: Queer Theory and the Death Drive*. Durham, NC: Duke University Press, 2003.

Edelmann, Claude. *The First Days of Life*. Paris: France Impressions, 1971.

Edsall, Thomas Byrne, with Mary D. Edsall. *Chain Reaction: The Impact of Race, Rights, and Taxes on American Politics*. New York: W. W. Norton, 1991.

Edwards, Lee. *Goldwater: The Man Who Made a Revolution*. Washington, DC: Regnery Press, 1995.

Egerton, John. *The Americanization of Dixie: The Southernization of America*. New York: Harper's Magazine Press, 1974.

Ehrlich, J. Shoshanna. *Who Decides?: The Abortion Rights of Teens*. Westport, CT: Praeger Publishers, 2006.

Eichstaedt, Peter H. *If You Poison Us: Uranium and Native Americans*. Santa Fe, NM: Red Crane Books, 1994.

Emmens, Carol A. *The Abortion Controversy*. New York: Julian Messner, 1987.

Enke, Anne. *Finding the Movement: Sexuality, Contested Space, and Feminist Activism*. Durham, NC: Duke University Press, 2007.

Espín, Orlando O. "Mexican Religious Practices, Popular Catholicism, and the Development of Doctrine." In *Horizons of the Sacred: Mexican Traditions in U.S. Catholicism*, ed. Timothy Matovina and Gary Riebe-Estella. Ithaca, NY: Cornell University Press, 2002.

Evans, Dylan. *An Introductory Dictionary of Lacanian Psychoanalysis*. London: Routledge, 1996.

Evans, John H. "Polarization in Abortion Attitudes in U.S. Religious Traditions, 1972–1998." *Sociological Forum* 17, no. 3 (Sept. 2002): 397–422.

Evans, Sara M. *Tidal Wave: How Women Changed America at Century's End*. New York: Free Press, 2003.

Faggioli, Massimo. *Vatican II: The Battle for Meaning.* Mahwah, NJ: Paulist Press, 1989.

Fairbanks, Robert B. "The Failure of Urban Renewal in the Southwest: From City Needs to Individual Rights." *Western Historical Quarterly* 37 (Autumn 2006): 303–26.

Faludi, Susan. *Backlash: The Undeclared War Against American Women.* New York: Crown Publishing Group, 1991.

Feldman, Glenn. *The Great Melding: War, The Dixiecrat Rebellion, and the Southern Model for America's New Conservatism.* Tuscaloosa: University of Alabama Press, 2015.

Fermaglich, Kirsten. *American Dreams and Nazi Nightmares: Early Holocaust Consciousness and Liberal America, 1957–1965.* Waltham, MA: Brandeis University Press, 2006.

Fernlund, Kevin, ed. *The Cold War American West, 1945–1989.* Albuquerque: University of New Mexico Press, 1998.

Ferree, Myra Marx, William Anthony Gamson, Jürgen Gerhards, and Dieter Rucht. *Shaping Abortion Discourse: Democracy and the Public Sphere in Germany and the United States.* Cambridge, MA: Cambridge University Press, 2002.

Findlay, John. *Magic Lands: Western Cityscapes and American Culture After 1940.* Berkeley: University of California Press, 1992.

Flamm, Michael W. *Law and Order: Street Crime, Civil Unrest, and the Crisis of Liberalism in the 1960s.* New York: Columbia University Press, 2005.

Fletcher, John. *Preaching to Convert: Evangelical Outreach and Secular Activism in a Secular Age.* Ann Arbor: University of Michigan Press, 2013.

Flippen, J. Brooks. *Jimmy Carter, the Politics of Family, and the Religious Right.* Athens: University of Georgia Press, 2011.

Flipse, Scott. "Below-the-Belt Politics: Protestant Evangelicals, Abortion, and the Foundation of the New Religious Right, 1960–75." In *Conservative Sixties,* ed. David Farber and Jeff Roche. New York: Peter Lang, 2003.

Formisano, Ronald P. *Boston Against Busing: Race, Class, and Ethnicity in 1960s and 1970s.* Chapel Hill: University of North Carolina Press, 1991.

Frank, Gillian. "The Colour of the Unborn: Anti-Abortion and Anti-Bussing Politics in Michigan, United States, 1967–1973." *Gender & History* 26 (August 2014): 351–78.

Frank, Thomas. *What's the Matter with Kansas?: How Conservatives Won the Heart of America.* New York: Macmillan, 2005.

Frey, William H., and Rudy Teixeira. "America's New Swing Region: The Political Demography and Geography of the Mountain West." In *America's New Swing Region: Changing Politics and Demographics in the Mountain West,* ed. Rudy A. Teixeira. Washington, DC: Brookings Institution, 2012.

Furniss, Norman F. *The Mormon Conflict, 1850–1859.* New Haven, CT: Yale University Press, 1960.

Gaither, Milton. *Homeschool: An American History.* New York: Palgrave Macmillan, 2008.

Gallop, Jane. *Reading Lacan.* Ithaca, NY: Cornell University Press, 1985.

García, Mario T. *Católicos: Resistance and Affirmation in Chicano Catholic History.* Austin: University of Texas Press, 2008.

Garcia, Michelle. "Roundtable on the Religious Right and Communities of Color." *Third Force* 2, no. 4 (October 31, 1994).

Garfield, Daniel. "Don't Box Me In: The Unconstitutionality of Amendment 2 and English- Only Amendments." *Northwestern University Law Review* 89 (Winter 1995): 690–740.

Garrow, David J. *Liberty and Sexuality: The Right to Privacy and the Making of Roe v. Wade.* New York: Macmillan, 1994.

Geary, Daniel. *Beyond Civil Rights: The Moynihan Report and Its Legacy.* Philadelphia: University of Pennsylvania Press, 2015.

Gerhard, Jane. *Desiring Revolution: Second-Wave Feminism and the Rewriting of American Sexual Thought, 1920 to 1982.* New York: Columbia University Press, 2001.

Getty, Harry T. *Interethnic Relationships in the Community of Tucson.* Reprint, New York: Arno Press, 1976.

Gilens, Martin. "How the Poor Became Black: The Racialization of American Poverty in the Mass Media." In *Race and the Politics of Welfare Reform,* ed. Sanford F. Schram, Joe Soss, and Richard C. Fording. Ann Arbor: University of Michigan Press, 2003.

Gilgoff, Dan. *The Jesus Machine: How James Dobson, Focus on the Family, and Evangelical America Are Winning the Culture War.* New York: St. Martin's Press, 2007.

Gillis, Chester. "Vatican II." In *Religion and American Cultures Encyclopedia: An Encyclopedia of Traditions, Diversity and Popular Expression,* vol. 1, ed. Gary Laderman and Luis León. Santa Barbara, CA: ABC-CLIO, 2003.

Ginsburg, Faye D. *Contested Lives: The Abortion Debate Within an American Community.* Berkeley: University of California Press, 1998.

———. "Rescuing the Nation: Operation Rescue and the Rise of Anti-Abortion Militance." In *Abortion Wars: A Half Century of Struggle, 1950–2000,* ed. Rickie Solinger. Berkeley: University of California Press, 1998.

———. "Saving America's Souls: Operation Rescue's Crusade Against Abortion." In *Fundamentalisms and the State: Remaking Politics, Economies, and Militance,* ed. Martin Marty and R. Scott Appleby. Chicago, IL: University of Chicago Press, 1993.

Givens, Terryl. *The Latter-Day Saint Experience in America.* Westport, CT: Greenwood Press, 2004.

———. *People of Paradox: A History of Mormon Culture.* New York: Oxford University Press, 2006.

Glendinning, Chellis. *Chiva: A Village Takes on the Global Heroin Trade.* Gabriola Island, Canada: New Society Publishers, 2005.

Goldberg, Michelle. *Kingdom Coming: The Rise of Christian Nationalism.* New York: W. W. Norton, 2007.

Goldberg, Robert Allan. *Barry Goldwater.* New Haven, CT: Yale University Press, 1995.

Goldberg, Suzanne B. "Gay Rights through the Looking Glass: Politics, Morality, and the Trial of Colorado's Amendment 2." *Fordham Urban Law Review* 21 (Summer 1994): 1057–81.

Goldstein, Arnold P., Leonard Krasner, and Sol L. Garfield, eds. *Posttraumatic Stress Disorder.* New York: Macmillan, 1992.

Gómez, Arthur R. "Urban Imperialism in the Modern West: Farmington, New Mexico, vs. Durango, Colorado, 1945–1956." In *Essays in Twentieth-Century New Mexico History,* ed. Judith B. Demark. Albuquerque: University of New Mexico Press, 1994.

Gonzales, Phillip P. "Historical Poverty, Restructuring Effects, and Integrative Ties: Mexican American Neighborhoods in a Peripheral Sunbelt Economy." In *In the Barrios: Latinos and the Underclass Debate,* ed. Joan Moore and Raquel Pinderhughes. New York: Russell Sage Foundation, 1993.

Goodson, Patricia, and Elizabeth Edmundson. "The Problematic Promotion of Abstinence: An Overview of *Sex Respect.*" *Journal of School Health* 64 (May 1994): 205–10.

Gordon, Linda. *Woman's Body, Woman's Right: Birth Control in America.* Rev. ed. 1976; New York: Penguin Books, 1990.

Gordon, Sarah Barringer. *The Mormon Question: Polygamy and Constitutional Conflict in Nineteenth Century America.* Chapel Hill: University of North Carolina Press, 2002.

Gorney, Cynthia. *Articles of Faith: A Frontline History of the Abortion Wars.* New York: Simon and Schuster, 2000.

Gottlieb, Robert, and Peter Wiley. *America's Saints: The Rise of Mormon Power.* New York: G. P. Putnam's Sons, 1984.

Gould, Deborah B. *Moving Politics: Emotion and ACT UP's Fight Against AIDS.* Chicago, IL: University of Chicago Press, 2009.

Graham, Gael. *Young Activists: American High School Students in the Age of Protest.* DeKalb: Northern Illinois University Press, 2006.

Grainger, Brett. *In the World but Not of It: One Family's Militant Faith and the History of Fundamentalism in America.* New York: Walker and Co., 2008.

Greenbaum, Susan D. *Blaming the Poor: The Long Shadow of the Moynihan Report on Cruel Images about Poverty.* New Brunswick, NJ: Rutgers University Press, 2015.

Greenhouse, Linda. *Becoming Justice Blackmun: Harry Blackmun's Supreme Court Journey.* New York: Henry Holt and Co., 2005.

Greenhouse, Linda, and Riva B. Siegel. *Before Roe v. Wade: The Voices that Shaped the Abortion Debate Before the Supreme Court's Ruling.* New York: Kaplan Publishing, 2010.

Gregory, James N. *American Exodus: The Dust Bowl Migration and Okie Culture in California.* New York: Oxford University Press, 1989.

———. *The Southern Diaspora: How the Great Migrations of Black and White Southerners Transformed America*. Chapel Hill: University of North Carolina Press, 2005.

Gutiérrez, Elena R. *Fertile Matters: The Politics of Mexican-Origin Women's Reproduction*. Austin: University of Texas Press, 2008.

Gutiérrez, Ramón. *When Jesus Came, the Corn Mothers Went Away: Marriage, Sexuality, and Power in New Mexico, 1500–1846*. Stanford, CA: Stanford University Press, 1991.

Haag, Bernadine. *SHAM: Social Change Through Contrived Crises*. Sahuarita, AZ: Sahuarita Press, 1993.

Haffner, Debra W., and James Wagoner. "Vast Majority of Americans Show Support for Sexuality Education." *SEICUS Report* 27, no. 6 (August/September 1999): 22–23.

Haines, Herbert A. *Against Capital Punishment: The Anti-Death Penalty Movement in America, 1972–1994*. New York: Oxford University Press, 1996.

Hall, Jacquelyn Dowd. *Revolt Against Chivalry: Jesse Daniel Ames and the Women's Campaign Against Lynching*. New York: Columbia University Press, 1979.

Hallett, Paul H. *Witness to Permanence: Reflections of a Catholic Journalist*. San Francisco, CA: Ignatius Press, 1987.

Hamburg, David A. Foreword. In *Post-Traumatic Therapy and Victims of Violence*, ed. Frank M. Ochberg. New York: Brunner/Mazel, 1988.

Hancock, Ange-Marie. *The Politics of Disgust: The Public Identity of the Welfare Queen*. New York: New York University Press, 2004.

Hansen, Klaus J. *Mormonism and the American Experience*. Chicago, IL: University of Chicago Press, 1981.

Haraway, Donna. *Modest-Witness@Second_Millennium_FemaleMan_Meets_OncoMouse*. New York: Routledge, 1997.

Harding, Susan Friend. *The Book of Jerry Falwell: Fundamentalist Language and Politics*. Princeton, NJ: Princeton University Press, 2000.

Harmon, Katherine E. *There Were Also Many Women There: Women in the Liturgical Movement in the United States, 1926–59*. Collegeville, MN: Liturgical Press, 2012.

Hartmann, Andrew. *A War for the Soul of America: A History of the Culture Wars*. Chicago, IL: University of Chicago Press, 2015.

Haugeberg, Karissa. *Women Against Abortion: Inside the Largest Moral Reform Movement of the Twentieth Century*. Urbana: University of Illinois Press, 2017.

Heltzel, Peter G. *Jesus and Justice: Evangelicals, Race, and American Politics*. New Haven, CT: Yale University Press, 2009.

Hendershot, Heather. *Shaking the World for Jesus: Media and Conservative Evangelical Culture*. Chicago, IL: University of Chicago Press, 2004.

Henold, Mary J. "'This is Our Challenge! We Will Pursue It': The National Council of Catholic Women, the Feminist Movement, and the Second Vatican Council, 1960–1975." In *Empowering the People of God: Catholic Action Before and After Vatican II,* ed. Jeremy Bonner, Mary Beth Fraser Connelly, and Christopher Denny. New York: Fordham University Press, 2014.

Hevly, Bruce, and John Findlay, eds. *The Atomic West.* Seattle: University of Washington Press, 1998.

Hewitt, Nancy. *Southern Discomfort: Women's Activism in Tampa, Florida, 1880s–1920s.* Urbana: University of Illinois Press, 2001.

Higginbotham, Evelyn Brooks. *Righteous Discontent: The Woman's Movement in the Black Baptist Church, 1880–1920.* Cambridge, MA: Harvard University Press, 1994.

Hoffmann, Stefan-Ludwig, ed. *Human Rights in the Twentieth Century.* New York: Cambridge University Press, 2010.

Holland, Jennifer L. "'Salt Lake City Is Our Selma': The Equal Rights Amendment and the Transformation of the Politics of Gender in Utah." MA thesis, Utah State University, 2005.

Hornsby, Alton, Jr. *Black America: A State by State Historical Encyclopedia,* vol. 2. Santa Barbara, CA: ABC-CLIO, 2011.

Hudson, Deal W. *Onward Christian Soldiers: The Growing Political Power of Catholics and Evangelicals in the United States.* New York: Threshold Editions, 2008.

Hughes, Richard L. "'The Civil Rights Movement of the 1990s?': The Anti-Abortion Movement and the Struggle for Racial Justice." *Oral History Review* 33 (Summer/Autumn 2006): 1–23.

Hulbert, Ann. *Raising America: Experts, Parents, and a Century of Advice About Children.* New York: Vintage Books, 2003.

Hunner, Jon. *Inventing Los Alamos: The Growth of an Atomic Community.* Norman: University of Oklahoma Press, 2004.

Hunter, James Davison. *Culture Wars: The Struggle to Define America.* New York: Basic Books, 1991.

Hunter, James Glenn. "A Religious Rhetoric of Abortion: LDS Views of Over One Hundred Years." PhD dissertation, University of Wyoming, 1991.

Hussey, Laura S. "Crisis Pregnancy Centers, Poverty, and the Expanding Frontiers of American Abortion Politics." *Politics and Policy* 41, no. 6 (December 2013): 985–1011.

Ianora, Terry. *Crisis Pregnancy Centers: The Birth of a Grassroots Movement.* Bloomington, IN: AuthorHouse, 2009.

Iriye, Akira, Petra Goedde, and William I. Hitchcock, eds. *The Human Rights Revolution: An International History.* New York: Oxford University Press, 2012.

Irvine, Janice M. *Talk About Sex: The Battles of Sex Education in the United States.* Berkeley: University of California Press, 2002.

Iverson, Peter. *Barry Goldwater: Native Arizonian.* Norman: University of Oklahoma Press, 1997.

———. *Diné: A History of the Navajo.* Albuquerque: University of New Mexico Press, 2002.

Jacobs, Margaret. *White Mother to a Dark Race: Settler Colonialism, Maternalism, and the Removal of Indigenous Children in the American West and Australia, 1880–1940.* Lincoln: University of Nebraska Press, 2009.

Jacoby, Karl. *Shadows at Dawn: An Apache Massacre and the Violence of History.* New York: Penguin Press, 2008.

Jacoby, Kerry N. *Souls, Bodies, and Spirits: The Drive to Abolish Abortion Since 1973.* Westport, CT: Praeger, 1998.

Jameson, Elizabeth. *All That Glitters: Class, Community, and Conflict in Cripple Creek.* Urbana: University of Illinois Press, 1998.

Jeffris, Jennifer. *Armed for Life: The Army of God and Anti-Abortion Terror in the United States.* Santa Barbara, CA: ABC-CLIO, 2011.

Johnson, Eithne. "Dr. Dobson's Advice to Christian Women: Strategic Motherhood." *Social Text* 57 (Winter 1998): 55–82.

Johnson, Emily Suzanne. *This is Our Message: Women's Leadership in the New Christian Right.* New York: Oxford University Press, 2019.

Jones, Sondra. *The Trial of Don Pedro León Luján: The Attack Against Indian Slavery and Mexican Traders in Utah.* Salt Lake City: University of Utah Press, 2000.

Joyce, Kathryn. *The Child Catchers: Rescue, Trafficking, and the New Gospel of Adoption.* New York: PublicAffairs, 2013.

Kandel, Lenore. *Collected Poems of Lenore Kandel.* Berkeley, CA: North Atlantic Books, 2012.

Kanowitz, Leo. "Love Lust in New Mexico and the Emerging Law of Obscenity." *Natural Resources Journal* 10 (April 1970): 339–52.

Karrer, Robert. "The National Right to Life Committee: Its Founding, Its History, and the Emergence of the Pro-Life Movement Prior to *Roe v. Wade.*" *The Catholic Historical Review* 97 (2011): 527–57.

Kelly, Kimberly. "In the Name of the Mother: Renegotiating Conservative Women's Authority in the Crisis Pregnancy Center Movement." *Signs* 38, no. 1 (Autumn 2012): 203–30.

Kelman, Ari. *A Misplaced Massacre: Struggling Over the Memory of Sand Creek.* Cambridge, MA: Harvard University Press, 2013.

Kerns, James. *The Speaker's Guide to 40 Years of General Conference.* Springville, UT: Cedar Fort Inc., 2010.

King, Alveda C. Foreword. In Sonya Howard, *Almost Wasn't: A Memoir of My Abortion and How God Used Me.* Philadelphia, PA: Xlibris, 2011.

———. *How Can the Dream Survive if We Murder Children?* Bloomington, IN: AuthorHouse, 2008.

Kintz, Linda, and Julia Lesage, eds. *Media, Culture, and the Religious Right.* Minneapolis: University of Minnesota Press, 1998.

Kissack, Terrance. "Freaking Fag Revolutionaries: New York's Gay Liberation Front, 1969– 71." *Radical History Review* 62 (Spring 1995): 105–34.

Klatch, Rebecca E. *Women of the New Right.* Philadelphia: Temple University Press, 1987.

Kline, Wendy. *Bodies of Knowledge: Sexuality, Reproduction, and Women's Health in the Second Wave.* Chicago, IL: University of Chicago Press, 2010.

Kluchin, Rebecca M. *Fit to Be Tied: Sterilization and Reproductive Rights in America, 1950–1980.* New Brunswick, NJ: Rutgers University Press, 2004.

Knack, Martha C. *Boundaries Between: The Southern Paiutes, 1775–1995.* Lincoln: University of Nebraska Press, 2004.

Koonz, Claudia. *Mothers in the Fatherland: Women, the Family, and Nazi Politics.* New York: St. Martins Press, 1987.

Kruse, Kevin M. "Beyond the Southern Cross: The National Origins of the Religious Right." In *The Myth of Southern Exceptionalism,* ed. Mathew D. Lassiter and Joseph Crepino. New York: Oxford University Press, 2010.

———. *White Flight: Atlanta and the Making of Modern Conservatism.* Princeton, NJ: Princeton University Press, 2005.

Kunzman, Robert. "Homeschooling and Fundamentalism." *International Electronic Journal of Elementary Education* 3, no. 1 (October 2010): 17–28.

Laderman, Gary, and Luis León, eds. *Religion and American Cultures Encyclopedia: An Encyclopedia of Traditions, Diversity and Popular Expression,* vol. 1. Santa Barbara, CA: ABC-CLIO, 2003.

Lancaster, Roger N. *Sex Panic and the Punitive State.* Berkeley: University of California Press, 2011.

Landy, David J., Lisa Kaeser, and Cory L. Richards. "Abstinence Information and the Provision of Information about Contraception in Public School District Sexuality Education Policies." *Family Planning Perspectives* 31, no. 6 (Nov.-Dec. 1999): 280–86.

Lang, Robert E., Mark Muro, and Andrea Sarzynski. "Mountain Megas: America's Newest Metropolitan Places and a Federal Partnership to Help Them Prosper." Brookings Institution, July 20, 2008.

Lassiter, Matthew D. "Big Government and Family Values." In *Sunbelt Rising: The Politics of Space, Place, and Region,* ed. Michelle M. Nickerson and Darren Dochuk. Philadelphia: University of Pennsylvania Press, 2011.

———. "Inventing Family Values." In *Rightward Bound: Making America Conservative in the 1970s,* ed. Bruce J. Schulman and Julian E. Zelizer. Cambridge, MA: Harvard University Press, 2008.

———. *The Silent Majority: Suburban Politics in the Sunbelt South.* Princeton, NJ: Princeton University Press, 2006.

Lawrence, Jane. "The Indian Health Service and the Sterilization of Native American Women." *American Indian Quarterly* 24, no. 3 (2000): 400–19.

Leary, Jaelyn deMaria. "Urban Homeland: An Exploration of Albuquerque's Santa Barbara/Martineztown Neighborhood." PhD diss., University of New Mexico, 2004.

Lee, Ellie. *Abortion, Motherhood, and Mental Health: Medicalizing Reproduction in the United States and Britain.* New York: Adeline De Gruyter, 2003.

Lesage, Julia. "Christian Media." In *Media, Culture and the Religious Right,* ed. Linda Kintz and Julia Lesage. Minneapolis: University of Minnesota Press, 1998.

Lieberman, Robert C. *Shifting the Color Line: Race and the American Welfare State.* Cambridge, MA: Harvard University Press, 2001.

Lindley, Susan Hill. *You Have Stept Out of Your Place: A History of Women and Religion in America.* Louisville, KY: Westminister John Knox Press, 1996.

Link, William A. "Time Is an Elusive Companion: Jesse Helms, Barry Goldwater, and the Dynamic of Modern Conservatism." In *Barry Goldwater and the Remaking of the Political Landscape,* ed. Elizabeth Tandy Shermer. Tucson: University of Arizona Press, 2013.

Lira, Natalie. "'Of Low Grade Mexican Parentage': Race, Gender and Eugenic Sterilization in California Institutions for the Feeble-Minded, 1920–1950." PhD dissertation, University of Michigan, 2015.

Littlefield, Alice. "Indian Education and the World of Work, 1893–1933." In *Native Americans and Wage Labor: Ethnohistorical Perspectives,* ed. Alice Littlefield and Martha Knack. Norman: University of Oklahoma Press, 1996.

Logan, Michael F. *Fighting Sprawl and City Hall: Resistance to Urban Growth in the Southwest.* Tucson: University of Arizona Press, 1995.

LoRusso, James Dennis. "'The Puritan Ethic on High': LDS Media and the Mormon Embrace of Free Enterprise in the Twentieth Century." In *Out of Obscurity: Mormonism since 1945,* ed. Patrick Q. Mason and John G. Turner. New York: Oxford University Press, 2016.

Lowe, Lisa. *Immigrant Acts: On Asian American Cultural Politics.* Durham, NC: Duke University Press, 1996.

Lucas, J. Anthony. *Common Ground: A Turbulent Decade in the Lives of Three America Families.* New York: Vintage Books, 1986.

Luckingham, Bradford. *Minorities in Phoenix: A Profile of Mexican American, Chinese American, and African American Communities, 1860–1992.* Tucson: University of Arizona Press, 1994.

———. *Phoenix: The History of a Southwestern Metropolis.* Tucson: University of Arizona Press, 1989.

———. *The Urban Southwest: A Profile History of Albuquerque, El Paso, Phoenix and Tucson.* El Paso: Texas Western Press, 1982.

Luhr, Eileen. *Witnessing Suburbia: Conservatives and Christian Youth Culture.* Berkeley: University of California Press, 2009.

Luker, Kristen. *Abortion and the Politics of Motherhood.* Berkeley: University of California Press, 1984.

———. *Dubious Conceptions: The Politics of Teen Pregnancy.* Cambridge, MA: Harvard University Press, 1996.

MacCarthy, Esther. "Catholic Women and War: The National Council of Catholic Women, 1919–1946." *Peace and Change* 5 (1978): 23–32.

Magee, Carole. *Africa in the American Imagination: Popular Culture, Racialized Identities, and African Visual Culture.* Chapel Hill: University of North Carolina Press, 2012.

Maines, David R., and Michael J. McCallion. *Transforming Catholicism: Liturgical Change in the Vatican II Church.* Lanham, MD: Lexington Books, 2007.

Major, Brenda. "Psychological Implications of Abortion—Highly Charged and Rife with Misleading Research." *Canadian Medical Association Journal* 168 (May 13, 2003): 1257–58.

Major, Brenda, Catherine Cozzarelli, M. Lynne Cooper, Josephine Zubek, Caroline Richards, Michael Wilhite, and Richard Gramzow. "Psychological Responses of Women after First-Trimester Abortion." *Archive of General Psychiatry* 57, no. 8 (August 2008): 777–84.

Manning, Christel J. "Women in a Divided Church: Liberal and Conservative Catholic Women Negotiate Changing Gender Roles." *Sociology of Religion* 58 (Winter 1997): 375–90.

Manuelito, Kathryn. "The Role of Education in American Indian Self-Determination: Lessons from the Ramah Navajo Community School." *Anthropology and Education Quarterly* 36, no. 1 (March 2005): 73–87.

Marchant-Shapiro, Theresa, and Kelly D. Patterson. "Partisan Change in the Mountain West." *Political Behavior* 17, no. 4 (1995): 359–78.

Markusan, Anne, Peter Hall, Scott Campbell, and Sabina Deitrick. *The Rise of the Gunbelt: The Military Remapping of Industrial America.* New York: Oxford University Press, 1991.

Marley, David John. "Riding in the Back of the Bus: The Christian Right's Adoption of Civil Rights Movement Rhetoric." In *The Civil Rights Movement in American Memory,* ed. Renee C. Romano and Leigh Raiford. Athens: University of Georgia Press, 2006.

Marsden, George M. *Reforming Fundamentalism: Fuller Seminary and the New Evangelicalism.* Grand Rapids, MI: William B. Erdmans Publishing Co., 1987.

Mart, Michelle. "The 'Christianization' of Israel and Jews in 1950s America." *Religion and American Culture: A Journal of Interpretation* 14, no. 1 (Winter 2004): 109–47.

Martin, William. *With God on Our Side: The Rise of the Religious Right in America.* New York: Broadway Books, 1996.

Mason, Carol. *Killing for Life: The Apocalyptic Narrative of Pro-Life Politics.* Ithaca, NY: Cornell University Press, 2002.

Mason, Elsie W. "Bishop C.H. Mason, Church of God in Christ." In *African American Religious History: Documentary Witness,* ed. Milton C. Sernett, 2d ed. Durham, NC: Duke University Press, 1999.

Massa, Mark S. *The American Catholic Revolution: How the Sixties Changed the Church Forever.* New York: Oxford University Press, 2010.

Mathews, Donald G., and Jane Sherron De Hart. *Sex, Gender, and the Politics of ERA: A State and the Nation.* New York: Oxford University Press, 1990.

Matovina, Timothy M. *Guadalupe and Her Faithful: Latino Catholics in San Antonio, from Colonial Origins to the Present.* Baltimore, MD: Johns Hopkins University Press, 2005.

———. *Latino Catholicism: Transformation of America's Largest Church.* Princeton, NJ: Princeton University Press, 2012.

———. "Lay Initiatives in Worship on the Texas *Frontera,* 1830–1860." *U.S. Catholic Historian* 12, no. 4 (Fall 1994): 107–20.

Mauss, Armand L. *The Angel and the Beehive: The Mormon Struggle with Assimilation.* Urbana: University of Illinois Press, 1994.

Mayberry, Maralee, J. Gary Knowles, Brian Ray, and Stacey Marlow. *Homeschooling: Parents as Educators.* Thousand Oaks, CA: Corwin Press, 1995.

Maynard-Moody, Steven. *The Dilemma of the Fetus: Fetal Research, Medical Progress, and Moral Politics.* New York: St. Martin's Press, 1995.

Mayo, Cris. *Disputing the Subject of Sex: Sexualities and Public School Controversies.* Lanham, MD: Rowman and Littlefield, 2004.

Maxwell, Elder Neil A. "A More Determined Discipleship: An Address Delivered at Brigham Young University, 10 October 1978." *Ensign,* February 1979.

McBride, Dorothy E. *Abortion in the United States: A Handbook.* Santa Barbara, CA: ABC-CLIO, 2008.

McCallum, Dennis, ed. *Death of Truth: Responding to Multiculturalism, the Rejection of Reason, and the New Postmodern Diversity.* Minneapolis, MN: Bethany House Publishers, 1996.

McDannell, Colleen. "Creating the Christian Home: Home Schooling in Contemporary America." In *American Sacred Space,* ed. David Chidester and Edward T. Linenthal. Bloomington: Indiana University Press, 1995.

———. *Spirit of Vatican II: A History of Catholic Reform in America.* New York: Basic Books, 2011.

McGirr, Lisa. *Suburban Warriors: The Origins of the New American Right.* Princeton, NJ: Princeton University Press, 2001.

McGreevy, John T. *Catholicism and American Freedom.* New York: W. W. Norton, 2003.

McIntosh, William Alex, Letitia T. Alston, and John P. Alston. "The Differential Impact of Religious Preference and Church Attendance on Attitudes Towards Abortion." *Review of Religious Research* 20, no. 2 (Spring 1979): 195–213.

McPherson, Robert S. *Navajo Land, Navajo Culture: The Utah Experience in the Twentieth Century.* Norman: University of Oklahoma Press, 2001.

Medina, Lara. *Las Hermanas: Chicana/Latina Religious-Political Activism in the U.S. Catholic Church.* Philadelphia, PA: Temple University Press, 2004.

Melcher, Mary S. *Pregnancy, Motherhood, and Choice in 20th Century Arizona.* Tucson: University of Arizona Press, 2012.

Meyerowitz, Joanne, ed. *Not June Cleaver: Women and Gender in Postwar America, 1945-1960.* Philadelphia: Temple University Press, 1994.

Middendorf, J. William, III. *Glorious Disaster: Barry Goldwater's Presidential Campaign and the Origins of the Conservative Movement.* New York: Basic Books, 2006.

Miller, Patricia. *Good Catholics: The Battle Over Abortion in the Catholic Church.* Berkeley: University of California Press, 2014.

Miller, Steven P. *The Age of Evangelicalism: America's Born Again Years.* New York: Oxford University Press, 2014.

Mitchell, Pablo. *Coyote Nation: Sexuality, Race, and Conquest in Modernizing New Mexico, 1880–1930.* Chicago, IL: University of Chicago Press, 2005.

Mohr, James C. *Abortion in America: The Origins and Evolutions of National Policy, 1800–1900.* New York: Oxford University Press, 1978.

Montoya, Maria. *Translating Property: The Maxwell Land Grant and the Conflict over Land in the American West, 1840–1900.* Berkeley: University of California Press, 2002.

Mooney, Bernice Maher, and J. Terrance Fitzgerald. *Salt of the Earth: The History of the Catholic Church in Utah, 1776–2007.* Salt Lake City: University of Utah Press, 2008.

Moore, Deborah Dash. *GI Jews: How World War II Changed a Generation.* Cambridge, MA: Harvard University Press, 2004.

Moore, Michele C., and Caroline M. de Costa. *Just the Facts: Abortion A to Z.* Victoria, Canada: Trafford, 2007.

Moran, Jeffrey P. *Teaching Sex: The Shaping of Adolescence in the 20th Century.* Cambridge, MA: Harvard University Press, 2000.

Moreton, Bethany. *To Serve God and Wal-Mart: The Making of Christian Free Enterprise.* Cambridge, MA: Harvard University Press, 2009.

Morgan, Lynn Marie. *Icons of Life: A Cultural History of Human Embryos.* Berkeley: University of California Press, 2009.

Morgan, Lynn Marie, and Meredith W. Michaels, eds. *Fetal Subjects, Feminist Positions.* Philadelphia: University of Pennsylvania Press, 1999.

Moskowitz, Eva S. *In Therapy We Trust: America's Obsession with Self-Fulfillment.* Baltimore, MD: John Hopkins University Press, 2001.

Mueller, Max Perry. *Race and the Making of the Mormon People.* Chapel Hill: University of North Carolina Press, 2017.

Muncy, Robyn. *Creating a Female Dominion in American Reform, 1890–1935.* New York: Oxford University Press, 1991.

Munson, Ziad W. *The Making of Pro-Life Activists: How Social Movement Mobilization Works.* Chicago, IL: University of Chicago Press, 2012.

Nash, Gerald D. *The Federal Landscape: An Economic History of the Twentieth Century West.* Tucson: University of Arizona Press, 1999.

Nathanson, Constance. *Dangerous Passage: The Social Control of Sexuality in Women's Adolescence.* Philadelphia, PA: Temple University Press, 1991.

Needle, Rachel, and Lenore Walter. "Is There a Post Abortion Syndrome?" *Abortion Counseling: A Clinician's Guide to Psychology, Legislation, Politics, and Competency.* New York: Springer Publishing Co., 2008.

Neito-Phillips, John M. *The Language of Blood: The Making of Spanish-American Identity in New Mexico.* Albuquerque: University of New Mexico Press, 2004.

Nelson, Jennifer. *More than Medicine: The History of the Feminist Women's Health Movement.* New York: New York University Press, 2015.

———. *Women of Color and the Reproductive Rights Movement.* New York: New York University, 2003.

Newman, Karen. *Fetal Positions: Individualism, Science, Visuality.* Stanford, CA: Stanford University Press, 1996.

Newman, Louise Michele. *White Women's Rights: The Racial Origins of Feminism in the United States.* New York: Oxford University Press, 1999.

Nickerson, Michelle M. *Mothers of Conservatism: Women and the Postwar Right.* Princeton, NJ: Princeton University Press, 2012.

Nickerson, Michelle M., and Darren Dochuk, eds. *Sunbelt Rising: The Politics of Space, Place, and Region.* Philadelphia: University of Pennsylvania Press, 2011.

Noll, Mark A. *God and Race in American Politics: A Short History.* Princeton, NJ: Princeton University Press, 2008.

Novick, Peter. *The Holocaust in American Life.* Boston: Houghton Mifflin, 1999.

Ochberg, Frank M. *Post-Traumatic Therapy and Victims of Violence.* New York: Brunner/Mazel, 1988.

O'Malley, John W. *Tradition and Transition: Historical Perspectives on Vatican II.* Lima, OH: Academic Renewal Press, 2002.

O'Neil, Daniel J. *Church Lobbying in a Western State: A Case Study on Abortion Legislation.* Tucson: University of Arizona Press, 1970.

———. "Public Hearings and Public Preferences: The Case of the White House Conference on Families." *Public Opinion Quarterly* 46, no. 4 (Winter 1982): 488–502.

O'Neill, Colleen. *Working the Navajo Way: Labor and Culture in the Twentieth Century.* Lawrence: University Press of Kansas, 2005.

Odem, Mary E. *Delinquent Daughters: Protecting and Policing Adolescent Female Sexuality in the United States, 1885–1920.* Chapel Hill: University of North Carolina Press, 1995.

Olson, Joel. "Whiteness and the Polarization of American Politics." *Political Research Quarterly* 61 (Dec. 2008): 704–18.

Otero, Lydia R. *La Calle: Spatial Conflicts and Urban Renewal in a Southwest City.* Tucson: University of Arizona Press, 2010.

Pascoe, Peggy. *Relations of Rescue: The Search for Female Moral Authority in the American West, 1874–1939.* New York: Oxford University Press, 1990.

———. *What Comes Naturally: Miscegenation Law and the Making of Race in America.* New York: Oxford University Press, 2009.

Pasternak, Judy. *Yellow Dirt: A Poisoned Land and the Betrayal of the Navajos.* New York: Free Press, 2011.

Patterson, James T. *Freedom Is Not Enough: The Moynihan Report and America's Struggle over the Black Family from LBJ to Obama.* New York: Basic Books, 2010.

Peck, Gunther. *Reinventing Free Labor: Padrones and Immigrant Workers in the North American West.* Cambridge, MA: Cambridge University Press, 2000.

Pehl, Matthew. "'Wherever They Mention His Name': Ethnic Catholicism on an Industrial Island." In *Catholicism in the American West: Rosary of Hidden Voices,* ed. Roberto R. Treviño and Richard V. Fracanviglia. Arlington: University of Texas at Arlington Press, 2007.

Pellegrini, Ann. "'Signaling Through the Flames': Hell House Performance and Structures of Religious Feeling." *American Quarterly* 59, no. 3 (2007): 911–35.

Perignotti, Maria Serenella, and Gianpaolo Donzelli. "Perinatal Care at the Threshold of Viability: An International Comparison of Practical Guidelines for the Treatment of Extremely Preterm Births." *Pediatrics* 121, no. 1 (January 1, 2008): 193–98.

Perlstein, Rick. *Before the Storm: Barry Goldwater and the Unmaking of the American Consensus.* New York: Hill and Wang, 2001.

Perry, Luke, and Christopher Cronin. *Mormons and American Politics: From Persecution to Power.* Santa Barbara, CA: Praeger, 2012.

Petchesky, Rosalind. *Abortion and a Woman's Choice.* New York: Longman, 1984.

Petit, Jeanne. "'Organized Catholic Womanhood': Suffrage, Citizenship, and the National Council of Catholic Women." In *Remapping the History of American Catholicism in the United States,* ed. David J. Endres. Washington, DC: Catholic University of America Press, 2017.

Pierce, James E. *Making the White Man's West: Whiteness and the Creation of the American West.* Boulder: University Press of Colorado, 2016.

Planty, Micheal, William Hussar, Thomas Snyder, Grace Kena, Angelina KewalRamani, Jana Kemp, Kevin Bianco, and Rachel Dinkes. *The Condition of Education 2009.* Washington, DC: National Center for Education Statistics, Institute of Education Sciences, U.S. Department of Education, 2009.

Powell, Allan Kent, ed. *Utah History Encyclopedia.* Salt Lake City: University of Utah Press, 1994.

Prince, Gregory A., and W. M. Robert Wright. *David O. McKay and the Rise of Modern Mormonism.* Salt Lake City: University of Utah Press, 2005.

Quadagno, Jill. *Color of Welfare: How Racism Undermined the War on Poverty.* New York: Oxford University Press, 1994.

Queen, Edward L., II, Stephen F. Prothero, and Gardiner H. Shattuck, Jr., eds., *Encyclopedia of American Religious History,* vol. 1. New York: Facts on File, 2009.

Quigley, Christine. *Modern Mummies: The Preservation of the Human Body in the Twentieth Century.* Jefferson, NC: McFarland and Co., 1998.

Quinn, D. Michael. "Exporting Utah's Theocracy since 1975: Mormon Organizational Behavior and America's Culture Wars." In *God and Country: Politics in Utah,* ed. Jeffrey E. Sells. Salt Lake City, UT: Signature Books, 2005.

———. "The LDS Church's Campaign Against the Equal Rights Amendment." *Journal of Mormon History* 20 (Fall 1994): 85–155.

Reagan, Leslie J. *Dangerous Pregnancies: Mothers, Disabilities, and Abortion in Modern America.* Berkeley: University of California Press, 2010.

———. *When Abortion Was a Crime: Women, Medicine, and Law in the United States, 1867–1973.* Berkeley: University of California Press, 1997.

Reardon, David. *Aborted Women: Silent No More.* Chicago, IL: Loyola University Press, 1987.

Reese, William J. *America's Public Schools: From the Common School to "No Child Left Behind."* Baltimore, MD: John's Hopkins University Press, 2005.

Reeve, W. Paul. *Religion of a Different Color: Race and the Mormon Struggle for Whiteness.* New York: Oxford University Press, 2015.

Reeves, Shawna Renee. "The Development of Post-Abortion Syndrome within the Crisis Pregnancy Center Movement in America: A Historical-Theoretical Study: A Project Based upon an Independent Investigation." MA thesis, Smith College, 2003.

Reyhner, Jon, and Jeanne Eder. *American Indian Education: A History.* Norman: University of Oklahoma Press, 2004.

Rich, Myra. *A History of Planned Parenthood of the Rocky Mountains.* Denver: Planned Parenthood, 1994.

Ridgeley, Susan B. *Practicing What the Doctor Preached: At Home with Focus on the Family.* New York: Oxford University Press, 2016.

Risen, James, and Judy L. Thomas. *Wrath of Angels: The American Abortion War.* New York: Basic Books, 1998.

Roberts, Dorothy. *Killing the Black Body: Race, Reproduction and the Meaning of Liberty.* New York: Pantheon Books, 1997.

Roberts, Keenan. *The Hell House Outreach Manual.* Thornton: New Destiny Christian Center of the Assemblies of God, 2008.

Robinson, Carin. "From Every Tribe and Nation? Blacks and the Christian Right." *Social Science Quarterly* 87 (August 2006): 591–601.

Rodriguez, Jeanette. *Our Lady of Guadalupe: Faith and Empowerment among Mexican-American Women.* Austin: University of Texas Press, 1994.

Rodríguez, Richard T. *Next of Kin: The Family in Chicano/a Cultural Politics.* Durham: Duke University Press, 2009.

Roessel, Robert A. *Navajo Education, 1948–1978.* Rough Rock, AZ: Navajo Curriculum Center, Rough Rock Demonstration School, 1979.

Rogers, Brent M. *Unpopular Sovereignty: Mormons and the Federal Management of Early Utah Territory.* Lincoln: University of Nebraska Press, 2017.

Romero, Tom I., Jr. "Of Race and Rights: Legal Culture, Social Change, and the Making of a Multiracial Metropolis, Denver 1940–1975." PhD diss., University of Michigan, 2004.

Ruíz, Vicki L. *Out of the Shadows: Mexican Women in the Twentieth Century.* New York: Oxford University Press, 1998.

Rymph, Catherine E. *Republican Women: Feminism and Conservatism from Suffrage through the Rise of the New Right.* Chapel Hill: University of North Carolina Press, 2006.

Sale, Kirpatrick. *Power Shift: The Rise of the Southern Rim and its Challenge to the Eastern Establishment.* New York: Random House, 1975.

Sánchez, George I. *"The People": A Study of the Navajo.* Lawrence, KS: U.S. Indian Service, 1948.

Sandler, Lauren. *Righteous: Dispatches from the Evangelical Youth Movement.* New York: Penguin Books, 2006.

Sartre, John-Paul. *The Imaginary: The Phenomenology Psychology of the Imagination,* 3d ed. 1940; New York: Routledge, 2004.

Saurette, Paul, and Kelly Gordon. *The Changing Voice of the Anti-Abortion Movement: The Rise of "Pro-Woman" Rhetoric in Canada and the United States.* Toronto: University of Toronto Press, 2016.

Schackel, Sandra. *Social Housekeepers: Women Shaping Public Policy in New Mexico, 1920–1940.* Albuquerque: University of New Mexico Press, 1992.

Scheidler, Joseph M. *Closed: 99 Ways to Stop Abortion*, rev. ed. 1985; Rockford, IL: Tan Books and Publishers, 1993.

Schoen, Johanna. *Abortion After Roe*. Chapel Hill: University of North Carolina Press, 2015.

———. *Choice and Coercion: Birth Control, Sterilization and Abortion in Public Health and Welfare*. Chapel Hill: University of North Carolina Press, 2005.

Schulman, Bruce J. *The Seventies: The Great Shift in American Culture, Society, and Politics*. New York: Free Press, 2001.

Schultz, Kevin M. *Tri-Faith America: How Postwar Catholics and Jews Held America to its Protestant Promise*. New York: Oxford University Press, 2011.

Schumaker, Katy. *Troublemakers: Students' Rights and Racial Justice in the Long 1960s*. New York: New York University Press, 2019.

Self, Robert O. *All in the Family: The Realignment of American Democracy since the 1960s*. New York: Hill and Wang, 2012.

———. *American Babylon: Race and the Struggle for Postwar Oakland*. Princeton, NJ: Princeton University Press, 2003.

Shapiro, Ian, ed. *Abortion: The Supreme Court Decisions, 1965–2007*. 3d ed. Indianapolis, IN: Hackett Publishing, 2007.

Sheahan, Margot. *The Whole Parent: Book One: 12 Steps to Serenity for Unwed Parents (A Practical Life Guide)*. Los Angeles, CA: VCA Publishing, 2001.

Sheldon, Rebekah. *The Child to Come: Life After the Human Catastrophe*. Minneapolis: University of Minnesota Press, 2016.

Shepherd, Gary, and Gordon Shepherd. *Binding Earth and Heaven: Patriarchal Blessings in the Prophetic Development of Early Mormonism*. University Park: Pennsylvania State University Press, 2012.

Sheridan, Thomas E. *Arizona: A History*. Tucson: University of Arizona Press, 1995.

———. *Los Tucsonenses: The Mexican Community in Tucson, 1854–1941*. Tucson: University of Arizona Press, 1986.

Shermer, Elizabeth Tandy, ed. *Barry Goldwater and the Remaking of the American Political Landscape*. Tucson: University of Arizona Press, 2013.

———. *Sunbelt Capitalism: Phoenix and the Transformation of American Politics*. Philadelphia: University of Pennsylvania Press, 2013.

Shipps, Jan. *Mormonism: The Story of a New Religious Tradition*. Urbana: University of Illinois Press, 1985.

Siegel, Reva. "The Right's Reasons: Constitutional Conflict and the Spread of Woman- Protective Antiabortion Argument." *Duke Law Journal* 57 (April 2008): 1641–92.

Sikkink, David. "Public Schooling and Its Discontents: Religious Identities, Schooling Choices for Children, and Civic Participation." PhD diss., University of North Carolina-Chapel Hill, 1998.

Silk, Mark. "Notes on the Judeo-Christian Tradition in America." *American Quarterly* 34, no.1 (Spring 1984): 65–85.

Silk, Mark, and Andrew Walsh. *One Nation, Divisible: How Regional Religious Differences Shape American Politics.* Lanham, MD: Rowman and Littlefield, 2008.

Singular, Stephen. *The Wichita Divide: The Murder of Dr. George Tiller and the Battle Over Abortion.* New York: St. Martin's Press, 2011.

Smith, Andrea. *Conquest: Sexual Violence and American Indian Genocide.* Cambridge, MA: South End Press, 2005.

Smith, Christian, and David Sikkink. "Is Private Schooling Privatizing?" *First Things* 92 (April 1999): 16–20.

Smith-Rosenberg, Carol. *Disorderly Conduct: Visions of Gender in Victorian America.* New York: Knopf, 1985.

Solinger, Rickie, ed. *Abortion Wars: A Half Century of Struggle, 1950–2000.* Berkeley: University of California Press, 1998.

———. *Beggars and Choosers: How the Politics of Choice Shapes Adoption, Abortion, and Welfare in the United States.* New York: Hill and Wang, 2001.

———. *Pregnancy and Power: A Short History of Reproductive Politics in America.* New York: New York University, 2005.

———. *Wake Up Little Susie: Single Pregnancy and Race before Roe v. Wade.* New York: Routledge, 1992.

Speckhard, Anne. *Post-Abortion Counseling: Manual for Christian Counseling.* Falls Church, VA: Post-Abortion Counseling and Education, 1987.

———. "The Psycho-Social Aspects of Stress Following Abortion: A Thesis." PhD diss., University of Minnesota, 1985.

Stabile, Carol A. "The Traffic in Fetuses." In *Fetal Subjects, Feminist Positions,* ed. Meredith M. Michaels and Lynn M. Morgan. Philadelphia: University of Pennsylvania Press, 1999.

Staub, Michael. "'Negroes Are Not Jews': Race, Holocaust Consciousness, and the Rise of Jewish Neoconservatism." *Radical History Review* 75 (Fall 1999): 3–27.

———. *Torn at the Roots: The Crisis of Jewish Liberalism in Postwar America.* New York: Columbia University Press, 2002.

Stein, Marc. *Sexual Injustice: Supreme Court Rulings from Griswold to Roe.* Chapel Hill: University of North Carolina Press, 2010.

Steiner, Mark Allen. *The Rhetoric of Operation Rescue: Projecting the Christian Pro-Life Message.* New York: T & T Clark, 2006.

Steinhoff, Patricia G., and Milton Diamond. *Abortion Politics: The Hawaii Experience.* Honolulu: University of Hawaii Press, 1977.

Stephenson, Jill. *Women in Nazi Germany.* New York: Longman, 2001.

Stephenson, Lisa P. *Dismantling the Dualisms for American Pentecostal Women in Ministry: A Feminist-Pneumatological Approach.* Leiden, Netherlands: Brill, 2012.

Stern, Alexandra Minna. *Eugenic Nation: Faults and Frontiers of Better Breeding in Modern America.* Berkeley: University of California Press, 2005.

Stern, Alexandra Minna, and Natalie Lira. "Mexican Americans and Eugenic Sterilization: Resisting Reproductive Injustice in California, 1920–1950." *Aztlan: Journal of Chicano Studies* 39 (Fall 2014): 9–34.

Stevens, Mitchell L. *Kingdom of Children: Culture and Controversy in the Home-schooling Movement.* Princeton, NJ: Princeton University Press, 2001.

Stevens-Arroyo, Anthony M. "The Latino Religious Resurgence." *Annals of the American Academy of Political and Social Science* 558 (July 1998): 163–77.

———. "Pious Colonialism: Assessing a Church Paradigm for Chicano Identity." In *Mexican American Religions: Spirituality, Activism, and Culture,* ed. Gastón Espinosa and Mario T. García. Durham, NC: Duke University Press, 2008.

Stormer, Brian. *Articulating Life's Memory: U.S. Medical Rhetoric about Abortion in the Nineteenth Century.* Lanham, MD: Lexington Books, 2002.

Strub, Whitney. *Perversion for Profit: The Politics of Pornography and the Rise of the New Right.* New York: Columbia University Press, 2011.

———. "Pornography, Heteronormativity, and the Genealogy of New Right Sexual Citizenship in the United States." In *Inventing the Silent Majority in Western Europe and the United States: Conservatism in the 1960s and 1970s,* ed. Anna Von Der Goltz and Britta Waldschmidt-Nelson. Cambridge: Cambridge University Press, 2017.

Sugrue, Thomas J. *The Origins of the Urban Crisis: Race and Inequality in Postwar Detroit.* Princeton, NJ: Princeton University Press, 1996.

Summerhill, Louise. *The Story of Birthright: An Alternative to Abortion,* 11th ed. Toronto: Birthright International, 2006.

Szasz, Ferenc Morton. *Larger than Life: New Mexico in the Twentieth Century.* Albuquerque: University of New Mexico Press, 2006.

———. *Religion in the Modern American West.* Tucson: University of Arizona Press, 2000.

Taranto, Stacie. *Kitchen Table Politics: Conservative Women and Family Values in New York.* Philadelphia: University of Pennsylvania Press, 2017.

Tatalovich, Raymond, and Byron W. Daynes. *The Politics of Abortion: A Study of Community Conflict in Public Policymaking.* New York: Praeger, 1981.

Taylor, Janelle S. *The Public Life of the Fetal Sonogram: Technology, Consumption, and the Politics of Reproduction.* New Brunswick, NJ: Rutgers University Press, 2008.

Taylor, Quintard. *In Search of the Racial Frontier: African Americans in the American West.* New York: W.W. Norton, 1998.

Tentler, Leslie Woodcock. *Catholics and Contraception: An American History.* Ithaca, NY: Cornell University Press, 2004.

Theobald, Brianna. *Reproduction on the Reservation: Pregnancy, Childbirth, and Colonialism in the Long Twentieth Century.* Chapel Hill: University of North Carolina Press, 2019.

Thompson, Hildegard. *The Navajos' Long Walk for Education: A History of Navajo Education.* Tsaile, AZ: Navajo Community College Press, 1975.

Tobias, Henry J. *Jews in New Mexico since World War II.* Albuquerque: University of New Mexico Press, 2008.

Torpy, Sally J. "Native American Women and Coerced Sterilization: On the Trail of Tears in the 1970s." *American Indian Culture and Research Journal* 24, no. 2 (2000): 1–22.

Trennert, Robert. *The Phoenix Indian School: Forced Assimilation in Arizona, 1891–1935.* Norman: University of Oklahoma Press, 1988.

Treviño, Roberto R. *The Church in the Barrio: Mexican American Ethno-Catholicism in Houston.* Chapel Hill: University of North Carolina Press, 2006.

Tribe, Laurence H. *Abortion: A Clash of Absolutes.* New York: W.W. Norton, 1992.

Trudell, Bonnie, and Mariamne Whatley. "Sex Respect: A Problematic Public School Sexuality Curriculum." *Journal of Sex Education and Therapy* 17, no. 2 (1991): 125–40.

Trujillo, Michael L. *Land of Disenchantment: Latina/o Identities and Transformations in Northern New Mexico.* Albuquerque: University of New Mexico Press, 2009.

Tymkovich, Timothy M., John Daniel Dailey, and Paul Farley. "A Tale of Three Theories: Reason and Prejudice in the Battle Over Amendment 2." *University of Colorado Law Review* 68 (Spring 1997): 287–333.

United States Catholic Conference. *Respect Life!: Respect Life Week, October 1–7, 1972.* Washington, DC: United States Catholic Conference, 1972.

Vigil, Ernesto B. *The Crusade for Justice: Chicano Militancy and the Government's War on Dissent.* Madison: University of Wisconsin Press, 1999.

Vinovskis, Maris. *An "Epidemic" of Adolescent Pregnancy? Some Historical and Policy Considerations.* New York: Oxford University Press, 1998.

Watkins, Elizabeth Siegal. *On the Pill: A Social History of Oral Contraceptives, 1950–1970.* Baltimore, MD: John Hopkins University Press, 1998.

Weaver, Mary Jo. *New Catholic Women: A Contemporary Challenge to Traditional Religious Authority.* San Francisco, CA: Harper and Row, 1988.

Weaver, Mary Jo, and R. Scott Appleby, eds. *Being Right: Catholic Conservatives in America.* Bloomington: Indiana University Press, 1995.

Weiss, Jessica. *To Have and to Hold: Marriage, the Baby Boom, and Social Change.* Chicago, IL: University of Chicago Press, 2000.

Welshimer, Kathleen J., and Shirley E. Harris. "A Survey of Rural Parents' Attitudes Towards Sexuality Education." *Journal of School Health* 64, no. 9 (November 1994): 347–52.

Weslin, Norman. *The Gathering of the Lambs.* Boulder, CO [no publisher], 2000.

West, Elliott. *The Contested Plains: Indians, Goldseekers, and the Rush to Colorado.* Lawrence: University of Kansas Press, 1998.

Wexler, Laura. *Tender Violence: Domestic Visions in an Age of U.S. Imperialism.* Chapel Hill: University of North Carolina Press, 2000.

White, O. Kendall, Jr. "A Review and Commentary on the Prospects of a Mormon New Christian Right Coalition." *Review of Religious Research* 28, no. 2 (December 1986): 180–88.

Whittaker, Mathew C. *Race Work: The Rise of Civil Rights in the Urban West.* Lincoln: University of Nebraska Press, 2005.

Wilcox, Clyde. "Evangelicals and Abortion." In *A Public Faith: Evangelicals and Civic Engagement,* ed. Michael Cromartie. Lanham, MD: Rowman and Littlefield, 2003.

Wilcox, Clyde, and Carin Robinson. *Onward Christian Soldiers? The Religious Right in American Politics,* 4th ed. Boulder, CO: Westview Press, 2010.

Williams, Daniel K. *Defending the Unborn: The Pro-Life Movement before Roe v. Wade.* New York: Oxford University Press, 2016.

———. *God's Own Party: The Making of the Christian Right.* New York: Oxford University Press, 2010.

———. "Sex and Evangelicals: Gender Issues, the Sexual Revolution, and Abortion in the 1960s." In *American Evangelicals in the 1960s,* ed. Axel R. Schafer. Madison: University of Wisconsin Press, 2013.

Willke, Dr., and Mrs. J[ohn] C. Willke. *Handbook on Abortion.* Cincinnati, OH: Hiltz Publishing Co., 1972.

———, with Marie Willke Meyers, M.D. *Abortion and the Pro-Life Movement: An Inside View.* West Conshohocken, PA: Infinity Publishing, 2014.

Wilson, Chris. *The Myth of Santa Fe: Creating a Modern Regional Tradition.* Albuquerque: University of New Mexico Press, 1997.

Wilson, John P., and Beverley Raphael, eds. *International Handbook of Traumatic Stress Syndromes.* New York: Plenum Press, 1993.

Wisenale, Steven K. "Family Policy at the End of the 20th Century." In *Redefining Family Policy: Implications for the 21st Century,* ed. Joyce M. Mercier, Steven B. Garasky, and Mack C. Shelley II. Hoboken, NJ: Wiley-Blackwell, 2000.

Withycombe, Shannon K. *Lost: Miscarriage in Nineteenth-Century America.* New Brunswick, NJ: Rutgers University Press, 2018.

Wittman, Laura. *The Tomb of the Unknown Soldier, Modern Mourning, and the Reinvention of the Mystical Body.* Toronto: University of Toronto Press, 2011.

Wood, Robert Turner. *The Postwar Transformation of Albuquerque, New Mexico, 1945–1972.* Santa Fe, NM: Sunstone Press, 2014.

———. "The Transformation of Albuquerque, 1945–1972." PhD diss., University of New Mexico, 1980.

Young, Neil J. *We Gather Together: The Religious Right and the Problem of Interfaith Politics.* New York: Oxford University Press, 2016.

Ziegler, Mary. *After Roe: The Lost History of the Abortion Debate.* Cambridge, MA: Harvard University Press, 2015.

MOVIES

Cowan, Reed, and Steven Greenstreet, directors. *8: The Mormon Proposition.* David v. Goliath Films, 2010.

Dabner, Jack Duane. *The Silent Scream.* American Portrait Films, 1984.

Edelmann, Claude, and Jim Baufle, directors. *The First Days of Life.* Cinema Medica, 1971.

Matter of Choice: A 28-Minute Documentary on Abortion. American Portrait Films, 1982.

Ratliff, George, director. *Hell House.* Greenhouse Pictures, 2001.

INDEX

Page numbers in italics refer to illustrations

American Medical Association (AMA), 26–28, 137

American Psychiatric Association (APA), 137, 253n73

American West: abortion access in, 147; and Catholic Church, 107; and Church of Jesus Christ of Latter-day Saints (Mormon, LDS), 97; and race, 33, 124, 133–34; and rise of anti-abortion movement, 1, 3, 5, 7–12, 25–26, 28, 34, 38, 53, 79–80, 109, 117, 205; sex education in, 162, 180; shifting politics in, 34, 36–38, 209, 214n20; Southern Baptists in, 101

Anti-abortion films, 1–4, 14, 45–48, 68–69, 79, 93, 102–3, 127, 129–30, 143, 149, 154–57, 171–72

Anti-abortion funerals/memorial services and cemeteries, 3, 76, 79–82, *81,* 86, 90, 116

Anti-abortion movement, origins of, 6, 15, 21–29, 216n33

Anti-abortion photos, 3, 60, 65, 67–71, 73, 76, 78, 81, 85–86, 93, 121, 127, 131, 143, 152–54, 160, 177, 179–80, 189, 207

Anti-abortion women activists, 6–7, 34–35, 62–63; as moral mothers, 121–35

Anti-feminism. *See* Gender transgression/change

Arizona: abortion access in, 147, 207; Arizona State University, 34; Catholic Church in, 34, 37, 90–93, 95; Council of Catholic Women in, *32,* 31–33, 35–36, 44, 61, 52; crisis pregnancy centers in, 126, 129, 130, 138–39; Diocese of Phoenix, 90, 93; Diocese of Tucson, 43, 49, 91; ecumenical coalitions in, 109, 113–15; evangelicals in, 101; and Barry Goldwater, 7–10; informed consent laws in, 146–47; Phoenix First Assembly of God, 101; protest of abortion providers in, 113–15, *114,* 189; race in, 82, 84, 198, 207; rise of anti-abortion movement in, 1, 3, 7–10, 24–29, 32, 49–51, 54, 62, 166, 185; sex education in, 154–56,158–59, 162; shifting partisan politics in, 34, 37–38, 221n53; Sugar Hill neighborhood in Tucson, 121, 124–25; Women Exploited

by Abortion (WEBA) in, 139, 143–45. *See also* Conservation of Human Life; Gerster, Carolyn; Jakubcyzk, John; Reachout; Seader, Phil and Helen

Arizona Conference on Families, 198

Arizona Register, 43

Arizona Right to Life, 1, 7, 27–28, 34, 93, 145, 155–56, 158, 166, 180, 185, 189

Arnold, Jack, 28, 37, 45

Bauer, Gary, 204

Biological or medical arguments, use of, 26–28, 58–60, 62–63, 67–69, 127–31, 164

Birthright, 121, 124–28, 143. *See also* Crisis pregnancy centers (CPCs)

Black, Richard H., *208*

Bond, Mary, 194–95

Capital punishment, 75–76, 234n83

Carenet, 126, 134, 140, 161–62. *See also* Crisis pregnancy centers (CPCs)

Carlin, Leonard, 63

Casti Connubii encyclical, 29

Catholic Church/Catholics, 9, 11; abortion as central issue of, 90–97, 100; anti-pornography activism and, 43–48; and Church of Jesus Christ of Latter-day Saints (Mormons, LDS), 67–70, 76; Colorado Catholic Conference, 57; and contraception, 11, 29, 31, 39–40; and crisis pregnancy centers, 124–25, 145; debate on abortion, 29–33, 91–94, 104–9; ecumenical coalitions including, 109–17; ethnic Mexicans and anti-abortion movement, 35–36, 104–9, 123, 127, 134; funerals/memorial services and cemeteries for fetuses, 79–82, 86; moral middle and, 95–6, 100, 103–4, 149, 180, 185, 209; Pastoral Plan for Pro-Life Activities, 94–95; and race, 11, 35–36, 39–43, 73–74, 82, 104–9, 145; Respect Life week, 79; rise of anti-abortion movement, 23–24, 27, 29–33, 38–45, 49, 52, 55, 57–58, 61–68, 87–88; schools, 154. *See also* Abortion, as a religious issue; Catholic Council of Nurses; Catholic Lawyers Guild; *Casti*

Connubii encyclical; Council of Catholic Women (CCW); *Humanae Vitae* encyclical; Knights of Columbus; National Conference of Catholic Bishops; Vatican II (Second Vatican Council)

Catholic Council of Nurses, 31

Catholic Lawyers Guild, 31, 63

Chastity, 33, 157, 164, 180, 185–90, 195, 205

Chicano/a, 36, 78, 82–83, 85, 106–9, 195. *See also* Latinx; ethnic Mexicans

Children and young adults, 80, 82, 131–33, 148–80, 202, 230n36, 241n22, 236n91, 262n93, 263n103; books for, 163–64, 172; in schools, 150–62, 167–69; as symbols, 148–50, 174–80, 202, 210n36, 262n91, 262n93, 263n103. *See also* Abstinence education; Adolescent Family Life Act (AFLA); Sex education in schools; Teen pregnancy

Christian Action Council, 140

Christian Coalition, 168, 204

Christian Family Movement, 31, 35

Christian identity, 87–104, 210

Church of God in Christ, 79

Church of Jesus Christ of Latter-day Saints (LDS, Mormon), 9–11, 25; and contraception, 10–11, 215n29; and crisis pregnancy centers, 250n7; and ensoulment, 69–70; and gender, 97, 100–101, 117; joining the moral middle, 91, 95–97, 104, 110–12, 149, 180, 209; race and, 66, 97, 234n76; and Utah's abortion politics, 65–76, 97–101, 117. *See also* Abortion as a religious issue; Relief Society; Utah Anti-Abortion League

Citizens for Decent Literature, 43, 45, 48

Civil disobedience, 13–14, 22, 122, 174–77, 216–17n39, 263n100. *See also* Freedom of Access to Clinic Entrances (FACE) Act; Operation Rescue; Racketeer Influenced and Corrupt Organizations Act (RICO)

Civil rights rhetoric, 2, 4–7, 11, 16, 22–24, 41–43, 55, 66, 76–79, 83–6, 118, 149–50, 153, 173, 176, 178, 183, 197–98, 204, 207, 209–10

Clements, Virginia (Ginny), 26

Clergy Consultation Service (CCS), 87, 240n4

Colorado: access to abortion in, 77, 147; anti-birth control movement in, 39–41, 43, 223n76, 225n103; Catholic Lawyers Guild of Denver, 63; Colorado Catholic Conference, 57; Columbine High School shooting, 206–7; crisis pregnancy centers in, 124–25, 134; evangelicals in, 101, 103; Heritage Christian Center (Denver), 101; mothers on welfare, 229n9; and Operation Rescue, 176–77, *178;* and race, 41, 82, 85; rise of anti-abortion movement in, 1, 3, 8–10, 15, 21, 26, 33–34, 52, 56–65, 87–88, *89,* 92, 94, 96, 117; sex education in, 151, 154, 156. *See also* Dolan, Ruth; Focus on the Family; Lamm, Richard; Our Lady of Guadalupe (Denver); Sebesta, Margaret

Colorado Joint Council on Medical and Social Legislation, 62, 217n7

Colorado Right to Life, 61, 110, 125, 206

Colorado Springs Right to Life, 34, 94–96

Concerned Women for America, 168

Conservation of Human Life, 121. *See also* Reachout

Contraception, 10–11, 15, 23–24, 29–31, 33, 38–41, 43, 48–51, 53, 56, 58, 64, 71, 73, 75, 84, 91, 105, 131–32, 134, 144, 157–58, 162, 169, 186, 193, 197, 215n29, 219n47, 225n103, 231n31

Council of Catholic Women (CCW), 31–33, *32,* 353–56, 44, 61, 52

Crisis Pregnancy Center (Phoenix), 128, 137

Crisis pregnancy centers (CPCs), 1–3, 15, 64, 110, 121–47, *130,* 154, 158, 161–62, 181, 184, 188–89, 203, 207, 210. *See also* Aid to Women; Birthright; Carenet; Post-abortion syndrome; Reachout

DeConcini, Dennis, 7, 51–52

DeConcini, Ora, 25, 51–52

Democratic Party, 3, 21–24, 36–38, 41, 52–53, 56, 64–65, 107, 191, 209. *See also* Party politics

Relief Society, 98–99, 243n50
Republican Party/GOP, 4, 7, 11–12, 15, 22, 24, 37–38, 53, 56, 105, 146, 203–6, 208–10. *See also* Party politics
Right to Life: Arizona, 1, 7, 27–28, 34, 93, 145, 155–56, 158, 166, 180, 185, 189; Colorado, 61, 110, 125, 206; Colorado Springs, 34, 94–96; Georgia, 84; National, 8, 34, 57, 69, 84, 100, 110, 125–27, 148, 151, 154, 166, 171, 180; New Mexico, 76–83, 93, 154; Utah, 29–30, 67, 219n31
Robertson, Pat, 103
Roe v. Wade, 2, 12, 29, 67, 71–73, 76–77, 79, 90, 99–100, 102, 137, 148, 150–51, 153, 177, 183, 185, 208, 210, 216n34, 231n47
Rubella, 58, 230n20
Rue, Vincent, 136, 254n85. *See also* Post-abortion syndrome
Ruiz, Libby, 25, 35–36, 38, 108, 217n7, 226n130, 234n76, 235n91, 240n4. *See also* Ethnic Mexicans

Sanger, Margaret, 10
Schaeffer, Francis, 102, 140
Scheidler, Joseph, 115
Seader, Phil and Helen, 34, 62, 109, 126, 129, 132–34, 143, 181–82
Sebesta, Margaret (pseudonym), 21–22, 24, 34–36, 52–53, 59, 62, 85, 92, 124–25, 151
Sex education in schools, 36, 51, 68, 92, 150–53, 155–57, 162, 167–68, 192, 194. *See also* Abstinence education; Children and young adults
Sex Respect (education program), 158. *See also* Abstinence education
Sexual immorality, concern over, 43, 52, 63–64, 88, 90, 124, 132, 158. *See also* Gender transgression/change, concern over
Sheahan, Margot, 185–90. *See also* Unwed Parents Anonymous
Silent No More Awareness Campaign, 84
Single or unwed mothers, 141, 185–90, 202–3, 205, 223n76. *See also* Unwed Parents Anonymous

Slavery rhetoric, 2, 11, 55–6, 65–66, 71, 73–6, 85, 153, 207. See also *Dred Scott* decision
Social imaginary, 213n113, 228n4
Southern Baptist, 87, 101–2, 240n6; Baptists for Life, 102; Southern Baptist Convention, 29, 102
Spousal consent/notification laws, 185, 189–90
Sterilization, 10, 82–83, 229n9
Stewart, Robert, *59*, 58–62, 85

Teen pregnancy, 132–35, 138, 157, 172, 185–90. *See also* Children and young adults; Single or unwed mothers
Terry, Randall, 13, 176
Thalidomide, 49, 229–30n17
Tiller, George, 174–75
Touch of Life dolls, 165, 172. *See also* Ephemera/fetal imagery; Fetus dolls /models
Traditional family, 181–205

Ultrasounds, 128, 203
Unitarian Universalists, 87
United Farm Workers (UFW), 106, 246n88
United Methodists, 87, 240n6
United Parents Under God, 152–54
University of Arizona, 126, 144
Unplanned pregnancy, 2, 6, 110, 121, 153, 159, 186
Unwed Parents Anonymous, 184–90, 203, 205. *See also* Sheahan, Margot
Utah: access to abortion, 147; Catholics in, 29–30; crisis pregnancy centers in, 124, 250n7; history of abortion in, 37, 65–76, *72*, 97; race in, 8–10, 37–38, 66, 73–76, 82, 97, 234n76; rise of anti-abortion movement in, 1, 8–11, 24, 29–30, 93, 148. *See also* Church of Jesus Christ of Latter-day Saints (LDS, Mormon)
Utah Anti-Abortion League, 30, 67
Utah Right to Life, 29–30, 67, 219n31

Vatican II (Second Vatican Council), 31, 42, 91, 105, 108–9. *See also* Catholic Church/Catholics

Founded in 1893,
UNIVERSITY OF CALIFORNIA PRESS
publishes bold, progressive books and journals
on topics in the arts, humanities, social sciences,
and natural sciences—with a focus on social
justice issues—that inspire thought and action
among readers worldwide.

The UC PRESS FOUNDATION
raises funds to uphold the press's vital role
as an independent, nonprofit publisher, and
receives philanthropic support from a wide
range of individuals and institutions—and from
committed readers like you. To learn more, visit
ucpress.edu/supportus.

Printed in Great Britain
by Amazon

15466614R00185